Advances in Biochemistry and Biotechnology

The Editors

Dr. Biplab Sarkar, Ph.D., is presently working as Senior scientist at National Institute of Abiotic Stress Management (Deemed University), Baramati, Pune, Maharashtra under Indian Council of Agricultural Research (ICAR), Govt. of India. Previously, he worked as faculty of biotechnology at KIIT University, Bhubaneswar, Odisha and Amity University, Noida, Uttar Pradesh. He has already completed fourteen years of research and eight years of teaching. He published fifteen international peer reviewed paper, six papers in national journal, thirty conference papers, six book chapters and guided several research students in post graduate dissertation thesis. He was awarded Young Scientist by DST,Govt. of India and got a project as principal investigator. He is acting as a reviewer of some national and international peer reviewed journal. He worked as a Senior Research Fellow assessment, at Central Institute of Freshwater Aquaculture (CIFA), Bhubaneswar on pesticide impact analysis in fish and on pheromones. He visited Asian Institute of Technology (AIT), Bangkok, Thailand on department of nanotechnology, for a collaborative research work. His future research interest is to apply nanotechnology tools for aquaculture development.

Dr. Chiranjib Chakraborty, Ph.D., is currently professor at Department of Bio-informatics, Galgotias University, India. After obtaining his Ph.D., he worked as Visiting Research Professor-National Sun Yat Sen University, Taiwan; Sr. Visiting Scholar-Institute of Animal Science, Beijing; Associate Professor- VIT University, Vellore, India; Visiting Scientist-Machine Intelligence Unit, Indian Statistical Institute, Kolkata, India; Visiting Scholar- Department of Computer Science, Hong Kong Baptist University, Hong Kong. He published more than 65 SCI papers, 5 books and 2 edited books and he is editorial board member of several internal journals.

Advances in Biochemistry and Biotechnology

— *Volume 2* —

(Special Issue on Animal and Aquaculture Biotechnology)

Edited by
Dr. Biplab Sarkar
Senior Scientist,
National Institute of Abiotic Stress Management (Deemed University)
(Indian Council of Agricultural Research)
Malegaon, Baramati – 413 115, Pune, Maharashtra, India

Dr. Chiranjib Chakraborty
Professor,
Department of Bio-informatics,
School of Computer and Information Sciences, Galgotias University,
Greater Noida, Uttar Pradesh, India

2014
Daya Publishing House®
A Division of
Astral International Pvt. Ltd.
New Delhi – 110 002

ISBN **9789351302742**

Published by : **Daya Publishing House®**
A Division of
Astral International Pvt. Ltd.
– ISO 9001:2008 Certified Company –
4760-61/23, Ansari Road, Darya Ganj
New Delhi-110 002
Ph. 011-43549197, 23278134
E-mail: info@astralint.com
Website: www.astralint.com

Laser Typesetting : **Classic Computer Services**, Delhi - 110 035

Printed at : **Thomson Press India Limited**

PRINTED IN INDIA

— *Dedicated to* —
"Sri Ramakrishna Paramhansha"

Preface

It is our immense pleasure that we have completed the Second Volume of *Advances in Biochemistry and Biotechnology*. First volume was published by Daya Publishing House which was edited by second editor, Dr. Chiranjib Chakraborty in 2005. In this second volume, we, the two researcher friends (Dr. Biplab Sarkar and Dr. Chiranjib Chakraborty), have edited this volume which is a specialized version of Animal Biotechnology and Aquaculture Biotechnology.

The book on *"Advances in Biochemistry and Biotechnology, Volume 2"* has been written, compiled and edited with a view to focus the frontiers and recent development in aquaculture and animal biotechnology research. In current years, this sector is showing one of the highest productivity and growth and has multifaceted potential to grow. Here, some of the new innovations and discoveries from these segment has been shortlisted and highlighted to ignite young researchers and students. Nanotechnology is the world of subatomic material which could rewrite the behavior and property of matters but unforeseen world of nanotoxicity is a new menace to biota and environment. Among nanomaterials, silver has touched new commercial taboo but toxicity threat is creating buzz. Cancer and tuberculosis are old disease with unsolved therapeutics and drug targets. Conventional Indian phytochemicals can be one of the best drug alternative for cancer and microRNA can be utilized as biomarker. Delivery of small peptides can be another drug candidate against pathogenesis of tuberculosis. On the other hand, AIDS is a fatal disease and students should know about its current research scenario. In aquaculture, algae can be applied to use as a source of bioenergy where fish waste material will be a good source of therapeutic proteins. Knowledge of innate immunity can be elucidated and engineered for a healthy, disease free aquaculture. Moreover, concept of cell free DNA, point care diagnostics, and synthetic biology are new innovative concepts of modern era.

The book contains fifteen chapters. Out of these, seven chapters are dedicated towards aquaculture biotechnology and another seven are written on animal biotechnology. Topics of the texts are informative, nonconventional, and paves the way for some interesting future innovation and technology development.

In this juncture of publication, we would like to pay our thanks and gratitude to Mr. Anil Mittal, Managing Director, Astral International (P) Limited, New Delhi for accepting our noble concept of publishing book on these current frontiers of aquatic and animal biotechnology. We appreciate his mission to disseminate the new scientific resource to young students and researchers. We would like to acknowledge the blessings and motivation of Dr. S. Ayyappan, DG ICAR and Secretary (DARE) behind this book. We like to express our gratitude to Dr. P. S. Minhas, Director, NIASM, Baramati, Pune for his continuous encouragement and support. We would like to remember the motivation and support from the directors of KIIT University, Bhubaneshwar and VIIT University, Vellore. We would like appreciate the cooperation and support from all the authors who have contributed in our book. We would like to thanks Dr. Subhendu Sarkar for his cooperation in editing.

If our book will create a bit ripple on the mind of young and budding scientists, we would feel the pulse of success of our current endeavours.

Biplab Sarkar
Chiranjib Chakraborty

Contents

List of Contributors

Amulya Moha
Department of Biology and Health Promotions, St. Francis College, 180 Remsen Street, Brooklyn, New Your City, NY 11201, USA.

Anchal Singh
Amity Institute of Biotechnology, Amity University Uttar Pradesh, Sector-125, Noida –201 303, U.P., India

Ashis Saha
Central Institute of Freshwater Aquaculture, Bhubaneswar, Orissa, India

Ashish Swarup Verma
Amity Institute of Biotechnology, Amity University Uttar Pradesh, Sector-125, Noida –201 303, U.P., India

Avinash Sonawane
School of Biotechnology, Campus-11, KIIT University, Bhubaneswar – 751 024, Orissa, India

Biplab Sarkar
National Institute of Abiotic Stress Management (Deemed University) (Indian Council of Agricultural Research) Malegaon, Baramati – 413115 (Pune) Maharashtra, India

Chanakya Nath Kundu
KIIT School of Biotechnology, KIIT University, Campus-11, Patia, Bhubaneswar – 751 024, Orissa,
India

Chiranjib Chakraborty
Department of Bio-informatics, School of Computer and Information sciences, Galgotias University,
Greater Noida, India
Hallym University, College of Medicine, South Korea
Visiting Research Professor-National Sun Yat Sen University, Taiwan
Department of Computer Sciences, Hong Kong Baptist University, Kowloon Tong, Hong Kong

Dibyajyoti Banerjee
Department of Experimental Medicine and Biotechnology, Postgraduate Institute of Medical Education
and Research, Chandigarh – 160 012, India

Dipon Das
KIIT School of Biotechnology, KIIT University, Campus-11, Patia, Bhubaneswar – 751 024, Orissa,
India

Indarchand Gupta
Department of Biotechnology, SGB Amravati University, Amravati – 444 602, Maharashtra, India

Jaya Kumari
Norwegian College of Fishery Science, Faculty of Biosciences, Fisheries and Economics University of
Tromsø, N-9037 Tromsø, Norway

Jogeswar Satchidananda Purohit
Department of Zoology, Smt. C.H.M. College, (University of Mumbai) Ulhasnagar, Thane, Maharashtra,
India
School of Biotechnology, Campus-11, KIIT University, Bhubaneswar – 751 024, Orissa, India

Kirtimaan Syal
Department of Experimental Medicine and Biotechnology, Postgraduate Institute of Medical Education
and Research, Chandigarh – 160 012, India
Current: Molecular Biophysics Unit, Indian Institute of Science, Bangalore – 560 012, India

Madan Mohan Chaturvedi
Department of Zoology, University of Delhi, North Campus, New Delhi, India

Mahendra Rai
Department of Biotechnology, SGB Amravati University, Amravati – 444 602, Maharashtra, India

Mrinal Samanta
Fish Health Management Division, Central Institute of Freshwater Aquaculture, Kausalyaganga,
Bhubaneswar – 751 002, Orissa

Nitish Nagpal
Department of Experimental Medicine and Biotechnology, Postgraduate Institute of Medical Education
and Research, Chandigarh – 160 012, India

Ole Sorensen
Department of Clinical Sciences, BMC, B14, Tornavagen 10, SE-221 84, University of Lund, Sweden

Pragnya Panda
School of Biotechnology, Campus-11, KIIT University, Bhubaneswar – 751 024, Orissa, India

Prangya Paramita Tripathy
Research Scientist, School of Biotechnology, KIIT University Bhubaneswar, Orissa, India

Purusottam Mohapatra
KIIT School of Biotechnology, KIIT University, Campus-11, Patia, Bhubaneswar – 751 024, Orissa, India

Rajasri Bhattacharyya
Department of Experimental Medicine and Biotechnology, Postgraduate Institute of Medical Education and Research, Chandigarh – 160 012, India

Ranjan Preet
KIIT School of Biotechnology, KIIT University, Campus-11, Patia, Bhubaneswar – 751 024, Orissa, India

Rinu Sharma
University School of Biotechnology, Guru Gobind Singh Indraprastha University, Sector-16C, Dwarka, New Delhi – 110 075, India

S.C. Rath
Central Institute of Freshwater Aquaculture, Bhubaneswar, Orissa, India

S.S. Giri
Central Institute of Freshwater Aquaculture, Bhubaneswar, Orissa, India

Sanjay Kumar Ojha
School of Biotechnology, KIIT University, Bhubaneswar – 751 024, Odisha

Shakti Ranjan Satapathy
KIIT School of Biotechnology, KIIT University, Campus-11, Patia, Bhubaneswar – 751 024, Orissa, India

Shishir Agrahari
Amity Institute of Biotechnology, Amity University Uttar Pradesh, Sector-125, Noida –201 303, U.P., India

Shruti Rastogi
Amity Institute of Biotechnology, Amity University Uttar Pradesh, Sector-125, Noida –201 303, U.P., India

Snehasish Mishra
School of Biotechnology, KIIT University, Bhubaneswar – 751 024, Odisha

Soumitra Mohanty
School of Biotechnology, Campus-11, KIIT University, Bhubaneswar – 751 024, Orissa, India

Subendu Sarkar
Calcutta National Medical College, 32 Gorachand Road, Kolkata – 700 014, West Bengal, India

Surya Prakash Netam
School of Biotechnology, Campus-11, KIIT University, Bhubaneswar – 751 024, Orissa, India

Trilochan Swain
Shree-Kshetramohan Biocomplex, Jagatsinghpur, Orissa, India

U.K. Maurya
National Institute of Abiotic Stress Management, Malegaon, Baramati – 413 115 Pune, Maharashtra, India

2014, Advances in Biochemistry and Biotechnology Volume 2

Edited by: Dr. Biplab Sarkar and Dr. Chiranjib Chakraborty

Published by: DAYA PUBLISHING HOUSE

Pages 1-4

1

Current Changing Scenario of Biochemistry and Biotechnology in the Perspective of Aquaculture and Animal Biotechnology

Biplab Sarkar[1] and Chiranjib Chakraborty[2]

[1]National Institute of Abiotic Stress Management (Deemed University)
(Indian Council of Agricultural Research) Malegaon, Baramati – 413 115, Pune, Maharashtra, India
[2]Department of Bio-informatics, School of Computer and Information Sciences,
Galgotias University, Greater Noida, India

The current scenario of biochemistry and biotechnology is changing very quickly throughout the world. This book review series presents current trends in changing scenario of biochemistry and biotechnology. The aim is to cover all aspects of interdisciplinary technology of biochemistry and biotechnology. In 2005, the first volume of this book was published with an aim to cover pharmaceutical, biomedical as well as environmental biotechnology (Chakraborty, 2005a). In that time, in developing India, those subjects were gained the highest magnitude (Chakraborty, 2005b). Now, we have completed the second volume to capture the changing scenario of biochemistry and biotechnology especially aquaculture and animal biotechnology segment.

Aquaculture technology has crossed its long journey from conventional practices of capture and culture to a new world of productivity, food science and innovation through biotechnological manipulation and intervention (Floros *et al.*, 2010). Biotechnological methods has helped to consolidate and tracking out answers of many genuine problems in almost all frontiers and branches of aquaculture like production technology,breeding, nutrition, genetics, health management etc. But fisheries and aquaculture biotechnology is a dynamic process and should bring forth new ideas with the fast changing pace of biological science. In this book, we are presenting some chapters in aquaculture biotechnology which are new in ideas and innovative in expression. Another important topics, Zebrafish as an animal model getting popularity in all field like medical science, nano-technology etc. (Hsu *et al.*, 2007; *Chakraborty et al.*, 2009; Chakraborty and Agoramoorthy, 2010) which has also been highlighted.

Bioactive peptides, which can be collected from fishery waste, have plenty of medicinal potential. So, other than food, fishery and its byproduct can be applied for pharmaceutical sector as therapeutics. Finding for alternative source of energy is a long pursuit.Potentiality of aquatic micro algae as an alternate source of energy can be explored as it contains high amount of lipids. Innate and adaptive immunity are the basis of immune surveillance in fish but modulator approach in this immunological pattern can be helpful for efficacious fish health management. Impact of nanotechnology in aquaculture should be explored but at the same time, nanoparticle based toxicity can be studied in zebra fish model to investigate the safe level concentration of this nanoparticle in water and fish. The innate immune response is the first line of defense against invading pathogens and is the most universal, rapidly acting, and by some appraisals, the most important type of immunity. But innate immunity is not properly elucidated in fish. Pattern recognition receptors are the key players in the mechanism of this immune response. So, discussion on the various types of these receptors will help us to study the signaling mechanism behind this immune response. On the other side, adaptive immunity in fish is also partially explored. So, a comparative profiling between these two sectors of immunity can help us to assess the health management pattern in fish.

In animal biotechnology, tools and innovations for the management of animal health including human health is cynosure of all researchers around the globe (Gaskell and Bauer,2001; Faber *et al.*, 2003). From time immemorial, animal healthcare methods has taken an undulating routes with the challenges from conventional diseases and outbreak of new diseases.Some of the diseases like cancer are still unanswered, few needs innovations as therapeutic targets has been changed with the advent of multi drug resistance phenomenon or antibiotic resistivity like tuberculosis and some new pathogen has appeared with unknown characteristics with horror and fatality. These veracity and versatility has always kept the room open for innovative diagnostics and therapeutics as well as new management pattern in biomedical aspects of animal biotechnology. In this book, we are trying to highlight these enigmas of health management aspects with an approach to provide solution with modern biotechnological tools and approach.

As cancer diagnostics and therapeutics are still inclusive, we have tried to highlight a herbal based therapeutics against cancer which is a old but unexplored therapy. Micro RNA is an astonishing molecule, but how this miRNA can be used as a molecular based biomarker for cancer has been elucidated in other chapter. Tuberculosis is a chronic disease which affects a sizable amount of poor people in third world countries, but did not get attention as pharmaceutical corporate are more concern over diseases of elite. Here, we have tried to put forward a holistic picture of tuberculosis and some new drug targets against tuberculosis. AIDS is also a deadly disease and here, chapter has been prepared on biotechnological basis of AIDS control. Synthetic biology is the latest addition of animal biotechnology. A theoretical format of synthetic biology, its origin, evolution and potentiality has been elucidated to familiarize the readers with this modern day's scientific fiction. Nanotechnology is the science of twenty-first century and role of silver nanoparticle as an antimicrobial therapeutics are a promising area. Cell free DNA is a potential subject which is not properly unleashed. So, historical perspective of cfDNA, its sources, sequential analysis and methods of quantification, with special emphasis on clinical significance of cfDNA in various pathological conditions has been narrated.

Color Type	Area of Biotech
Red	Health, Medical, Diagnostics
Yellow	Food Biotechnology, Nutrition Science
Blue	Aquaculture, Coastal and Marine Biotech
Green	Agricultural, Environmental Biotechnology – Biofuels, Biofertilizers, Bioremediation, Geomicrobiology
Brown	Arid Zone and Desert Biotechnology
Dark	Bioterrorism, Biowarfare, Biocrimes, Anticrop warfare
Purple	Patents, Publications, Inventions, IPRs
White	Patents, Publications, Inventions, IPRs(White)
Gold	Bioinformatics, Nanobiotechnology
Grey	Fermentation and Bioprocess Technology

Figure 1.1: Colours of Biotechnology.

Though field of laboratory medicine has grown tremendously, yet sample transport requirement in a classical clinical laboratory is a routine practice round the globe. So, point care diagnostic should be technique of the future.

However, presently, ten colours have been proved in total biotechnology sector (Figure 1.1). One colour is indicating each sector(s) of the biotechnology. These sectors has been provided over time to understand the biotech applications for the cause of science, development, and the current and post human future of humankind (DaSilva, 2004;DaSilva, 2012). The color index below may be a useful guide with further additions to understand the reader. Now, the reader will further decide about the chapter's position where each chapter of this book is belonging in the table. We are providing this work to the reader.

References

Chakraborty C (2005a). Advances in biochemistry and biotechnology (Vol.1) (ISBN 81-7035-362-9) Daya Publishing House, Delhi. India; p.283.

Chakraborty C (2005b). From editor desk: Current changing scenario of biotechnology and biochemistry advances in biochemistry and biotechnology (Vol.1) *(ISBN 81-7035-362-9) Daya Publishing House, Delhi.* India; p.1-9.

Chakraborty C, Hsu CH, Wen ZH, Lin CS, Agoramoorthy G (2009). Zebrafish: A complete animal model for *in vitro* drug discovery and development. Current Drug Metabolism. 10(2): 116-24.

Chakraborty C, Agoramoorthy G (2010). Why zebrafish? Rivista Di Biologia/Biology Forum 103(1) 25-28.

DaSilva EJ (2012). The Colours of Biotechnology: Science, Development and Humankind. *Electronic Journal of Biotechnology*, 7(3).

DaSilva E J (2004). The colours of biotechnology: science, development and humankind. *Electronic Journal of Biotechnology*, 7(3), 01-02.

Faber D C, Molina JA, Ohlrichs CL, Vander Zwaag DF, Ferre L B (2003). Commercialization of animal biotechnology. *Theriogenology*, 59(1), 125-138.

Floros J D, Newsome, R., Fisher, W., BarbosaCánovas, G. V., Chen, H., Dunne, C. P, Ziegler, G. R. (2010). Feeding the world today and tomorrow: the importance of food science and technology. *Comprehensive Reviews in Food Science and Food Safety*, 9(5), 572-599.

Gaskell G, Bauer M W (2001). *Biotechnology, 1996-2000: The Years of Controversy*. NMSI Trading L.

Hsu CH, Wen ZH, Lin CS, Chakraborty C (2007). Zebrafish model: use in studying cellular mechanisms for a spectrum of clinical disease entities. Current Neurovascular Research, 4: 111-120.

2014, Advances in Biochemistry and Biotechnology Volume 2   *Pages 5-20*

Edited by: Dr. Biplab Sarkar and Dr. Chiranjib Chakraborty

Published by: DAYA PUBLISHING HOUSE

2

Potential Applications of Bioactive Peptides Derived from Fish Waste

*Prangya Paramita Tripathy**

Research Scientist, School of Biotechnology, KIIT University Bhubaneswar, Orissa, India

ABSTRACT

Bioactive peptides (BAP) are specific sequences of amino acids which remain inactive within the original protein, and exhibit defined properties when they are released by enzymatic hydrolysis. Many peptides of plant and animal origin with relevant bioactive potential have been discovered. The proteins restraining such masked biological activities are found in milk, eggs, meat and fish as well as in different plant protein sources such as soy, wheat, rice etc. Varied health effects have been exemplified to bioactive peptides, including antimicrobial properties, blood pressure-lowering (ACE inhibitory) effects, cholesterol-lowering ability, antithrombotic and antioxidant activities, enhancement of mineral absorption and/or bioavailability, cyto- or immunomodulatory effects, and opioid activities. At present, India's

* *Corresponding E-mail:* prangya_tripathy@rediffmail.com

total annual fish production is about 6.65 million tons with estimated potential based on the present levels of productivity is about 8.4 million tons. The production is associated with enormous fish waste generation. In this chapter the possible utility of fish wastes for bioactive peptide production and their potential applications are discussed.

Keywords: Bioactive peptide, ACE inhibitory, Immunomodulatory, Opioid, Antithrombotic.

Introduction

There are references of aquaculture in India in Kautilya's *Arthashastra* (321–300 B.C.) and King Someswara's *Manasoltara* (1127 A.D.). The traditional practice of fish culture in small ponds in eastern India is known to have existed for hundreds of years. Significant advances were made in the state of West Bengal in the early nineteenth century with the controlled breeding of carp in *bundhs* (tanks or impoundments where river conditions are simulated). Fish culture received notable attention in Tamil Nadu (formerly the state of Madras) as early as 1911, subsequently; states such as Bengal, Punjab, Uttar Pradesh, Orissa, Mysore and Hyderabad established Fisheries Departments for pisciculture practices. The three Indian major carps, namely catla (*Catla catla*), rohu (*Labeo rohita*) and mrigal (*Cirrhinus mrigala*) contribute the bulk of production with over 1.8 million tonnes (FAO 2003); followed by silver carp, grass carp and common carp forming a second important group. Average national production from still water ponds has increased from 0.6 tonnes/ha/year in 1974 to 2.2 tonnes/ha/year by 2001–2002 (Tripathi 2003), with several farmers even demonstrating production levels as high as 8–12 tonnes/ha/year. This huge production is associated with enormous amount of fish waste generation. The utilisation of fishery waste for value added products would thus essential for many reasons. The intention is to increase the use in foods, functional foods and biochemical products for human consumption. When the fish is gutted, headed and further processed - either on-board in fishing vessels, in processing plants on shore, or during household consumption, lot of by-products have been generated. By-products from fisheries include viscera (liver, stomachs, etc.), heads, backbones, cuts and rejected fish from processing. Today most of the by-products are used as raw materials for feed production; such as fishmeal, silage and feed for farm animals. Still a sizeable amount of waste was thrown both from household consumption and from fish industry. If we succeed to utilise more of the by-products as food for humans and as ingredients in foodstuff, health foods, pharmacy, cosmetics etc., the value adding may increase by 4-5 fold. Several reports suggested that the proteins in meat and fish having latent biological activity (*i.e.* bioactive peptide retaining ability). The present chapter discusses the possibility of extraction of various bioactive peptides derived from fish waste and their applications.

Plausible Utilisation of Fish Waste

Fish resources come out as huge and by-products were looked upon as valueless garbage in the early period of developed fisheries. Norway government was first recognized it as a serious problem in 1970s and initiated an applied research program for value addition of fishery by-products. Subsequently this programme spreads to the other parts of the world. From this programme a new technology was developed for fish viscera silage processing where a highly nutritious hydrolysate concentrate, very suitable as a protein supplement in animal feed could be recovered (Raa *et al.,* 1982). By minor modifications this technology could also be used to recover crude fish pepsins and the low molecular weight peptone fraction by ultrafiltration (Gildberg *et al.,* 1977; Gildberg *et al.,* 1986; Gildberg

1992). Pepsins from cold water fish are active at low temperature (Gildberg, 1988) and suitable for gentle enzymatic processing of some fishery products (Gildberg, 1993). The hydrolysate fraction has a high nutritional value and also contains immuno-stimulating peptides (Almas 1990; Gildberg *et al.,* 1996). There is an urgent need for better recovery and utilization of the by-products as raw materials for foods and nutraceuticals and also for pharmaceutical and biotechnological applications is essential (Venugopal and Shahidi 1995; Haard 2000; Shahidi and Janak-Kamil 2001).

It has been documented that peptides from the digests of fish muscle possesses potent inhibitory activity against angiotensin I-converting enzyme (ACE) (Galardy *et al.,* 1984; Kohama *et al.,* 1996; Matsufuji *et al.,* 1994; Yohshikawa *et al.,* 2000; Sorensen *et al.,* 2004). They possess potent antihypertensive activities. Fish silages also can be fermented with the *Lactobacillus* sp. for various fermented products which could be used as potential source of bioactive peptides. Hasan (2003) reported successful preparation of fermented silage using fermentation starters of *L. pentosus, L. plantarum,* liquid of fermented bamboo shoot and aged silage, which is attractive to be used as animal feed. These bacteria offer possible future application for silage preparation for tropical fish. However BAP from such fermented product is still in its infancy and intensive research is required in this field.

Bioactive Peptides: Types and Functions

Bioactive peptides are specific sequences of amino acids which remain inactive within the original protein, and exhibit defined properties when they are released by enzymatic hydrolysis. These peptides might have target oriented hormone like action and may affect the major body systems– namely, the cardiovascular, digestive, immune and nervous systems. Accordingly they are classified in Table 2.1.

Table 2.1: Classification of Bioactive Peptides according to their Targeted Function.

Systems Influenced	Name of Peptides	
Gastrointestinal system	Antimicrobial	
	Mineral binding	Also affect gastro-intestinal and immune system
	Anti appetizing	
Cardiovascular system	Antihypertensive BAP	
	Antioxidative	
	Antithrombotic	
	Hypocholesterolemic	
Nervous System	Opioid agonist	
	Opioid antagonist	
Immune system	Immunomodulatory	

The proteins containing these latent biological activities are found in milk, eggs, meat and fish as well as in different plant protein sources such as soy, wheat, and so on (Table 2.2). Such peptides can be released in three ways: (a) through hydrolysis by digestive enzymes, (b) through hydrolysis by proteolytic microorganisms and (c) through the action of proteolytic enzymes derived from microorganisms or plants. It is now well established that bioactive peptides are produced from several food proteins during gastrointestinal digestion and fermentation of food materials with lactic acid bacteria. The production and properties of bioactive peptides have been reviewed recently by many experts (FitzGerald *et al.,* 2003; Korhonen *et al.,* 2003).

Table 2.2: Examples of some Bioactive Peptides (Origin, sequence and references).

Effect	Origin	Encrypting Protein(s)	Name/Sequence (in single-letter code)	References
ACE Inhibitory/ Hypotensive	Soy	Soy protein	NWGPLV	Kodera et al., 2006
	Fish	Fish muscle protein	LKP, IKP, LRP (derived from sardine, bonito, tuna, squid)	Nagai et al., 2006
	Meat	Meat muscle protein	IKW, LKP	Vercruysse et al., 2005
	Milk	α – LA, β - LG	Lactokinins (e.g. WLAHK, LRP, LKP)	Murray et al., 2007
		α-, β-, k-CN	Casokinins (e.g. FFVAP, FALPQY, VPP)	Mizushima et al., 2004
		β-CN	Ser-Lys-Val-Tyr-Pro-Phe-Pro-Gly Pro-Ile	Ashar et al., 2004
		β-CN	Ser-Lys-Val-Tyr-Pro	Ashar et al., 2004
	Egg	Ovotransferrin Ovalbumin Ovokinin	KVREGTTY Ovokinin (FRADHPPL)	Lee et al., 2006
			Ovokinin (2–7) (KVREGTTY)	Miguel et al., 2006
	Wheat	Wheat giladin	IAP	Motoi et al., 2003
	Broccoli	Plant protein	YPK	Lee et al., 2006
Immunomodulatory	Rice	Rice albumin	Oryzatensin (GYPMYPLR)	Takahashi 1994
	Egg	Ovalbumin	Peptides not specified	Mine et al., 2006
	Milk	α-, β-, k-CN, α – LA	Immunopeptides (e.g. α S1-immunocasokinin) (TTMPLW)	Meisel 2005
	Wheat	Wheat gluten	Immunopeptides	Horiguchi et al., 2005
Cytomodulatory	Milk	α-, β- CN	α-Casomorphin (HIQKED(V)), β-casomorphin-7 (YPFPGPI)	Kampa et al., 1997
Opioid agonist	Wheat	Wheat gluten	Gluten-exorphins A4, A5 (GYYPT), B4, B5, and C (YPISL)	Takahashi et al., 2000; Fukudome et al., 1993
	Milk	α -LA, β -LG	α-Lactorphins,β -lactorphins	Silva et al., 2005
		α-, β- CN	Casomorphins	Silva et al., 2005
Opiod antagonist	Milk	Lactoferrin	Lactoferroxins	Clare et al., 2000
		k-CN	Casoxins	Clare et al., 2000
Antimicrobial	Egg	Ovotransferrin	OTAP-92 (f109–200)[a]	Mine et al., 2006
		Lysozyme	Peptides not specified	
	Milk	Lactoferrin	Lactoferricin	McCann et al., 2006
		α -, β -, k-CN	Casecidins, Isracidin, Kappacin	Hayes et al., 2006
Antithrombotic	Milk	k-CN (glycomacro-peptide)	(f106–116)a, casoplatelin	Chabance et al., 1995
Mineral binding, anticarcinogenic	Milk	α-, β- CN	Caseinophosphopeptides	Walker et al., 2006
Hypocholesterolemic	Soy	Glycinin	LPYPR	Wang et al., 1995

Contd...

Table 2.2–*Contd...*

Effect	Origin	Encrypting Protein(s)	Name/Sequence (in single-letter code)	References
	Milk	β -LG	IIAEK	Nagaoka *et al.*, 2001
	Soy	Soy protein hydrolysate	High molecular weight fraction of soy protein digested by microbial proteases	Sugano *et al.*, 1990
Antioxidant	Fish	Sardine muscle	MY	Erdmann *et al.*, 2006
	Wheat	Wheat germ protein	Peptides not specified	Zhu *et al.*, 2006
	Milk	α -LA, β -LG	MHIRL, YVEEL, WYSLAMAASDI	Hernandez-Ledesma *et al.*, 2005
	Fish	Seal protein hydrolysates	Peptides not specified	Shahidi *et al.*, 1996

CN: Casein; LA: Lactalbumin; LG: Lactoglobulin; ᵃf: Fragment.

It may be inferred that the potential of distinct dietary peptide sequences lies by promoting the human health by reducing the risk of chronic diseases or boosting natural immune protection.

A) Peptides that Influence Gastrointestinal System

Bioactive peptides may involve in important functions such as regulation of digestive enzymes and modulation of nutrient absorption in the intestinal tract before hydrolysis to amino acids and subsequent absorption (Shimizu, 2004). These include

(a) Mineral Binding

(b) Antimicrobial

(c) Anti appetizing

(a) Mineral Binding

Casein-derived phosphorylated peptides, caseinophosphopeptides (CPPs) was first suggested by Mellander in 1950 (first reference for bioactive peptides). These peptides enhanced vitamin D-independent bone calcification in infants affected with rickets. Caseinophosphopeptides (CPPs) yielded by the tryptic digestion of the N terminus polar region of the casein proteins (Cross *et al.*, 2005). These regions contain clusters of phosphorylated seryl residues. These phosphoseryl clusters might have been responsible for the interaction between the caseins and calcium phosphate that leads to the formation of casein micelles. CPPs have the capability of stabilizing calcium and phosphate ions through the formation of complexes, thus enhancing their general bioavailability. Since CPPs can bind and solubilize minerals, they have been considered physiologically beneficial in the prevention of osteoporosis, dental caries, hypertension and anemia. In a study, Narva *et al.* (2004) demonstrated that *L. helveticus* fermented whey and the tripeptides VPP and IPP stimulated the proliferation of osteoblasts in vitro, whereas sour-milk whey and calcium had no effect. More cell culture and human studies are, however, necessary to demonstrate the potential of CPPs and other peptides to enhance dietary mineral bioavailability and to modulate bone formation (Bouhallab *et al.*, 2004). CPPs are also associated with the mucosal immunity which is supported by a study of Otani, Kihara and Park (2000) that showed the oral administration of a commercial CPP preparation enhanced the intestinal IgA levels of piglets. CPPs may have a role on anticariogenic effect by promoting recalcification of tooth enamel, whereas glycomacropeptide (GMP) derived from kappa-casein seems to contribute to the anticaries effect by inhibiting the adhesion and growth of plaque-forming bacteria on oral mucosa (Brody 2000; Malkoski *et al.*, 2001). Various dental care products containing CPPs and/or GMP have been launched on the market in some countries. Although fish is a rich source of calcium, the reports related to CPP production from fishery by product is scanty. Thus there will be immense scope for research in this field.

(b) Antimicrobial

Lactoferricins, the most studied antimicrobial peptides have been derived from bovine and human lactoferrin (Kitts *et al.*, 2003; Wakabayashi *et al.*, 2003). These peptides exhibit antimicrobial activity against various Gram-positive and -negative bacteria, *e.g. Escherichia, Helicobacter, Listeria, Salmonella* and *Staphylococcus, Bacillus,* Yeasts and filamentous fungi. The antibacterial mechanism of lactoferricins lies in the disruption of the normal membrane permeability. *In vivo,* they have the capability to modulate the intestinal microflora (Shimizu 2004). However, these peptides are strain specific that means, they are produced from milk only when fermented with specific cultures of *Lactobacillus.* When scanned with more than fifty lactobacillus cultures isolated from different sources of milk and milk products of Orissa, only two lactobacillus cultures showed antimicrobial peptide producing ability (Tripathy *et al.*, 2011, unpublished data, Figure 2.1). These peptides will definitely find exciting applications in the field of food safety and as pharmaceuticals (Fitzgerald *et al.*, 2006). These peptides can also be isolated from fishery by-products and the same can be applied against fish pathogens.

(c) Anti-appetizing

Anti-appetizing properties mainly played by glycomacropeptide (GMP) and cytomodulatory peptide (CMP). The role of CMP includes inhibition of gastric secretions, delaying of stomach contractions and helps in the liberation of cholecystokinin (CKK) (the satiety hormone involved in controlling food intake and digestion in the duodenum of animals and humans contractions) (Brody 2000; Pihlanto *et al.*, 2003; Manso *et al.*, 2004; Yvon *et al.*, 1994). But, on the other hand, it has also been experimented that glycomacropeptide (GMP) can be absorbed as intact and partially digested into the blood circulation of adult humans after milk or yoghurt ingestion (Chabance *et al.*, 1998). Furthermore

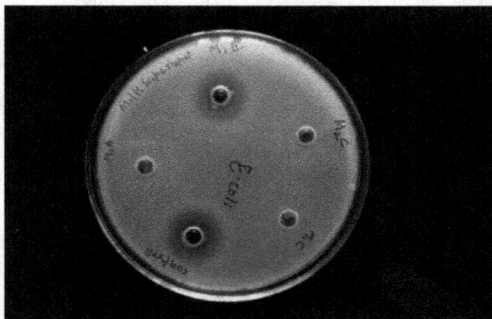

Figure 2.1: Antimicrobial Peptides Produced by *Lactobacillus* sp. Isolated from Indigenous Fermented Product of Orissa Showing Zone of Inhibition Against *E. coli.*

due to its carbohydrate (mainly sialic acid) content, GMP may have a beneficial role in modulating the gut microflora, as this macropeptide is known to promote the growth of bifidobacteria (Manso *et al.*, 2004). Little evidence is available with regard to anti-appetizing peptide from the fishery waste.

B) Peptides that Affect the Cardiovascular System

- (a) Antihypertensive BAP
- (b) Antithrombotic
- (c) Hypocholesterolemic
- (d) Antioxidative

(a) Antihypertensive BAP

Hypertension affects about a quarter of the world's population and has become a major health problem in India, yet controllable, risk factor in cardiovascular disease and related complications. Angiotensin-converting enzyme (EC 3.4.15.1) (ACE) is known to play a leading role in the regulation of blood pressure in animals, including humans. Angiotensin-converting enzyme (EC 3.4.15.1) (ACE) inhibitory peptide is the major antihypertensive agent found in milk and milk products (Murray *et al.*, 2007; Mizushima *et al.*, 2004). Also this is the most studied peptide found in fish, fishery waste and meat (Nagai *et al.*, 2006; Vercruysse *et al.*, 2005). The enzyme converts angiotensin I into angiotensin II, the former being an inert peptide (propeptide) and the latter being an active agent. The enzyme is also responsible for the breakdown of bradykinin, which is a sluggish peptide. The enzyme is thus an obvious drug target in treatment of certain cardiovascular diseases, including hypertension. Lactic acid bacteria are known to produce inhibitors of the enzyme in various amounts during fermentation (Xu 1998). The inhibitors are formed by the bacterial proteinases when the lactic acid bacteria hydrolyze milk proteins, mainly casein, into peptides, which can be used as nitrogen sources necessary for growth. The IC_{50} value (inhibitor concentration leading to 50 per cent inhibition) is used to estimate the effectiveness of different ACE inhibitory peptides. However, it is not always directly related to the in vivo hypotensive effect. Some peptides can be susceptible to degradation or modification in the gut, the vascular system and the liver. By contrast, hypotensive activity of a long-chain candidate peptide can be caused by peptide fragments generated by gastrointestinal enzymes (Meisel *et al.*, 2006). All of the ACE inhibitors known to date that are formed in milk during fermentation are peptides that act as competitive inhibitors, such as Ile-Pro-Pro and Val-Pro-Pro (Meisel 2005). After oral administration in spontaneously hypertensive rats (SHR) it has been reported that fermented milk rich in inhibitory substances can lower systolic blood pressure (Fuglsang *et al.*, 2003).

Several researchers reported that peptides from the digests of fish muscle possesses potent inhibitory activity against angiotensin I-converting enzyme (ACE) (Galardy *et al.*, 1984; Kohama *et al.*, 1996; Matsufuji et al.1994; Yohshikawa *et al.*, 2000; Sorensen *et al.*, 2004). They possess potent antihypertensive activities. A comparative study was performed for assessment of relative antihypertensive activities of two peptides from fish to that of captopril (a common drug). For this purpose they were orally administered to rats. When compared on molar basis the two fish peptides accounted for 66 per cent and 91 per cent relative to that of captopril. Interestingly these peptides wield remarkably higher antihypertensive activities *in vivo* despite weaker *in vitro* ACE inhibitory effects, which were determined by using captopril as the reference drug. Such peptides may be regarded as healthy components of fish muscles and may be produced as ingredients or diet supplements (Sorensen *et al.*, 2004). Recently it has been shown that protein hydrolysates from *Alaska pollack*, shrimp waste, cod head and sardine had some inhibitory effect on angiotensin I converting enzyme (Byun *et al.,* 2001; Bordenave *et al.,* 2002).

(b) Antithrombotic BAP

Milk derived antithrombotic peptides are known as casoplatelins. They come from the C-terminal fragment of bovine-casein (glycomacropeptide) and they are the inhibitors of platelet aggregation activated by adenosine di phosphate. The major antithrombotic peptides occurring in bovine-casein are its fragments: 106-116, 106-112, 112-116 and 113-116, (MAIPPKKNQDK; fragment 106-116) (Fiat *et al.,* 1993). Such peptides can be detected in the plasma of five days old human after breastfeeding or ingestion of cow milk-based infant formulae and also in bovine newborns (Chabance *et al.,* 1995). However, the physiological effects of these antithrombotic peptides remain unclear. These peptides were also found in enzymatically hydrolyzed fish muscle. These results have suggested the capability of fish peptides to inhibit coagulation factors in the intrinsic pathway of coagulation (Rajapakse *et al.,* 2005). There is also scope for obtaining such peptides from fish muscle with suitable cultures of *Lactobacillus* species.

(c) Hypocholesterolemic BAP

Hypercholesterolemia is one of the most important risk factors during the development of cardiovascular diseases (Kannel *et al.,* 1971). Various synthetic drugs and natural extracts with cholesterol-lowering effect have been explored for their potential in prevention and treatment of hypercholesterolemia. Literature indicates that proteins from soybean can reduce blood cholesterol level in experimental animal models as well as in human subjects (Kim *et al.,* 1980; Potter 1995). A daily intake of 25 g of soybean protein is recommended by the U.S. Food and Drug Administration (FDA 1999) for maintaining the lower level of serum cholesterol level and reduction in the risk of cardiovascular diseases. Milk is another important source of bioactive peptides with cholesterol-lowering effect. A hypocholesterolemic peptide was isolated from milk β-lactoglobulin tryptic hydrolysate, which was identified to be IIAEK (Nagaoka *et al.,* 2001). Those authors demonstrated that this peptide inhibited the absorption of micellar cholesterol in Caco-2 cells in vitro and exhibited greater hypocholesterolemic activity than the medicine β-sitosterol in rats. The suppression of cholesterol absorption in Caco-2 cells by IIAEK using both artificial micelles and pig bile-derived natural micelle was also evaluated by (Kirana *et al.,* 2005). Pork protein hydrolysate prepared with papain has also been shown to exert a hypocholesterolemic effect in cholesterol-fed rats (Morimatsu *et al.,* 1996). However little reports are available for these kind of peptides of fish origin.

(d) Antioxidative BAP

Recent studies have shown that antioxidative peptides can be released from caseins in hydrolysis by digestive enzymes and in fermentation of milk with proteolytic LAB strains (Korhonen *et al.,* 2003). Most of the identified peptides are derived from α_{s1}-casein and have been shown to possess free radical-scavenging activities and to inhibit enzymatic and non-enzymatic lipid peroxidation (Rival *et al.,* 2001; Rival *et al.,* 2001; Suetsuna *et al.,* 2000). Efforts are also made to make nutraceuticals from milk and Indian herbs for potential use in functional dairy foods (Singh *et al.,* 2009). In the future, antioxidative peptides may find applications as ingredients in different fields *e.g.* in the prevention of oxidation in fat-containing foodstuffs, cosmetics and pharmaceuticals. More studies are needed to demonstrate the potential health benefits of the antioxidative peptides formed during milk fermentation.

Aquatic species and by-products from aquaculture industry are probably the most extensively investigated source of antioxidative peptides. Four peptide fractions have been separated from protein hydrolysates of capelin with one fraction possessing notable antioxidant activity, another two, a weak antioxidant efficacy, and the fourth exerting a pro-oxidant effect (Amarowicz *et al.,* 1997). Synergistic effects of capelin protein hydrolysates with synthetic antioxidants, butylated hydroxylanisole (BHA), butylated hydroxyltoluene (BHT), and tert-butylhydroquinone (TBHQ) were monitored (Amarowicz *et al.,* 2002) recently. Protein hydrolysates prepared from mussel and fermented mussel sauce have shown antioxidant activity (Rajakapse *et al.,* 2005). Marine mammal protein hydrolysates have been explored for potential antioxidant activity. Shahidi and Amarowicz (1996) evaluated the antioxidant effectiveness of harp seal protein hydrolysates and found that the hydrolysates displayed antioxidant property at certain concentrations while a pro-oxidant property was observed at higher concentrations. Recently, a variety of fish processing waste such as protein hydrolysates from tuna backbones (J.Y *et al.,* 2007), *Alaska pollack* frame and skin (Kim *et al.,* 2001; J.Y *et al.,* 2007), hoki frame (Kim *et al.,* 2007), and other marine wastes (Guerard *et al.,* 2005) has been considered for potential source of peptides with antioxidant potential.

Peptides of Nervous System

Peptides with opioid activity (both agonist and antagonistic activities) have been identified in various casein fractions hydrolyzed by digestive enzymes (Brantl *et al.,* 1979; Pihlanto-Leppa la *et al.,* 1994; Teschemacher 2003). Opioid receptors are located in the nervous, endocrine and immune systems as well as in the gastrointestinal tract of mammals and can interact with their endogenous ligands and with exogenous opioids and opioid antagonists. Thus, orally administered opioid peptides may modulate absorption processes in the gut and influence the gastrointestinal function in two ways: first, by affecting smooth muscles, which reduces the transit time, and second, by affecting the intestinal transport of electrolytes, which explains their anti-secretory properties. The actual physiological effects of milk-derived opioid peptides remain unclear. Reports of opoid peptides from fish protein hydrolysate (FPH) however not available till date.

Immunomodulatory BAP

The bioactive peptides generated during milk fermentation with lactic acid bacteria have been found to modulate the proliferation of human lymphocytes, to down-regulate the production of certain cytokines and to stimulate the phagocytic activities of macrophages (Matar *et al.,* 2003; Meisel *et al.,* 2003). Immunomodulatory milk peptides may lessen allergic reactions in atopic humans and enhance mucosal immunity in the gastrointestinal tract (Korhonen *et al.,* 2003). Recently it was demonstrated that commercial whey protein isolates contain immunomodulating peptides can be released by enzymatic digestion (Mercier *et al.,* 2004). This information is of high relevance when developing infant formulas with optimized immunomodulatory properties. Immunopeptides are also having the contribution for antitumor activities as observed in many studies with fermented milks (Matar *et al.,* 2003). Meisel and FitzGerald (2003) studied that caseinophosphopeptides (CPPs) are having cytomodulatory activity as they inhibit the cancer cell growth and rouse the activity of immunocompetent and neonatal intestinal cells. Glycomacropeptide (GMP) and its derivatives exhibiting a variety of immunomodulatory functions, such as immunosuppressive effects on the production of IgG antibodies (Monnai *et al.,* 1998; Manso *et al.,* 2004) and immunoenhancing effects on proliferation and phagocytic activities of human macrophage like cells U937 (Li *et al.,* 2004). In an *in vivo* study, Matar *et al.* (2003) demonstrated that lactic acid bacterial peptides are having important immunomodulating properties, *e.g.,* proliferation of human lymphocytes, down-regulation of certain cytokines production and stimulation of the phagocytic activities of the macrophages. Reports are also available regarding the benefit of treating the acquired immune deficiency syndrome by immunomodulatory bioactive peptides (Gottileb *et al.*, 1996).

Both in *vitro* and in *vivo* experiments with fish indicate that a low molecular weight peptide fraction (between 500-3000 Da) from silage of cod stomach stimulates non-specific immune response reactions and improves the disease resistance in fish (Gildberg *et al.*, 1996; Gildbcrg *et al.*, 1998). Similar results have been achieved with low molecular weight proteins from cod milt (Pedersen *et al.*, 2003). Both acidic and basic peptides often seem to be involved in immunostimulation.

Summary

Till date the following BAPs have been reported from fisheries.

☆ Reports are available regarding the antioxidative peptide from fish protein hydrolysates (FPH). Further studies should focus on the hydrolysis process in order to get more knowledge on how different fish species and fractions of raw materials influence the properties of the hydrolysates. The health effect of bioactive peptides from fish should be documented and different fractions of the hydrolysates should be studied and analysed for antioxidative bioactive potential. Antioxidative properties obtained with fish skin peptides (Kim *et al.*, 2001) indicate that protein hydrolysates from fish by-products may have a potential as supplements in nutraceuticals.

☆ Fish wastes also stimulate nonspecific immune response and involved in disease resistance as observed from *in vitro* and *in vivo* studies (Gildberg *et al.*, 1996).

☆ FPH from Alaska pollack, shrimp waste, cod head and sardine are having some inhibitory effect on angiotensin I converting enzyme (Byun *et al.*, 2001; Bordenave *et al.*, 2002). This indicates that application of such hydrolysates in food may reduce high blood pressure.

☆ Recently, stimulation of the proliferation of human white blood cells was obtained during *in vitro* cultivation with peptides from commercial Thai anchovy fish sauce (Thongthai *et al.*, 2003).

Future Research Potential

Since India is an important hub for both freshwater and marine fisheries, there will be enormous scope in this field, particularly for the production and development of new chemotheraupeutic agents. The advance in proteomics (Atmospheric pressure ionization triple quadrupole (API-III), Electrospray ionization (ESI-MS/MS), Matrix-assisted laser desorption ionization–time-of-flight (MALDI-TOF) methods may facilitate more exciting results in this field in future.

References

Almas KA (1990). Utilization of marine biomass for production of microbial growth media and biochemicals. In: Voigt MN and Botta JR (ed) Advances in fisheries technology and biotechnology for increased profitability, Technomic Publishing Co. Inc., Lancaster, pp. 361-372.

Amarowicz R, Shahidi F (1997). Antioxidant activity of peptide fractions of capelin protein hydrolysates. Food Chem 58: 355–359.

Amarowicz R, Karamac M, Weidner S *et al.* (2002). Antioxidant activity of caryopses and embryos extracts. J Food Lipids 9: 201-210.

Ashar MN, Chand R (2004). Fermented milk containing ACE inhibitory peptides reduces blood pressure in middle aged hypertensive subjects. Milchwissenschaft 59: 363–366.

Bordenave S, Fruitier I, Ballandier I *et al.* (2002). HPLC preparation of fish waste hydrolysate fractions. Effect on Guinea pig ileum and ACE activity. Prepar Biochem Biotechnol 32: 65-77.

Bouhallab S, Bougle D (2004). Biopeptides of milk: Caseinophosphopeptides and mineral bioavailability. Reprod Nutr Dev 44: 493–498.

Brantl V, Teschemacher H, Henschen A *et al.* (1979). Novel opioid peptides derived from casein (β-casomorphins). Isolation from bovine casein peptone. Hoppe-Seyler's Zeitschrift fur Physiologie und Chemie 360: 1211–1216.

Brody EP (2000). Biological activities of bovine glycomacropeptide. Br J Nutr 84: S39–S46.

Byun HG, Kim SK (2001). Purification and characterization of angiotensin I converting enzyme (ACE) inhibitory peptide from *Alaska pollack* (*Theragra chiiicogramma*) skins. Proc Biochem 36: 1155-1162.

Chabance B, Jolles P, Izquierdo C *et al.* (1995). Characterization of an antithrombotic peptide from kappa-casein in newborn plasma after milk ingestion. Br J Nutr 73: 583-590.

Chabance B, Marteau P, Rambaud JC *et al.* (1998). Casein peptide release and passage to the blood in humans during digestion of milk or yogurt. Biochimie 80: 155–165.

Clare DA, Swaisgood HE (2000). Bioactive milk peptides: a prospectus. J Dairy Sci 83: 1187-1195.

Cross KJ, Huq NL, Palamara JE *et al.* (2005). Physico-chemical characterization of casein phosphopeptide amorphous calcium phosphate nanocomplexes. J Biol Chem 280: 15362-15369.

Erdmann K, Grosser N, Schipporeit K *et al.* (2006). The ACE inhibitory dipeptide Met-Tyr diminishes free radical formation in human endothelial cells via induction of heme oxygenase-1 and ferritin. J Nutr 136: 2148-2152.

Fiat AM, Migliore-Samour D, Jolle's P *et al.* (1993). Biologically active peptides from milk proteins with emphasis on two examples concerning antithrombotic and immunomodulating activities. J Dairy Sci 76: 301–310.

Fuglsang A, Rattray FP, Nilsson D *et al.* (2003). Lactic acid bacteria: inhibition of angiotensin converting enzyme *in vitro* and *in vivo*. Antonie van Leeuwenhoek Intern J Gen Mol Microbiol 83: 27-34.

Fukudome S, Yoshikawa M (1993). Gluten exorphin-C–a novel opioid peptide derived from wheat gluten. FEBS Letters 316: 17-19.

Galardy R, Podhasky P, Olson KR (1984). Angiotensin-converting enzyme activity in tissues of the rainbow trout. J Exp Zoology 230: 155-158.

Gildberg A (1988). Aspartic proteinases in fish and aquatic invertebrates. Comp Biochem Physiol 91B: 425-435.

Gildberg A (1992). Recovery of proteinases and protein hydrolysates from fish viscera. Biores Technol 39: 271-276.

Gildberg A (1993). Enzymatiic processing of marine raw materials. Proc Biochem 28: I-IS.

Gildberg A, Bogvald J, Johansen A *et al.* (1996). Isolation of acid peptide fractions from a fish protein hydrolysate with strong stimulatory effect on Atlantic salmon head kidney leukocytes. Comp Biochem Physiol 114B: 97-101.

Gildberg A, Raa J (1977). Properties of a propionic acid/formic acid preserved silage of cod viscera. *J Sci Food Agriculture* 28: 647-653.

Gildherg A, Almas KA (1986). In: Food Engineering and Process Application. M. LeMaguer and P Jelen (ed) Utilization of fish viscera, Elsevier Appl Sci Publishers London, pp. 383-393.

Gildberg A, Mikkelsen H (1998). Effects of supplementing the feed to atlantic cod (*Gadus morhua*) fry with lactic acid bacteria and immunostimulating peptides during a challenge trial with *Vibrio anguillarum*. Aquaculture 167: 103-113.

Gottlieb AA, Sizemore RC, Gottlieb MS *et al.* (1996). Rationale and clinical results of using leucocyte-derived immunosupportive therapies in HIV disease. Biotherapy 9: 27-31.

Guerard F, Sumaya-Martinez MT, Linard B *et al.* (2005). Agro Food Industry Hi-Tech 16: 16–18.

Haard NF (2000). In: Seafood Enzymes. NF Haard and BK Simpson (ed) Seafood enzymes: The role of adaptation and other interspecific factors, Marcel Dekker, pp. 1-36.

Hasan B (2003). Fermentation of Fish Silage using *Lactobacillus pentosus*. Jurnal Natur Indonesia 6: 11-15.

Hayes A, Ross RP, Fitzgerald GF *et al.* (2006). Casein-derived antimicrobial peptides generated by *Lactobacillus acidophilus* DPC6026. Appl Environ Microbiol 72: 2260–2264.

Hernandez-Ledesma B, Davalos A, Bartolome B *et al.* (2005). Preparation of antioxidant enzymatic hydrolysates from alpha-lactalbumin and beta-lactoglobulin. Identification of active peptides by HPLC-MS/MS. J Agric Food Chem 53: 588-593.

Horiguchi N, Horiguchi H, Suzuki Y (2005). Effect of wheat gluten hydrolysate on the immune system in healthy human subjects. Biosci Biotechnol Biochem 69: 2445-2449.

Je JY, Park PJ, Kim SK (2005). Antioxidant activity of a peptide isolated from Alaska pollack (*Theragra chalcogramma*) frame protein hydrolysate. Food Res Intern 38: 45-50.

Je JY, Qian ZJ, Byun HG *et al.* (2007). Purification and characterization of an antioxidantpeptide from tuna backbone protein by enzymatic hydrolysis. Proc.Proc Biochem.Biochem 42, 840-846 (2007)42: 840-846.

Kampa M, Bakogeorgou E, Hatzoglou A *et al.* (1997). Opioid alkaloids and casomorphin peptides decrease the proliferation of prostatic cancer cell lines (LNCaP, PC3 and DU145) through a partial interaction with opioid receptors. Eur J Pharmacol 335: 255-265.

Kannel WB, Castelli WP, Gordon T *et al.* (1971). Serum cholesterol, lipoproteins and the risk of coronary heart disease. The Framingham Study. Ann Intern Med 74: 1-12.

Kim DN, Lee KT, Reiner JM *et al.* (1980). Increased steroid excretion in swine fed high-fat, high-cholesterol diet with soy protein. Exp Mol Pathol 33: 25–35.

Kim SK, Lee HC, Byun HG *et al.* (1996). Isolation and characterization of antioxidative peptides from enzymatic hydrolysates of yellow fin sole skin gelation. J Korean Fish Soc 29: 246-255.

Kim SK, Kim YK, Byun HK *et al.* (2001). Isolation and characterization of antioxidative peptides from gelatin hydrolysate of *Alaska pollack* skin. J Agric Food Chem 49: 1984-1989.

Kim SY, Je JY, Kim SK (2007). Purification and characterization of antioxidant peptide from hoki (*Johnius balengerii*) frame protein by gastrointestinal digestion. J Nutr Biochem 18: 31–38.

Kirana C, Rogers PF, Bennett LE *et al.* (2005). Rapid screening for potential cholesterol-lowering peptides using naturally derived micelle preparation. Aust J Dairy Technology 60: 163–166.

Kitts DD, Weiler K (2003). Bioactive proteins and peptides from food sources. Applications of bioprocesses used in isolation and recovery. Curr Pharmaceut Design 9: 1309–1323.

Kodera T, Nio N (2006). Identification of an angiotensin I-converting enzyme inhibitory peptides from protein hydrolysates by a soybean protease and the antihypertensive effects of hydrolysates in spontaneously hypertensive model rats. J Food Sci 71: C164-C173.

Kohama Y, Kuroda T, Itoh S et al. (1996). Tuna muscle peptide, PTHIKWGD, inhibits leukocyte-mediated injury and leukocyte adhesion to cultured endothelial cells. Biol Pharmaceut Bull 19: 139-141.

Korhonen H, Pihlanto A (2006). Bioactive peptides: production and functionality. Int Dairy J 16: 945-960.

Korhonen H, Pihlanto A (2003). Food-derived bioactive peptides–opportunities for designing future foods. Curr Pharmaceut Design 9: 1297–1308.

Lee JE, Bae IY, Lee HG et al. (2006). Tyr-Pro-Lys, an angiotensin I-converting enzyme inhibitory peptide derived from broccoli (Brassica oleracea Italica). Food Chem 99: 143-148.

Lee NY, Cheng JT, Enomoto T et al. (2006). One peptide derived from hen ovotransferrin as pro-drug to inhibit angiotensin converting enzyme. J Food Drug Anal 14: 31-35.

Li EW, Mine Y (2004). Immunoenhancing effects of bovine glycomacropeptide and its derivatives on the proliferative response and phagocytic activities of human macrophage like cells, U937. J Agric Food Chem 52: 2704–2708.

Malkoski M, Dashper SG, O'Brien-Simpson NM et al. (2001). Kappacin, a novel antibacterial peptide from bovine milk. Antimicrob Agents Chemother 45: 2309–2315.

Manso MA, Lopez-Fandino R (2004). Kappa-Casein macropeptides from cheese whey: Physicochemical, biological, nutritional, and technological features for possible uses. Food Rev Intern 20: 329–355.

Matar C, LeBlanc JG, Martin L et al. (2003). Biologically active peptides released in fermented milk: Role and functions, Handbook of fermented functional foods. Functional foods and nutraceuticals series. In: E. R. Farnworth (ed) Biologically active peptides released in fermented milk: Role and functions, Handbook of fermented functional foods. Functional foods and nutraceuticals series, CRC Press, Florida, USA, pp. 177–201.

Matsufuji H, Matsui T, Seki E et al. (1994). Angiotensin I-converting enzyme inhibitory peptides in an alkaline protease hydrolyzate derived from sardine muscle. Biosci Biotechnol Biochem 58: 2244-2245.

McCann KB, Shiell BJ, Michalski WP et al. (2006). Isolation and characterisation of a novel antibacterial peptide from bovine αS1-casein. Int Dairy J 16: 316-323.

Meisel H, Walsh DJ, Murray BA et al. (2006). ACE inhibitory peptides. In: Mine V (ed) Nutraceutical Proteins and Peptides in Health and Disease, Taylor and Francis, pp. 269-315.

Meisel H (2005). Biochemical properties of peptides encrypted in bovine milk proteins. Curr Med Chem 12: 1905-1919.

Meisel H, FitzGerald RJ (2003). Biofunctional peptides from milk proteins: Mineral binding and cytomodulatory effects. Curr Pharmaceut Design 9: 1289-1295.

Mellander O (1950). The physiological importance of the casein phosphopeptide calcium salts II. Peroral calcium dosage of infants. Acta of the Society of Medicine of Uppsala 55: 247–255.

Mercier A, Gauthier SF, Fliss I (2004). Immunomodulating effects of whey proteins and their enzymatic digests. Int Dairy J 14: 175–183.

Miguel M, Aleixandre A (2006). Antihypertensive peptides derived from egg proteins. J Nutr 136: 1457-1460.

Mine Y, Kovacs-Nolan J (2006). New insights in biologically active proteins and peptides derived from hen egg. World's Poult Sci J 62: 87-95.

Mizushima S, Ohshige K, Watanabe J et al. (2004). Randomized controlled trial of sour milk on blood pressure in borderline hypertensive men. Am J Hyper 17: 701-706.

Monnai M, Horimoto Y, Otani H (1998). Immunomodificatory effect of dietary bovine k-caseinoglycopeptide on serum antibody levels and proliferative responses of lymphocytes in mice. Milchwissenschaft 53: 129-132.

Morimatsu F, Ito M, Budijanto S et al. (1996). Plasma cholesterol-suppressing effect of papain hydrolyzed pork meat in rats fed hypercholesterolemic diet. J Nutr Sci Vitaminol 42: 145–153.

Motoi H, Kodama T (2003). Isolation and characterization of angiotensin I-converting enzyme inhibitory peptides from wheat gliadin hydrolysate. Nahrung 47: 352-356.

Murray BA, FitzGerald RJ (2007). Angiotensin converting enzyme inhibitory peptides derived from food proteins: biochemistry, bioactivity and production. Curr Pharmaceut Design 13: 773–791.

Nagai T, Suzuki N, Nagashima T (2006). Antioxidative activities and angiotensin I-converting enzyme inhibitory activities of enzymatic hydrolysates from commercially available Kamaboko species. J Food Sci Technol 12: 335-346.

Nagaoka S, Futamura Y, Miwa K et al. (2001). Identification of novel hypocholesterolemic peptides derived from bovine milk betalactoglobulin. Biochem Biophys Res Commun 281: 11-17.

Narva M, Halleen J, Vaananen K et al. (2004). Effects of *Lactobacillus helveticus* fermented milk on bone cells in vitro. Life Sciences 75: 1727–1734.

National Heart Lung and Blood Institute: The seventh report of the joint national committee on prevention, detection, evaluation and treatment of high blood pressure. Publication No. 03-5233, Bethesda, MD, National Institutes of Health.

Singh RRB, Rastogi S (2011). Novel Approaches for Production of Nutraceuticals from Milk and Indian Herbs for Potential Use in Functional Dairy Foods. NAIP project report NDRI, Karnal, India.

Ondetti MA, Rubin B, Cushman DW (1977). Design of specific inhibitors of angiotensin-converting enzyme: new class of orally active antihypertensive agents. Science 196: 441-444.

Otani H, Kihara Y, Park M (2000). The immunoenhancing property of dietary casein phosphopeptide preparation in mice. Food Agric Immunol 12: 165–173.

Pedersen GM, Gildberg A, Steiro K et al. (2003). Histone-like proteins from Atlantic cod milt: Stimulatory effect on Atlantic salmon leucocytes *in vivo* and *in vitro*. Comp Biochem Physiol 34B: 407-416.

Pihlanto A, Korhonen H (2003). Bioactive peptides and proteins. In: SL Taylor (ed) Advances in food and nutrition research. Elsevier Inc, San Diego, USA, pp. 175 -276.

Pihlanto-Leppala A, Antila P, Mantsala P *et al.* (1994). Opioid peptides produced by *in vitro* proteolysis of bovine caseins. Int Dairy J 4: 291– 301.

Potter SM (1995). Overview of proposed mechanisms for the hypocholesterolemic effect of soy. J Nutr 125: 606S–611S.

Raa J, Gildberg A (1982). Fish silage: A review. CRC Critical Reviews F(X) dSci Nutr 16: 383-420.

Rajapakse N, Jung WK, Mendis E *et al.* (2005). A novel anticougulant purified from fish protein hydrolysate inhibits factor xiia and platelet aggregation. Life Sciences 76: 2607-2619.

Rival SG, Fornaroli S, Boeriu CG *et al.* (2001). Caseins and casein hydrolysates. Lipoxygenase inhibitory properties. J Agric Food Chem 4: 287–294.

Rival SG, Fornaroli S, Boeriu CG *et al.* (2001). Caseins and casein hydrolysates. Antioxidative properties and relevance to lipoxygenase inhibition. J Agric Food Chem 4: 295–302.

Shahidi F, Amarowicz R (1996). Antioxidant activity of protein hydrolyzates from aquatic species. J Am Oil Chem Soc (73): 1197-1199.

Shahidi F, Janak-Kamil YVA (2001). Enzymes from fish and aquatic invertebrates and their application in the food industry. Trends Food Sci Technol 12: 435-464.

Shimizu M (2004). Food-derived peptides and intestinal functions. BioFactors 21: 43–47.

Silva SV, Malcata FX (2005). Caseins as source of bioactive peptides. Int Dairy J 15: 1-15.

Sorensen R, Kildal E, Stepaniak L *et al.* (2004). Screening for peptides from fish and cheese inhibitory to prolyl endopeptidase. NAHRUNG 48: 53-56.

Suetsuna K, Ukeda H, Ochi H (2000). Isolation and characterization of free radical scavenging activities peptides derived from casein. J Nutr Biochem 11: 128-131.

Sugano M, Goto S, Yamada Y *et al.* (1990). Cholesterol-lowering activity of various undigested fractions of soybean protein in rats. J Nutr 120: 977-985.

Takahashi M, Fukunaga H, Kaneto H *et al.* (2000). Behavioral and pharmacological studies on gluten exorphin A5, a newly isolated bioactive food protein fragment in mice. Japanese J Pharmacol 84: 259-265.

Takahashi M, Moriguchi S, Yoshikawa M *et al.* (1994). Isolation and characterization of oryzatensin - a novel bioactive peptide with ileum-contracting and immunomodulating activities derived from rice albumin. Int J Biochem Mol Biol 33: 1151-1158.

Teschemacher H (2003). Opioid receptor ligands derived from food proteins. Curr Pharmaceut Design 9: 1331–1344.

Thongthai C, Gildberg A (2005). Asian Fish Sauce as a Source of Nutrition. In: John Shi, Chi-Tang Ho, and Fereidoon Shahidi(ed). Asian Functional Foods, by Marcel Dekker/CRC Press, ISBN 0-8247-5855-2, pp. 215-265.

Tripathi SD (2003). Inland Fisheries in India. In: Fish for All National Launch, 18–19 December 2003, Kolkata, India, pp. 33–57.

US Food and Drug Administration (1999). Federal Register Journal 64: 57688–57733.

Venugopal V, Shahidi F (1995). Value added products from underutilized fish species. Crit Rev Food Sci Nutr 35: 431-453.

Vercruysse L, Van Camp J, Smagghe G (2005). ACE inhibitor peptides derived from enzymatic hydrolysates of animal muscle protein: a review. J Agric Food Chem 53: 8106-8115.

Wakabayashi H, Takase M, Tomita M (2003). Lactoferricin derived from milk protein lactoferrin. Current Pharmaceutical Design 9: 1277–1287.

Walker G, Cai F, Shen P *et al.* (2006). Increased remineralization of tooth enamel by milk containing added casein phosphopeptide-amorphous calcium phosphate. J Dairy Res 73: 74-78.

Wang W, de Mejia EG (2005). A new frontier in soy bioactive peptides that may prevent age-related diseases. Compr Rev Food Sci Food Safety 4: 63-78.

Xu RJ (1998). Bioactive peptides in milk and their biological and health implications. Food Rev Intern 14: 1-16.

Yoshikawa M, Fujita H, Matoba N *et al.* (2000). Bioactive peptides derived from food proteins preventing lifestyle-related diseases. Biofactors 12: 143-146.

Yvon M, Beucher S, Guilloteau P *et al.* (1994). Effects of caseinomacropeptide (CMP) on digestion regulation. Reprod Nutr Dev 34: 527–537.

Zhu KX, Zhou HM, Qian HF (2006). Antioxidant and free radical scavenging activities of wheat germ protein hydrolysates (WGPH) prepared with alcalase. Proc Biochem 41: 1296-1302.

2014, Advances in Biochemistry and Biotechnology Volume 2   *Pages 21-56*

Edited by: Dr. Biplab Sarkar and Dr. Chiranjib Chakraborty

Published by: DAYA PUBLISHING HOUSE

3

Integrating Oilgae Technology to Aquaculture

*Sanjay Kumar Ojha and Snehasish Mishra**

Bioenergy Lab, School of Biotechnology, KIIT University,
Bhubaneswar – 751 024, Odisha

ABSTRACT

The role of microorganisms including algae as the primary producers and consumers in a pond ecosystem, particularly in the tropical region, is well known and documented often. Recent studies reveal that among all available green fuel options, algae stand apart to mass supply renewable energy to an extent that it has the potential to completely replace fossil fuels. Algal cells vary in compositions between strains or types. Some are protein-rich, whereas others are lipid-rich. Whereas the former type is the preferred candidate species for SCP production, the latter is undoubtedly positioned to revolutionise sourcing of eco-friendly, user-friendly and sustainable bioenergy. Microalgae yield up to 80 per cent oil by dry weight which means, a

* *Corresponding author.* E-mail: snehasish.mishra@gmail.com

hundred times more oil per acre than other common oil yielding crops. The chapter discusses the integration of biodiesel and aquaculture technology for profitable production, harvest, oil extraction, purification, transfer of technology, and thereby integration into the economy to adopt, replicate and commercialise, particularly at the fisheries or coastal rural community level.

Keywords: Oilgae, Alternate energy source, Integrated aquaculture, Rural entrepreneurship.

Role of Algology in Aquaculture

Algae are important since they are in the first ring of the food chain as primary producers in nature, especially in a pond ecosystem. Macro- and micro-algae are distributed in marine-, fresh- and brackish-water environments. Although the lipid-rich algae, particularly the marine microalgal species, have caught the attention of researchers for the third generation nonconventional biofuels in recent times (Mishra *et al.*, in press), owing to their pigment, protein, vitamins and minerals contents, they have been conventionally used as live food for terrestrial and aquatic organisms. They are also being employed in wastewater amelioration, and also as a fertiliser (De Groot 1991). Algae, with varying nutritional value, have tremendous potential as fish feed, particularly for crustaceans and fish larvae (Biedenbach *et al.*, 1990; Navarro *et al.*, 1998).

Nutrition is the important factor in keeping ornamental fish healthy. Species, variety, colouration and pattern variations attract home owners to keep ornamental fish in their house, out of which the colouration parameter allegedly plays a deciding factor. Following high demand and production of ornamental fish, the demand for natural fish-food has proportionally increased. Basic information on the nutrient requirement and chemical composition of feed ingredients in relation to their acceptability and the ability of fish to digest and utilise nutrients (feed conversion ratio) from various sources is required to develop efficient and economical feed formulations for aquaculture. Coloration, and therefore pigmentation, plays an important role in ornamental such as Goldfish and Koi, as well as food-fish such as salmon, trout, sea bream and prawns.

Importance of aquarium fish is not only for domestic aesthetic value but also for their immense commercial value in the global trade. Ideally, pigmentation is an accepted global parameter for ornamental fish 'quality'. Colour is one of the major factors, which determines the price of aquarium fish in the world market (Saxena 1994; Paripatananont *et al.*, 1999; Lovell 2000; Gouveia *et al.*, 2003). For instance, koi and goldfish with red-colouration are more attractive and thus priced at a premium in the Chinese, Taiwanese and Japanese markets, as they are considered more auspicious. Fish is fed pigments-fortified special diets to trigger and enhance colouration. An economical and practical way to achieve this is through feeding of pigment-enriched feeds. Fish gain its colour through natural diets like algae as they synthesise and provide carotenoids, the pigmentation precursors. Bicyclic carotenoids like β-carotene are xanthophylls are converted to the most commonly occurring carotenoids in aquatic animals, astaxanthins (Simpson *et al.*, 1981; Goodwin 1986; Torrissen, 1989). Algal feed enhance feed value in more than one way, promoting good health and strengthening immune system of aquaculture animals (Trinadha *et al.*, 2003) beside enhancing pigmentation.

Algae in Food Fisheries

The value of dried microalgae as feed ingredients for crustaceans and fish larvae has been well demonstrated (Biedenbach *et al.*, 1990; Navarro *et al.*, 1998). Successful maintenance of 'difficult' species is often influenced by the aquarist's success in obtaining or rearing specialised food items

(Floyd 2002). Algae are a diverse group of aquatic photosynthetic organisms, generally categorised as either macroalgae (such as seaweed) or microalgae (unicellular). Unlike terrestrial plants that require irrigated fertile land, microalgae can grow in a wide range of habitats (Raja, 2009). Algal genera like *Spirulina*, *Chlorella*, *Scenedesmus*, *Dunaliella* and *Nannochloropsis* are popular as feed for their high nutrition (Venkatraman 1980; Avron *et al.*, 1992; Lee 1997; Yamaguchi 1997). Some others, like *Skeletonema*, *Phaeodactylum*, *Chaetoceros*, *Pavlova*, *Isochrysis* and *Tetraselmis*, are employed for their high PUFA, DHA (Docosahexanoic acid) and EPA (Eicosapentanoic acid) contents (Benemann 1992; Becker 1994; Wang 2003; Kuncky *et al.*, 2005). Formulated algal feed must satisfy the nutritional requirements vis-à-vis high acceptability by fish. As microalgae have tremendous impact on growth and vitality of fish, several hundred algal genera have been tested over the last four decades, and less than forty of them could pass the test in aquaculture (Khatoon *et al.*, 2010). Supplementing fish feeds with algae has certain physiological merits such as vitamin precursors, growth promoters and essential fatty acids as discussed earlier. In spite of reported enhanced growth of certain food-fish such as silver carp, research on the use of algae as a protein source in formulated feed is scant (Appler *et al.*, 1983; Appler 1985; Nakagawa *et al.*, 1987; Chow *et al.*, 1990). Mustafa and Nakagawa (1995) reported enhanced growth, feed utilisation, lipid metabolism, body composition, disease resistance and carcass quality of a variety of food-fish fed macro- and micro-algae supplemented meal.

Fish culture ponds are normally turbid with algae that grow in response to allochthonous fertiliser inputs (Boyd 1990; Green *et al.*, 2002). Worldwide commercial algal biomass production is estimated to be 5 million kg/yr with a market value of about US$330/kg. About one-fifth of this is used in fish and shellfish culture (Feuga 2004). Successful commercial utilisation of microalgae has been established in the production of nutritional supplements, antioxidants, natural dyes, and PUFA (Spolaore *et al.*, 2006). Green alga *Ulva lactuca* (Chlorophyta) and red alga *Pterocladia capillacea* (Rhodophyta) are among the most abundant microalgae available in excessive amounts all year around. The importance of these algae, as possible alternative protein sources or supplement for cultured fish has been recently recognised (Mustafa *et al.*, 1995). Microalgae, being the predominant component of the first trophic level in the aquatic food chain, has immense value as aquaculture live-feed and is widely use in hatchery seed production of shell- and fin-fish (Benemann 1992; Feuga 2004). Blue-green algae including *Nostoc*, *Arthrospira* (*Spirulina*) and *Aphanizomenon* species have been used as human food for thousands of years (Jensen *et al.*, 2001), though their cultivation is only a few decades old (Borowitzka 1999). *Spirulina* is a photosynthetic filamentous, spiral shaped, multicellular form. *Spirulina platensis* has been largely studied due to its commercial importance as a source of proteins, vitamins, essential amino acids, and fatty acids (Cifferi *et al.*, 1985), and more recently, as a potential source of nutraceuticals (Borowitzka, 1995).

Microalgae feeds are currently used mainly for the culture of larvae and juvenile shell- and fin-fish, and raising the zooplankton to feed juvenile animals (Benemann 1992; Chen 2003; Chakraborty *et al.*, 2007). For zooplankton to grow and reproduce in the hatchery, algal food is provided to the newly-hatched rotifers until it reach the desired size, then a boost of algae just prior to harvesting. This increases the nutritional value of the target culture species feeding on it. Nile tilapia juveniles obtain major nutrition (more than 48 per cent) for growth from feeding only on algae (Elnady *et al.*, 2010). Sommer *et al.* (1992) reported enhanced growth in trouts by adding carotenoid-rich microalgae *Haematococcus pluvialis*. Boonyratpalin and Unprasert (1989) observed a positive effect of dietary carotenoid on the growth of red tilapia.

Spirulina is regarded as a super food for ornamental fish as it increases and promotes more uniform growth rates when fed at the recommended.5-2.0 per cent inclusion rate. It improves the intestinal flora and feed conversion ratio in fish by breaking down the otherwise indigestible feed components. The beneficial internal flora produce vitamins and displace harmful microbes which is why fish fed *Spirulina* have less intestinal compaction, slimmer abdomen, and better infection resistance. It stimulates the production of enzymes that transport fats within the fish body. The fish utilises the fat to power growth instead of just storing it and becoming flabby. It also enhances the colour - the carotenoid pigments improve and intensify colouration. This is especially important for koi and goldfish for commanding a higher market price. Its chlorophyll and phycocyanin also enhance the skin colours. It increases survival rates. Studies in Japan on marine yellowtail showed that fingerlings fed a ration of 0.5 per cent (5 ppt) *Spirulina* resulted in a significant gain in survival over the non-*Spirulina* fed group. Similar results were obtained from professional Discus fish breeders upon incorporation of *Spirulina* powder into the diet for newborn Discus fry. Including *Spirulina* in the diet allegedly reduced the amount of medication or therapeutics in fish. *Spirulina* also reduces toxicity due to medications Most disease treatments involve chemical 'water baths' and the fish must absorb the drug from the water. Unfortunately, the treatment water is often discharged down the drain into our environment and waterways thus chemically polluting it. Feeding a fish orally with a diet containing *Spirulina* as a prophylactic measure could effectively reduce or eliminate the need for bath treatments, thus effectively reducing environmental pollution, thereby eliminating costly treatment systems and increasing the efficacy of the existing systems (Brine shrimp direct 2010).

Algae in Ornamental Fisheries

Fish are naturally coloured, and the colouration fades under intensive culture conditions. Fish can't synthesise carotenoid and depend on dietary carotenoid content for colouration. Hence, a direct relationship between dietary carotenoids and pigmentation exists (Halten *et al.,* 1997). Body colours of fish are predominantly dependent on the presence of special cells in the tissue, called chromatophores. Carotenoids are a group of over 600 natural lipid soluble pigments primarily produced in phytoplankton, algae and plants. These are absorbed in animals through the diets, sometimes transform into other carotenoids, and incorporate into various tissues. Fish skin colours primarily depend on the presence of chromatophores (xanthophores and erythrophores) containing carotenoids (*e.g.,* astaxanthin, canthaxanthin, lutein, and zeaxanthin). Fish are unable to perform *de novo* synthesis of carotenoids, like in other animals (Goodwin 1984). They modify alimentary carotenoids and store them in the integument and other tissues. Different species have different carotenoids metabolism and storage.

Carotenoids also have excellent antioxidative characteristics (Anderson 2000). If colour-enhancement can be done by administering pigment enriched feed, it will definitely improve the quality and cost of the fish. Plant sources have been utilised for inducing pigmentation in fish. *Spirulina* has been used as a source of carotenoid pigments for rainbow trout and fancy carp (Choubert 1979; Boonyaratpalin *et al.,* 1986; Alagappan *et al.,* 2004), and the marigold petal meal for the tiger barb (Boonyaratpalin *et al.,* 1977). *Chlorella vulgaris* was found to be as efficient as synthetic pigments in rainbow trout *Oncorhynchus mykiss* (Gouveia *et al.,* 1996), gilthead seabream *Sparus aurata* (Gouveia *et al.,* 2002), koi carp *Cyprinus carpio* and goldfish *Carassius auratus* (Gouveia *et al.,* 2003; Gouveia *et al.,* 2005). They found that the dietary carotenoid supplementation increased total skin carotenoid content in koi carp (*Cyprinus carpio*; Kawari – red, Showa – black and red, and Bekko – black-and-white varieties) and goldfish (*Carassius auratus*) by feeding a dietary carotenoid supplement of *Chlorella vulgaris*, *Haematococcus pluvialis* and *Arthrospira maxima* (*Spirulina*). *C. vulgaris* was most effective in koi carp colouration, providing both maximum total carotenoid deposition and red hue for the three chromatic koi carp varieties. Best colouration in goldfish, as ascertained by total carotenoid content, was achieved using *C. vulgaris*, and a red hue was maximal with *H. pluvialis* supplementation (Gouveia *et al.*, 2003). Algal genera are used as a source of pigments like carotenoid, astaxanthin, lutein and zeaxanthin in fish farming especially for the coloured fishes (Hanaa *et al.*, 2003).

Chemically synthesised astaxanthin is a different stereoisomer from natural astaxanthin (Ako *et al.*, 2000) and is a costly proposition for the small grower to incorporate into fish diets. Carotenoids from *Spirulina platensis* and *Haematococcus pluvialis* (biotech algae) have been incorporated in coloured swordtails, rainbowfish and topaz cichlids. Similar were the cases in rosy barbs, 24K mollies, kissing gouramis (Ako *et al.*, 2000). Ornamental fish require between 50 and 400ppm of synthetic or natural carotenoids in their diet to develop colouration similar to those of fish eating live foods (Boonyaratpalin *et al.*, 1977; Fey *et al.*, 1980; Lovell 1992). *Dunaliella salina* is a microalgae occurring naturally in a number of locations worldwide. Though it appears green in its natural marine environment, in conditions of high salinity and light intensity, it turns red due to protective carotenoids production. The microalga has been introduced to aquaculture in two forms, liquid paste and dry powder. The paste is a *D. salina* concentrate with levels of high-carotenoids, minerals, vitamins, and fatty acids. The paste is spray dried to create the dry form (www.nutracol.com). This microalga has several applications including its potential in biofuel (oilgae) production (Mishra *et al.*, in press). Gouveia and Rema (2005) investigated the effect of different carotenoid sources concentrations and temperature on goldfish skin pigmentation, and found best results in *C. vulgaris* and 26-30°C, respectively. The best carotenoid concentrations were achieved with astaxanthin diets.

Zatkova *et al.* (2010) examined the effect of carotenoid-rich microalgal (*Scenedesmus, Chlorella* and *Haematococcus*) biomass as feed supplement (12-60 mg/kg feed) in an albinic form of wels catfish (*Silurus glanis*) and reported an increase in specific growth rate and physical condition index (weight/length) by 11-58 per cent and 6-26 per cent, respectively. Skin colouration evaluated from digital images indicated an intensive yellow or yellow-orange colouration in all alga diet-fed fish groups as the colour saturation increased 1.4-2.4 times within 20-40 days. Bagnara and Hadley (1973) studied the specificity of the carotenoid pattern of fish and the selectivity of carotenoids uptake and concluded that the carotenoids concentrated in the skin, ovary, liver, muscle and other tissues. Astaxanthin, like other carotenoids, has been shown to have biological and nutritional functions in fish (Torrissen 1984; Torrissen *et al.*, 1989; Torrissen *et al.*, 1995). Koi breeders carried out fish trials to determine the ability of koi to assimilate xanthophylls from *Haematococcus* (NatuRose) and observed a dark red coloration (Lorenz 2000). Lorenz (2000) reported a significant improvement in colour and pigmentation in freshwater and marine ornamental fish, such as tetras, cichlids, gouramis, goldfish, koi, danios, swordtails, Rosy Bards, rainbow fish, discus and clown anemone fish. *Spirulina* added in the diet of ornamental fish such as goldfish and fancy red carp enhanced pigmentation (Miki *et al.*, 1986; Borowitzka 1994). Gouveia *et al.* (2003) compared various microalgal biomass carotenoid sources (*Chlorella vulgaris, H. pluvialis* and *Spirulina maxima*) with synthetic astaxanthin (Carophyll Pink) and the found that microalgal biomass, especially *C. vulgaris*, may contribute to enhanced skin colour of koi and goldfish.

Other than pigmentation, studies indicate that carotenoids also have a biological function involved in growth and reproduction. Researchers have reported positive effects on growth for different fishes fed diets supplemented with carotenoids, especially astaxanthin (Torrisen 1984; Torrisen 1986; Christiansen *et al.*, 1994). Mobilisation of carotenoids from the flesh to the skin and ovaries during maturation also shows that carotenoids may have a function in reproduction. Torrissen and Torrissen (1985) detected a decrease in the carotenoids content of the flesh of Atlantic salmon about six months prior to spawning and proved the mobilisation of carotenoids from the flesh to the skin and ovaries during maturation. Torrissen (1984, 1989) showed the presence of astaxanthin and canthaxanthin in the plasma of feeding rainbow trout, indicating that the serum is the transport medium (Tan Phaik Shiang, 2006).

In ornamental fish, the colour is much more than a cosmetic effect. Consumers associate natural colouration with healthy and high quality products. Muscle pigmentation in farmed salmonids, for instance, is regarded as the most important quality parameter of freshness (Koteng 1992). Beside flesh pigmentation, vivid skin colouration of cultured red and yellow skinned fish such as red porgy, *Pagrus pagrus* (Basurco *et al.*, 1999), Japanese red sea bream, *Pagrus major* (Lin *et al.*, 1998), Australian snapper, *Pagrus auratus* (Booth *et al.*, 2004; Doolan *et al.*, 2004), and yellowtail, *Seriola quinqueradiata* (Miki *et al.*, 1985) are well appreciated, and lead to high market values. Skin colour is an important characteristic affecting market price and playing a major role in the overall appraisal in ornamental fish as well (Gouveia *et al.*, 2005). Freshwater microalga *Haematococcus pluvialis* has the ability to accumulate large amounts of astaxanthin, on 1.5-5.0 per cent w/w on a dry weight basis (Johnson *et al.*, 1995; Krishna *et al.*, 1998). *Haematococcus* primarily contains monoesters of astaxanthin linked to 16:0, 18:0, 18:2, and 18:1 (major) fatty acids (Restrom *et al.*, 1981), having the unesterified, mono- and di-esters (Grung *et al.*, 1992). Feeding *Chlorella vulgaris* also produced positive pigmentation in certain fish (Gouveia *et al.*, 1996; Gouveia *et al.*, 2002). Microalga *Chlorococcum* sp. seems to be a promising source of astaxanthin, canthaxanthin and adonixanthin (Higuera-Ciapara *et al.*, 2006). In fish, carotenoids have similar functions as vitamin A precursors as those reported in other animal species (Schiedt *et al.*, 1985; Guillou *et al.*, 1989; Christiansen *et al.*, 1994; White *et al.*, 2003a), markedly affecting reproduction performance (Craik 1985; Christiansen *et al.*, 1996; Verakunpiriya *et al.*, 1997; Chou *et al.*, 2001; Vassallo-Agius *et al.*, 2001a,b), as antioxidants (Bjerkeng *et al.*, 1995; Shimidzu *et al.*, 1996; Nakano *et al.*, 1999; Bell *et al.*, 2000), enhance immune system (Nakano *et al.*, 1995; Amar *et al.*, 2003), and affect the liver structure (Segner *et al.*, 1989; Page *et al.*, 2005). Although some authors claim that the biological functions of carotenoids in fish are still speculative (Choubert *et al.*, 2005), other consider these compounds as important micronutrients that fish are unable to synthesise and, therefore, must be included in the diet (Baker *et al.*, 2001).

Algal Biology

Algae represent a large group of different organisms from different phylogenetic groups, representing many taxonomic divisions. These are photosynthetic, aquatic organisms usually devoid of true roots, stems, leaves and vascular tissue, and have simple reproductive structures. They have worldwide distribution in virtually all aquatic environments, in the sea, in freshwater and in wastewaters. Most are unicellular and sub-microscopic (microalgae), but some are quite large including some marine forms exceeding 50 m in length (macroalgae). They have high photosynthesis efficiency and faster growth rate. Oleaginous microalgae are defined as algae which can utilise carbon sources such as CO_2, carbohydrates and fats, and convert them into ordinary lipids and fatty acids under defined conditions (Chiara 2002). As these are rich in resources and can grow in a variety of culture conditions, they have great potential to be mass-cultured. Microalgae have the potential to be a major source of biofuels worldwide and are unique in sequestering CO_2. Among other advantageous attributes, microalgae grow at a rapid pace, they are able to grow in very inhospitable conditions, land and water use for growing microalgae is typically not competitive with land and water required for conventional food production. Microalgae production for liquid fuels and carbon sequestering is a revolutionary renewable biofuel platform. As the fats derived from algae are rich in saturated and unsaturated long-chain fatty acids as in vegetable oils, these are good candidates for biofuel production.

Photosynthesis and Solar Conversion Efficiency

Apart from metabolomics approaches to increase lipid production, two other approaches for large-scale cultivation are, increasing the photosynthetic efficiency, and the strain selection and improvement for optimal growth, survival, and oil production using wastewaters and seawater resources. Increasing the photosynthetic efficiency will enhance biofuel production. As photosynthesis is about capturing solar energy and storing it as chemical energy (*e.g.* oil, starch), increasing the light capture efficiency would be a significant innovation in developing second generation biofuel production systems. Most wild-type microalgae have evolved genetic strategies to assemble large light-harvesting antenna complexes which capture sunlight and transfer the derived energy to PSI and PSII. The advantage of this strategy in nature is that it maximises light capture under low light conditions. The downside is that, as excess light damages the photosynthetic machinery, higher plants and algae had to evolve photo-protective mechanisms (Horton *et al.*, 1996; Pascal *et al.*, 2007). These typically dissipate most of the captured energy as fluorescence and heat which is a 'waste' (in context of biofuel production) (Polle *et al.*, 2002). This energy dissipation takes place largely in the light harvesting complexes associated with PSII (*i.e.* LHCII). Demonstrably, the overall light conversion efficiency of photobioreactors is markedly improved by reducing the number of the chlorophyll-binding LHC

Table 3.1: Some Popular Algal Forms Presently being Employed for Biodiesel Production.

Algal Type	Species	Growth Characteristics
Macroalgae	*Chaetomorpha linum*	Present in unattached form in both estuarine systems and eutrophicated coastal lagoons. It can live all the year and can reach high biomass values, estimated at around 3.5–5 kg_{fwt} m^{-2}
	Ulva laetevirens	Present in attached and unattached forms in estuaries and shallow eutrophic lagoons large free-floating thalli. During growing season it may reach 15–20 kg_{fwt} m^{-2}
	Gracilaria bursa-pastoris	One of the few Rhodophyceae that has the ability to live in eutrophic coastal lagoons, present in attached and unattached form in coastal lagoons in both the hemispheres. In some period of time it becomes the dominant species of the drifting bed
	Pterocladiella capillacea	Commonly lives on rocky hard substrata, often on vertical rock-faces, from the inter-tidal level to about 20 m depth, in wave-exposed areas. This species is widely distributed in the Mediterranean Sea, but is found in both hemispheres
	Codium vermilaria	Lives on hard horizontal substrata either in sheltered or lightly wave-exposed areas, at 0-50 m depth, in shady places; distributed in the boreal hemisphere from the North Atlantic Ocean to the Mediterranean Sea
Microalgae	*Spirulina*	Multicellular, filamentous blue-green algae. Various commercial production plants are currently in operation. It has a growth rate of 30 g/m^2·day dry weight, an optimal temperature between 35-37°C, and tolerates high pH changes
	Chlorella	Unicellular organism found in almost any water (freshwater and marine). It has a growth rate of 26 g/m^2·day dry weight, temperature regime of 35-37°C (depending on species)
	Dunaliella	A halophile microalgae especially found in sea and salty fields. It has a growth rate of 1.65 g/m^2·day dry weight. The temperature and pH regimes depend on species
	Haematococcus pluvialis	A freshwater species of Chlorophyta. It is usually found in temperate regions around the world, having a growth rate of 9-13 g/m^2·day dry weight

proteins in each cell (Mussgnug *et al.*, 2007; Polle *et al.*, 2002). This strategy can be used to carefully fine-tune and optimise light capture efficiency of the antenna systems specifically for oil production. Few of the algal forms which are (or have the potential to be) employed for biodiesel production are present in Table 3.1. Lipid content and productivity of various marine and freshwater microalgae which has been studied so far is summarised in Table 3.2.

Table 3.2: Lipid Content and Productivity of Various Marine and Freshwater Microalgae.

	Microalga Species	Lipid Content (per cent, w/w$_{DW}$)	Lipid Productivity (mg L^{-1} d^{-1})
Freshwater	Botryococcus sp.	25.0–75.0	–
	Chaetoceros muelleri	33.6	21.8
	Chaetoceros calcitrans	14.6–16.4/39.8	17.6
	Chlorella emersonii	25.0–63.0	10.3–50.0
	Chlorella protothecoides	14.6–57.8	1214
	Chlorella sorokiniana	19.0–22.0	44.7
	Chlorella vulgaris	5.0–58.0	11.2–40.0
	Chlorella sp.	10.0–48.0	42.1
	Chlorella pyrenoidosa	2.0	
	Chlorella sp.	18.0–57.0	18.7
	Chlorococcum sp.	19.3	53.7
	Ellipsoidion sp.	27.4	47.3
	Haematococcus pluvialis	25.0	–
	Scenedesmus obliquus	11.0–55.0	–
	Scenedesmus quadricauda	1.9–18.4	35.1
	Scenedesmus sp.	19.6–21.1	40.8–53.9
Marine	Dunaliella salina	6.0–25.0	116.0
	Dunaliella primolecta	23.1	–
	Dunaliella tertiolecta	16.7–71.0	–
	Dunaliella sp.	17.5–67.0	33.5
	Isochrysis galbana	7.0–40.0	–
	Isochrysis sp.	7.1–33	37.8
	Nannochloris sp.	20.0–56.0	60.9–76.5
	Nannochloropsis oculata	22.7–29.7	84.0–142.0
	Nannochloropsis sp.	12.0–53.0	60.9–76.5
	Neochloris oleoabundans	29.0–65.0	90.0–134.0
	Pavlova salina	30.9	49.4
	Pavlova lutheri	35.5	40.2
	Phaeodactylum tricornutum	18.0–57.0	44.8
	Spirulina platensis	4.0–16.6	–

Source: Mata *et al.*, 2010.

Proximate Composition of Algae

Algae are eukaryotic cells, with nuclei and organelles including plastids for photosynthesis. Various algal strains have different combinations of chlorophyll molecules. Some have only Chlorophyll A, some A and B, while other strains, A and C. Algae biomass contains proteins, carbohydrates and natural oil as three main components. The chemical compositions of various microalgae are shown in Table 3.3 (Um *et al.*, 2009).

Table 3.3: Chemical Composition of some Algae Expressed in per cent Dry Matter Basis.

Strain	Protein	Carbohydrate	Lipids	Nucleic Acid
Scenedesmus obliquus	50-56	10-17	12-14	3-6
Scenedesmus quadricauda	47	–	1.9	–
Scenedesmus dimorphus	8-18	21-52	16-40	–
Chlamydomonas rheinhardii	48	17	21	–
Chlorella vulgaris	51-58	12-17	14-22	4-5
Chlorella pyrenoidosa	57	26	2	–
Spirogyra sp.	6-20	33-64	11-21	–
Dunaliella bioculata	49	4	8	–
Dunaliella salina	57	32	6	–
Euglena gracilis	39-61	14-18	14-20	–
Prymnesium parvum	28-45	25-33	22-38	1-2
Tetraselmis maculata	52	15	3	–
Porphyridium cruentum	28-39	40-57	9-14	–
Spirulina platensis	46-63	8-14	4–9	2-5
Spirulina maxima	60-71	13-16	6-7	3-4.5
Synechoccus sp.	63	15	11	5
Anabaena cylindrica	43-56	25-30	4-7	–

Microalgae are the fastest growing photosynthesising unicellular organisms that can complete an entire growing cycle every few days. Some algae species have high Oil content (up to 60 per cent oil by weight) and can produce up to 15,000 gallons of oil/Acre/yr under optimum conditions.

One key reason to consider algae as feedstock for oil is their yields. Put simply, algae are the only bio feedstock that can theoretically replace all the petro-fuel consumption of today, and future. Owing to the fact that oil yields are much lower for other feed stocks when compared to those from algae, it will be very difficult for the first generation biodiesel feedstock such as soy or palm to produce enough oil to replace even a small fraction of petro-oil needs without displacing large percentages of arable land towards crops for fuel production. When compared to diesel fuel, algal oil has same characteristic like density, viscosity, heating value (Table 3.4).

Growing Algae Commercially

Producing microalgal oils requires light, CO_2, water and inorganic nutrients as inputs for the algal growth. The latter are mainly nitrates, phosphates, iron and some trace elements. Approximately half of the dry weight of the microalgal biomass is carbon, which is typically derived from CO_2.

Table 3.4: Comparison of Characteristics of Biodiesel from Microalgal Oil and Diesel Fuel.

Properties	Biodiesel from Microalgae Oil	Diesel Fuel
Density kg/l	0.864	0.838
Viscosity Pa s	5.2×10^{-4} (40ºC)	$1.9–4.1 \times 10^{-4}$ (40ºC)
Flash point ºC	65–115˙	75
Solidifying point ºC	−12	−50–10
Cold filter plugging point ºC	−11	−3.0 (−6.7 max)
Acid value mg KOH/g	0.374	0.5 max
Heating value MJ/kg	41	40–45
HC ratio	1.18	1.18

Source: Department of Biological Sciences and Biotechnology, Tsinghua University, Beijing, China (2004).

Therefore, producing 100 tons of algal biomass fixes roughly 183 tons of CO_2. This CO_2, which is often available at little or no cost, must be fed continually during the daylight hours (Chisti 2007). Optimal temperature for growing many microalgae is between 20 and 30C. A temperature outside this range could kill or otherwise damage the cells. Despite over 30 years of research, commercial growth of algae in open ponds is still only currently viable for three species, *Spirulina*, *Dunaliella* and *Chlorella*, through the suppression of growth of competitive species by use of highly selective environments (Huntley *et al.*, 2007). Currently, a majority of microalgal production occurs in outdoor ponds (Spolaore *et al.*, 2006). Concerns have also been expressed about the possible contamination of food from microalgae grown in open ponds (Becker 1994). Bioreactors are considerably more expensive than open ponds and their use will probably be restricted to very high value products (Becker 1994). It is argued that lower extraction costs, due to the higher algae content, can make bioreactors more competitive (Chisti 2007). A study on the production of the valuable fatty acid, EPA, found that 60 per cent of the costs arise from the recovery (downstream) process and the cost of algae biomass production in bioreactors is high and need to be reduced (Molina-Grima *et al.*, 2003). Although some products are now being produced in bioreactors commercially, the development of microalgae biotechnology has been slowed by the limited performance of bioreactors (Spolaore *et al.*, 2006). Open ponds are likely to remain the major means of production, but efficient closed bioreactors may be viable in the production for high value products where purity is essential or a 'sensitive' algal species is required. There are mainly three types of algal culturing systems, natural lagoons, open ponds and photobioreactors (closed systems).

Cultivation in Natural Lagoons

An economical way to culture algae is in natural lagoons or lakes. This type of cultivation has been practiced for many years, if not centuries, in several locations around the world, such as Mexico, Australia and Lake Chad in Africa. Essentially, the algae are allowed to grow as best they can without any mechanical stirring or agitation to improve CO_2 uptake and then, after an appropriate period of time, they are harvested by the simplest available technology. Such systems have been used to produce dry biomass of *Spirulina* (a cyanobacterium) which is used mainly as a feed supplement for domestic animals; the oil content of this biomass is less than 10 per cent and is almost entirely composed of complex membrane lipids associated with photosynthesis. This natural growth system is also used for the cultivation of the saline-tolerant alga, *Dunaliella salina* grown in sea lagoons in Australia. The alga has a strong selective advantage over other algae and even bacteria that might contaminate the biomass and also from protozoa that would consume the algal cells. Biomass from such a process is used as a source of β-carotene. The overall level of fatty acid-containing lipids is, however, relatively low at about 8–11 per cent of the biomass as nothing has been done to increase the level of CO_2 entering the water which is essential to ensure lipid accumulation.

Once the surface is covered with algal cells these would self-shade those underneath and biomass production is therefore, limited by the final surface density of the cells. Yields of biomass in lagoon systems are of the order of 0.1 $g/m^2/day$ and it will therefore take 1-2 months for the cultures to reach their maximum density. Allowing for seasonal variations in the temperature, annual yields of biomass would, therefore, be of the order of 200-400 kg/hectare. Given the low lipid content of these cells, they could not then be a realistic source of fatty acids for biodiesel or similar applications. Furthermore, cultivation of algae as a realistic source of biomass would require an extremely large area of lagoons which is far from being available.

Open Pond Culture System

Open ponds are the oldest and simplest systems for mass-culture of microalgae. The pond is designed in a raceway configuration, in which a paddlewheel circulates and mixes the algal cells and nutrients. The raceways are typically made from poured concrete, or they are simply dug into the earth and lined with a plastic liner to prevent the ground from soaking up the liquid. Baffles in the channel guide the flow around the bends in order to optimise space utilisation by preventing dead-space. The system is often operated in a continuous mode - fresh feed is added in front of the paddlewheel, and algal broth is harvested behind the paddlewheel after it has circulated through the loop.

The ponds are 'raceway' designs, in which the algae, water and nutrients circulate around a racetrack. Paddlewheels provide the flow. The algae are thus kept suspended in water. Algae are circulated back up to the surface on a regular frequency. The ponds are kept shallow because of the need to keep the algae exposed to sunlight and the limited depth to which sunlight can penetrate as much. The size of these ponds is measured in terms of surface area, since surface area is so critical to capturing sunlight. Their productivity is measured in terms of biomass produced/day/unit available surface area. Such algae farms would be based on the use of open, shallow ponds in which some source of waste CO_2 could be efficiently bubbled into the ponds to facilitate algal growth. Careful control of pH and other physical conditions for introducing CO_2 into the ponds allowed greater than 90 per cent utilisation of injected CO_2. Raceway ponds, usually lined with plastic or cement, are about 15-35 cm deep. They are typically mixed with paddlewheels, usually lined with plastic or cement, and are between 0.2 and 0.5 ha in size. Paddlewheels provide motive force and keep the algae suspended in the water. The ponds are supplied with water and nutrients, and mature algae are continuously removed at one end (Demirbas, 2011). The characteristics and performance of attached and suspended culture system for *Chlorella* spp. have been mention in Table 3.5.

Process Research

Algae Mass Cultivation

Algae require considerable amounts of water in order to grow and thrive, the organisms themselves being typically 80-85 per cent water (Burlew, 1953). Photosynthesis dissociates roughly one mole of water/mole of CO_2 (Williams *et al.*, 2010). This means that approximately 5-10 kg of water is consumed per kg of dry algae biomass produced. In addition to water incorporated within the cell, most algae grow and reproduce in aqueous suspension. When algae blooms are observed, it appears that there are copious amounts of biomass; indeed a thin suspension of *Chlorella* contains 2×10^{10} individual cells in a liter of water (Burlew 1953). However, the percentage of suspended solids is actually quite low, typically less than 0.5 per cent wet biomass (0.1 per cent dry). Thus, for every gram of dry algae biomass generated, more than a kilogram of non-cellular water is required to produce and support it. Water not only provides a physical environment in which the algae live and reproduce, it also delivers nutrients, removes waste products, and acts as a thermal regulator. Unlike natural environments, mass cultivation systems require that the water be acquired, contained, circulated, and pumped to and between desired locations. All of these activities entail inputs of energy, both direct and indirect, and the amount of energy expended is tightly coupled to the volume of water involved. The volume of water involved depends upon system geometries, losses from the system, and most importantly, the ability to reclaim and reuse water. The latter is affected by the efficiency of the separation process(s), the quality of the return water, and the sensitivity of the specific culture to changes and/or impurities in the return water, including the waste byproducts.

Table 3.5: Compared Performance of Attached and Suspended Culture System for *Chlorella* spp.

	Attached Culture	Suspended Culture
Biomass yield	25.65±3.25 (g DW/m²)	1.27±0.12 (g DW/L)
Total surface area of the culture system (m²)	0.0136	–
Total volume of the culture system (ml)	200	200
Total biomass produced (g)	0.34±0.03	0.25±0.02
TFA content (per cent DW)	9.01±1.98	8.98±1.11
Culture time when harvesting (days)	10	9
Biomass harvesting method	Scraping	Centrifuge
Water content of the harvested biomass (per cent)	93.75±0.30	92.14±1.14
Procedure of harvest methods	Easy and less expensive	Complex and more expensive

Source: Johnson *et al.*, 2010.

Control of Competitors, Grazers and Pathogens

Competitors and grazers play spoilsport in algal culture systems. Zooplankton grazers may be controlled through physical (filtration, centrifugation, low DO concentration/high organic loading) and chemical treatments (application of chemicals/invertebrate hormone mimics, increase in pH and free ammonia concentration) (Schluter *et al.*, 1981). As many zooplanktons are able to survive extended periods of low DO (Schluter *et al.*, 1981), pH adjustment up to a value of 11 is perhaps the most pragmatic method of control for most zooplankton (Benemann *et al.*, 1978). Especially, since wastewaters generally contain high ammonia levels (up to 30ppm) and the apparent toxic effects of elevated pH on zooplankton may actually be due to increased free ammonia levels at higher pH (Oswald, 1988). Presently there are no general treatments to control fungal infections.

Algae for Wastewater Treatment

Extensive works have explored the feasibility of using microalgae for wastewater treatment, especially for the removal of nitrogen and phosphorus from effluents (Mallick 2002; Aslan *et al.*, 2006; Hernandez *et al.*, 2006; Hameed MSA 2007; Lebeau *et al.*, 2003; Galvez-Cloutier *et al.*, 2006) which would otherwise result in eutriphication if dumped into lakes and rivers (Galvez-Cloutier *et al.*, 2006).

Ironically enough, it is algae in the lakes and rivers that cause this problem. Thus, it is a matter of allowing nitrogen and phosphorus consumption by microalgae in a controlled manner that benefits rather than deteriorates the environment. Levels of several contaminant heavy metals have also been shown to be reduced by microalgae cultivation (Munoz *et al.,* 2006). A major concern associated with using wastewater for microalgae cultivation is contamination (de la Noue *et al.,* 1988; Munoz *et al.,* 2006). This can be managed by using appropriate pretreatment technologies to remove sediment and to deactivate (sterilize) the wastewater. In addition to the apparent benefit of combining microalgal biomass, and therefore biofuel production and wastewater treatment, successful implementation of this strategy would allow minimising the use of precious freshwater, for biofuel production.

Production and Process Integration

Process Scale-up

As the reactor is the hardware part of the process, only a sophisticated operation (software) makes it viable at the end. Process management offers several options to further improve the performance of the system and lower energy demands. The impact of temperature control on the energy balance of the process is highly dependent on the applied reactor system, algae strain, but most of all the operating region of the plant. At warm, highly irradiated sites like southern USA or Australia, cooling of the cultures is likely to become a critical parameter of the process. Whether this problem is tackled by direct evaporation or a closed cooling system, excess heat must be actively taken out of the system, adding to the energy demand of the process. Spraying the outer wall of the reactor with water is a means but requires the availability of cooling water. One way to reduce heating problem is by avoiding IR radiation in sunlight. This part of the sunlight spectrum makes up 40 per cent of the total energy without being used by the algae. IR-reflecting glass or plastics are available (Holland *et al.,* 1958) and is used to reduce heat in parked cars or to reduce heat radiation from light bulbs. Photobioreactors usually are operated as batch or sequential batch (semi-continuous), where harvesting is done preferably in the afternoon.

Long-term Maintenance of Desired Strain in Culture

Microalgae can be grown either in open ponds or in photobioreactors. The culture in open ponds is more economically favourable, (photobioreactors are much more expensive to build than open ponds) but raises the issue of land cost and water availability, appropriate climatic conditions, nutrients cost, and production. In the open pond option, other cultivation aspects such as maintenance of long-term growth of the desired algae strain without interference by competitors, grazers, or pathogens should also be taken into consideration.

Hydrodynamics of Mixing

In continuous production cycle in open pond system, algae broth and nutrients are introduced in front of the paddlewheel and circulated through the loop to the harvest extraction point. The paddlewheel is in continuous operation to prevent sedimentation. The level of mixing in a PBR strongly contributes to the growth of microalgae. Mixing is necessary to prevent cells from settling, to avoid thermal stratification, to distribute nutrients and breakdown diffusion gradients at the cell surface, to remove photosynthetically generated O_2 and to ensure that cells experience alternating periods of light and darkness of adequate length (Tredici, 2004). The fluid dynamics of the culture medium and the type of mixing influences average irradiance and the light regimen to which the cells are exposed, which in turns determine productivity.

Evaluation of Local Water Supply for Algal Cultivation

Oil-rich marine algae may be grown in low-quality, non-potable water media such as saline, brackish, or brine extracted from groundwater or saltwater bodies, therefore reducing the demand on freshwater resources. Pretreatment of water, whether saltwater or freshwater, is an important step in successful microalgal culture. Culture water should be free of suspended solids, plankton (*e.g.* protozoans, ciliates and contaminating algae species), bacteria, unacceptably high concentrations of dissolved organic compounds (DOC), dissolved metals, and pesticides though detecting them can be complicated and costly. Activated carbon (charcoal) filtration is helpful in reducing DOC, while deionisation resins are effective in removing metals and hydrocarbons.

As discussed in the beginning, oilgae could be a source of carbon sequestration, require less land, and for some systems, could be produced in arid environments and other areas where their land use would not compete with food crops (Chisti, 2007). Due to the limited water resources in arid environments, water use by algae biofuel production facilities may be highly contentious from the perspective of environmentalists, communities, developers (policy-makers), politicians and land stewards.

CO$_2$ Supply

As discussed earlier, the concentration of atmospheric CO$_2$ is far too low to serve as carbon source in efficient algae cultivation. There are plenty of sources for higher concentrated waste CO$_2$ streams; practically any combustion plant emission contains the required concentration, and usually exhaust gas CO$_2$ concentrations exceed 5 per cent (Negoro *et al.*, 1991, Negoro *et al.*, 1993; Doucha *et al.*, 2005). NOx from fuel gases are reported to be used by the algae as nitrogen source. Here the quality of the exhaust gas is of major importance. While the combustion of natural gas is reported to be suitable for CO$_2$ supply, elevated levels of sulphur and nitrogen oxides as from coal-fired power plants could be damaging (Maeda *et al.*, 1995) and therefore require elaborate gas purification, which would add to the energy balance of the algal process. Additionally, although highly abundant, CO$_2$ from fossil energy sources prevents the biofuel process from being CO$_2$ neutral, which could be avoided by the use of CO$_2$ from combined heat and power units fueled by spare wood or biogas. In both cases, suitable sites for such plants may be a question: large power plants usually exist in densely populated areas with expensive land prices, whereas most wood- or biogas-fired plants are located in rural areas with fertile soil which may rather be used for agriculture than for algae production.

Oil Harvesting Technology

Photobioreactors usually are operated as batch or sequential batch (semi-continuous), where harvesting is done preferably in the afternoons. Maximum biomass concentration with highest mutual shading is reached with highest irradiation during daytime, while lowest biomass concentration in the night leads to lowest biomass loss by respiration. There are three well-known methods to extract the oil from algae, Expeller/Press, Solvent extraction with hexane, and Supercritical fluid extraction. A simple process is to use a press to extract a large percentage (70–75 per cent) of the oils out of algae. Alternately, it can be extracted using chemicals. The most popular chemical for solvent extraction is hexane, which is relatively inexpensive. Supercritical fluid extraction, another extraction technology, is far more efficient than traditional solvent separation methods.

Algal oil separated by extraction with organic solvent after freeze-drying and sonication may not suitable for large-scale operation owing to the cost factor. An effective method is liquefaction for separating hydrocarbons as liquid fuel from harvested algal cells with high moisture content.

Microalgae are directly liquefied and the oil from liquefaction products is extracted by dichloromethane (CH_2Cl_2). Liquefaction can be performed in an aqueous solution of alkali or alkaline earth salt at about 575 K and 10 MPa (Minowa, 1995) using a stainless steel autoclave with mechanical mixing. Hydrothermal technology for direct liquefaction of algal biomass by direct hydrothermal liquefaction at around 575 K and 10 MPa is another alternate viable technology. Minowa *et al.* (1995) reported an oil yield of about 37 per cent (organic basis) with a viscosity of 150–330 mPas and heating value of 36 MJ/kg from *Dunaliella tertiolecta*. A maximum oil yield of 64 per cent (dry wt. basis) was recovered from *Botryococcus braunii* by liquefaction at 575K catalysed by sodium carbonate (Sawayama *et al.,* 1995). A greater amount of oil than the content of hydrocarbons in *B. braunii*, a colony-forming microalga, was obtained with a yield of 57-64 wt. per cent (50 wt per cent db) at 575K upon liquefaction with and without sodium carbonate as a catalytic converter (Banerjee *et al.,* 2002). The oil was equivalent in quality to petroleum oil. Thus, it is reasonable to believe that, hydrothermal liquefaction is reportedly a more effective technique for extraction of microalgal biodiesel than using the supercritical carbon dioxide (Aresta *et al.,* 2005). Due to the level of limited information in the hydrothermal liquefaction of algae, there is a need for more research on this.

Extraction by Mechanical Methods

Mechanical methods employed for the purpose include, Expression/Expeller press, and Ultrasonic-assisted extraction. The simplest method is mechanical crushing. Often, mechanical crushing is used in conjunction with chemicals.

Expression/Expeller Press

Dried algae retain its oil content which then can be "pressed" out with an oil press. Since different strains of algae vary widely in their physical attributes, various press configurations (such as screw, expeller, piston, etc.) work better for specific algae. Many commercial manufacturers of vegetable oil use a combination of mechanical pressing and chemical solvents in extracting oil.

Ultrasonic-Assisted Extraction

A branch of sonochemistry, ultrasonication greatly accelerates extraction process. Using an ultrasonic reactor, ultrasonic wave cavitates bubbles in a solvent material, and when these bubbles collapse near the cell walls, it creates shock waves and liquid jets that cause the cell-walls to break and release the cellular contents into the solvent.

Extraction by Chemical Methods

Algal oil can be extracted using chemicals. Benzene and ether have been used, oil can also be separated by hexane extraction, which is widely used in the food industry and is relatively inexpensive. Using solvents for oil extraction is the dangers involved in working with the chemicals. Care must be taken to avoid exposure to vapors and direct contact with the skin, either of which can cause serious damage. Benzene is classified as a carcinogen. Chemical solvents also present the problem of being an explosion hazard. The chemical methods include hexane solvent method, soxhlet extraction, and supercritical fluid extraction.

Hexane Solvent Method

Algal oil can be extracted using chemicals. Benzene and ether have been used, but a popular chemical for solvent extraction is hexane, which is relatively inexpensive. Hexane solvent extraction can be used in isolation or it can be used along with the oil press/expeller method. After the oil has been extracted using an expeller, the remaining pulp can be mixed with cyclo-hexane to extract the remaining oil content. The oil dissolves in the cyclohexane, and the pulp is filtered out from the solution. The oil and cyclohexane are separated by means of distillation. These two stages (cold press and hexane solvent) together will be able to derive more than 95 per cent of the total oil present in the algae.

Soxhlet Extraction

Soxhlet extraction is an extraction method that uses chemical solvents. Oils from the algae are extracted through repeated washing, or percolation, with an organic solvent such as hexane or petroleum ether, under reflux in special glassware.

Supercritical Fluid Extraction

In supercritical fluid/CO_2 extraction, CO_2 is liquefied under pressure and heated to the point that it has the properties of both a liquid and a gas; this liquefied fluid then acts as the solvent in extracting the oil.

The lipids, once extracted and purified, present an excellent feedstock for a variety of liquid fuel production alternatives. Lipids extracted from biomass can be used directly as liquid fuel feedstocks, or they may have higher value uses such as ω^3 fatty acids. Biomass-derived lipids can be a viable feedstock to traditional refining operations producing products such as straight chain alkanes suitable as a direct replacement product to gasoline. Alternatively, triglyceride lipids are chemically-reacted to form esters and can selectively be utilised as biodiesel liquid fuel, replacing current edible oils being used to produce biodiesel (2nd generation biofuels).

Analysis of Algal Biofuels for Compliance with ASTM Standards

ASTM (American Society for Testing and Materials) International is a globally recognised leader in the development and delivery of international voluntary consensus standards. Today, some 12000 ASTM standards are used around the world to improve product quality, enhance safety, facilitate market access and trade, and build consumer confidence. On May 5, 2009, the Administrator of the EPA (Environmental Protection Agency) released proposed rules based on changes that the Energy Independence and Security Act (EISA), 2007 made to the Renewable Fuel Standard (RFS) which establish a new regulatory scheme (RFS 2) for renewable fuels under the Clean Air Act (the CAA).

As oilgae expands to be a viable alternative fuel to traditional petroleum based fuels, many forward-looking companies are starting to produce and distribute it. Quality and consistency of the finished product is of major concern because of the variety of production techniques and feedstock. Some of the selected, critical, key tests involved to determine the quality and consistency of the product include, free and total glycerin, cloud and pour point, cold soak filterability, viscosity, total acid number, flash point, water and sediment, sulphur, phosphorus, potassium, sodium, calcium, magnesium, distillation, and oxidative stability.

Economic Analysis

Many in the industry admit that the algae cultivation simply for biofuels may not be currently profitable by itself and that the industry must take advantage of markets for additional high-value co-products such as nutraceuticals, fertilisers, and also energy production from the leftover (waste) algal biomass (Donovan *et al.*, 2009). A recent economic model of the production of algal biofuel found that oil for biofuel production could represent a relatively small portion of algae-related revenue opportunities. The model assumed an algae strain with an oil content of 20 per cent and a nutraceutical content of 2 per cent. It concluded that harvesting and oil extraction technologies need to focus on the capture of all valuable algae materials and that the co-product markets must be rigorously analysed to assess the feasibility of realising revenue opportunities for non fuel products (Brown 2009). The oil content of algae can be high at over 70 per cent with oil levels of 20-50 per cent being reasonably common, but more typically 10-30 per cent when grown under nutrient replete conditions (Gavrilescu *et al.,* 2005; Campbell *et al.,* 2009). The NREL study found oil yields in certain species of up to 60 per cent, but maximum productivity levels were found at lower oil content (Sheehan *et al.,* 2008). A figure of 50 per cent oil content for commercial algae is suggestible, but this is considered higher than feasible by many and a lower figure of 20 per cent may be more realistic and is supported by initial large scale production trials (Campbell *et al.,* 2009). 50-80 per cent of the material produced from algae meant for biofuel production could, therefore, be from algal 'waste' biomass.

When algal biofuel production becomes a commercial reality the algal waste biomass could be very large, and for environmental, energy and commercial reasons it will be essential to be used effectively. The algal waste biomass thus, could be used in co-generation, but it may have a relatively low energy density. Problems with drying and handling may also be encountered. An alternative approach may be to use anaerobic digestion to produce biogas. A recent study has shown that the conversion of the algal waste biomass to methane can recover more energy than the extraction of lipid from algae. Further, when the lipid content is below 40 per cent anaerobic digestion of the entire biomass without lipid extraction may be the optimal strategy for energy recovery (Sialve *et al.,* 2009).

Potential for Value-Added Co-products

The absence of support structures, such as roots and stems, allows for a larger fraction of the microalgae to be used to create desired products compared to other types of biomass. There is a broad range of valuable products to harvest. The product type and quality obtained depends on microalgae species, growing conditions, and recovery methods implemented. Utilisation areas can be divided into three categories:

☆ Energy – production of substances such as hydrocarbons, hydrogen, methanol, etc.

☆ Foods and chemicals – proteins, oils and fats, sterols, carbohydrates, sugars, alcohols, etc.

☆ Other chemicals – dyes, perfumes, vitamins/supplements, etc.

Researchers have demonstrated that biomass can be used as an effective feed substitute for animals. Chae and co-authors (2006) reported *E. gracilis* microalgae as an especially effective feed source for broiler chicken (one broiler chicken can consume approximately 114gm of dried microalgae each day on an average). The edible species that have been studied extensively because of their many valuable products include, *Nostoc, Spirulina* and *Aphaniomenon*, which can be utilised raw (unprocessed) food as they are rich in carotenoid, chlorophyll, phycocyanin, amino acids, minerals and bioactive compounds. The compounds have immense medicinal values like, immune-stimulating, metabolism enhancing, cholesterol reducing, anti-inflammatory, and antioxidant properties, besides their nutritional value. Currently, there is a substantial market for various products created from biomass.

Another important aspect of microalgae is that they are rich in ω^3 fatty acids including docosahexaenoic acid and eicosapentanoic acid that have significant therapeutic importance as anti-inflammatory to treat heart disease. EPA prevents and treats various medical conditions, such as coronary heart disease, blood platelet aggregation, abnormal cholesterol levels, several carcinomas, and arresting and minimising tumour growth. It is also naturally found aplenty in fish oils; microalgal sources have significant advantages, including the lack of fishy smell, enhanced purity, low cholesterol content, and a less costly recovery process though. Concern regarding the contamination of fish oil with pesticides and heavy metals is also important. Microalgae are actually the primary producers of ω^3 polyunsaturated fatty acids, and fish usually obtains EPA *via* bioaccumulation in the food chain.

Economics of Algae Biodiesel Production

There are a few economic feasibility studies on microalgae oil (Richardson *et al.*, 2009). Currently, microalgae biofuel has not been deemed economically feasible compared to agricultural biomass (Carlsson *et al.*, 2007), *i.e.* second generation biodiesel. The associated critical and controversial issues are the potential biomass yield that can be obtained by algal culture, and the production costs of the biomass and derived products. The basis of the estimates is usually on three parameters: photosynthetic efficiency, assumptions on scale-up, and on long-term cultivation issues. The productivity of raceway ponds and photobioreactors is limited by a range of issues.

Typical productivity for microalgae in open ponds is 30-50 t/ha/year (Sheehan *et al.*, 1998; Benemann *et al.*, 1996). Several possible target areas to improve productivity in large-scale installations have been proposed (Grobbelaar 2000; Suh *et al.*, 2003; Torzillo *et al.*, 2003; Carvalho *et al.*, 2006). With a majority of the cost being contributed towards the cultivation expenses, harvesting is 20-30 per cent. Higher productivity may be possible in commercial photobioreactors though it may require 10 times capital investment than open pond systems. Genetic upgradation, developing low-cost harvesting processes, improving the photobioreactor and integrating coproduction of high-value products/processes are cost optimisation options (Chisti 2007). Harvested algae waste biomass can be biogasified to produce methane (biogas). Productivity for *Chlorella vulgaris* in photobioreactors is reportedly 13-150 t/ha/year (Pulz 2001).

The estimated algal production cost for open pond systems ($10/kg) and photobioreactors ($30–$70/kg) is two order magnitudes higher and almost three order magnitudes higher than conventional agricultural biomass respectively (Carlsson *et al.*, 2007). Assuming that biomass contains 30 per cent oil by weight and the CO_2 available at no additional cost, the estimated production cost for photobioreactors and raceway ponds could be $1.40 and $1.81/l oil, respectively. However, for microalgal biodiesel to be competitive with petro-diesel, algal oil price should be less than $0.48/l at current price (Chisti 2007). Comparing the potential of microalgal biodiesel with bioethanol from sugarcane on an equal energy basis, sugarcane bioethanol can be produced at a price comparable to that of gasoline (Gray *et al.*, 2007; Demirbas *et al.*, 2011). The best bioethanol yield from sugarcane in Brazil is 7.5 m^3/ha (Demirbas *et al.*, 2011). Bioethanol has only 64 per cent of the energy content of biodiesel. Therefore, if all the energy associated with 0.53 billion m^3 of biodiesel that the US needs annually (Chisti 2007) was to be provided by bioethanol, 828 million m^3 of bioethanol would be needed, which means planting sugarcane over an area of 111 million hectares or 61 per cent of the total available cropping area of the US.

Microalgal oil recovery and conversion to biodiesel are unaltered by production system (such as, open systems or photobioreactors). The cost of biomass production, therefore, is the only relevant factor for a comparative assessment of photobioreactors and raceways for producing microalgal biodiesel. Using economy of scale, if the annual biomass production capacity is increased to 10,000 t, the production cost/kg reduces to roughly $0.47 and $0.60 for photobioreactors and raceways, respectively. Biodiesel from palm oil costs roughly $0.66/l or 35 per cent more than petrodiesel, suggesting that the process of converting palm oil to biodiesel adds about $0.14/l to the price of oil. For palm oil sourced biodiesel to be competitive with petrodiesel, the price of palm oil should not exceed $0.48/l, assuming a tax exemption on biodiesel. Using the same analogy, a reasonable target competitive price for microalgal diesel is $0.48/l (Chisti 2007; Demirbas *et al.*, 2011).

The costs of producing algal oil range from $21,000/t using *P. carterae* to a conjectural price of approx. $800/t, assuming a productivity of 110 t oil/ha/yr. The costings include an annual minimal capital charge of 20 per cent which works out to $200/t, but not maintenance costs. Annual operating cost is estimated at about $15000/ha, which means a final cost in excess of $1100/t. The selling price (that should include an adequate financial return on investment) would therefore be about $1400/t. Considering that the best oilgae yield is a fifth of these projected values then a more realistic price would be five time higher than this, *i.e.* more than $7000/t.

In a critique of a Company that claims for efficient and cheap production of oilgae, Dimitrov (2007) expressed unlikelihood that the technology could be used to produce crude oil at less than $800/barrel. As there are approx. 7 barrels in a tonne (density-dependent), this gives a final cost of about $5600/t oil. Algal biomass with an oil content of 40 per cent could be produced at about $1750/t oil in a report from the Department of Energy, USA (Benemann *et al.,* 1998). Given the current state of technology it is an unrealistically low value. The best practical attainment to date indicates a price in considerable excess of this value, *i.e.* $21000/t. It opines, therefore, that even with the most propitious alga grown under near-ideal conditions, production at less than $5600-7000/t is unlikely, extraction cost excluded. The final costing, however, shall depend various factors, *viz.,* biomass yield, oil content, scale of operation and costs of recovery.

This infers that the current algal-oil production is still far more expensive than petroleum diesel fuels, which means the infeasibility of commercial algal-biofuel production. Algal oil as an economic activity for biofuel thus, is still highly dependent on the future petroleum prices. Assuming that algal oil has approx. 80 per cent of caloric energy value of crude petroleum, Chisti (2007) propounded an equation to estimate the algal oil cost to be competitive to petroleum diesel: $C_{algal oil} = 6.9 \times 10^{-3} C_{petroleum}$, where $C_{algal oil}$ is the price of microalgal oil per gallon, and $C_{petroleum}$ is the price of crude oil per barrel. Thus, with petroleum priced at $80/barrel, the competitive oilgae cost should be less than $0.55/gallon.

Enhancement of Economic Feasibility of Biofuels from Microalgae

Even though the world is facing financial crises but the energy demand is continuously rising. Major sector which accounts for highest oil consumption is transport. India is the third largest in road network with its 1.9 million miles roadways. According to the International Energy Agency (IEA), coal/peat account for nearly 40 per cent of India's energy consumption, followed by nearly 27 per cent for combustible renewables and wastes. Oil accounts for nearly 24 per cent, natural gas 06 per cent, hydroelectric power almost 02 per cent, nuclear nearly 01 per cent, and other renewables less than 0.5 per cent. According to Oil and Gas Journal (OGJ), India had approximately 5.6 billion barrels of oil reserves as of January 2010; the second-largest amount in the Asia-Pacific region (Anon., 2011b) even though nearly 30 per cent of the total energy needs are met through imports (IEA 2010). Microalgae are best substitute for a developing country like India to meet such a large burning up of fuel. Along with employment to its huge population, it can have its own technology for renewable energy, and cutting off the CO_2 emission comes as bonus.

Molecular and Biochemical Aspect of Oilgae Production

Metabonomics, the statistical identification of differences in metabolite levels due to genetic or environmental changes using NMR spectroscopy or mass spectrometry (in combination with chromatography techniques) followed by chemometric analysis (Nicholson *et al.,* 1999, 2002; Lindon *et al.,* 2004) allows determination of accumulated metabolic end products and intermediates. The biosynthesis of algal lipids requires acetyl-CoA as the starting point. Acetyl CoA carboxylase and other enzymes of the lipid biosynthesis pathway have been used as targets to improve oil production (Ratledge 2004). Lipid metabolism and the biosynthesis of fatty acids, glycerolipids, sterols, hydrocarbons and ether lipids in eukaryotic algae have been recently reviewed in the context of optimisation for biodiesel production (Metzger *et al.*, 2005; Guschina *et al.*, 2006). While *C. reinhardtii* serves as a model organism to study lipid biosynthesis in green algae (Riekhof *et al.*, 2005), some unusual hydrocarbons and ether lipids from *Botryococcus braunii* have been described (*e.g.* n-alkadienes, trienes, triterpenoid botryococcenes, methylated squalenes, tetraterpenoids; lycopadiene (Achitouv *et al.*, 2004; Metzger *et al.*, 2005). Transcriptomics and proteomics offer the additional possibility of identifying differentially expressed genes and proteins that are either directly involved in lipid biosynthesis and degradation or that are coordinately regulated. For example, identification of key regulatory genes and their proteins, such as transcription factors, kinases and phosphatases, and their over- or under-expression in transgenic cells can efficiently alter whole physiological pathways (Anderson *et al.*, 2004; McGrath *et al.*, 2005; Dombrecht *et al.*, 2007). Fatty acid production and composition has been altered in a number of plants by metabolic engineering using transgenes encoding for different enzymatic steps in fatty acid biosynthesis/modification pathways, most notably in canola (Dehesh *et al.*, 1996; Eccleston *et al.*, 1998; Um *et al.*, 2009).

R&D Focus Areas

Biorefinery: The High Value Co-product Strategy

Biorefinery term was coined to describe the integration of bioprocessing and appropriate eco-friendly chemical technologies to produce a wider range of chemicals and fuels from biomass in a cost effective and environmentally sustainable manner Chisti (2007). Such examples include, the two-phase conversion of fructose to 5-hydroxymethylfurfural, fermentative production of ethanol from sugars derived from cellulose and semi-cellulose (ABC Ltd, 2007) and bio-oils and/or biosyngas by the pyrolysis/gasification of woods or other biomasses (Mohan *et al.*, 2006). Microalgae also have the capacity to produce an array of high-value bioactive compounds, having use in health foods, pharma and as pigments (Oh *et al.*, 2003; Jiang 2000). Some well-studied examples include acetylic acids, β-carotene (Del Campo *et al.*, 2007), vitamin B (He *et al.*, 2005), ketocarotenoid astaxanthin (Ip *et al.*, 2005), polyunsaturated fatty acids (Wen *et al.*, 2003; Jiang *et al.*, 2004), and lutein (Shi *et al.*, 2002) (refer to Table 3.6). The economic feasibility of microalgal fuel production should be significantly enhanced by a high-value coproduct strategy, which would conceptually involve sequentially the cultivation of microalgae in a microalgal farming facility (CO_2 mitigation), harvesting the biomass, extracting bioactive products, thermal processing (pyrolysis, liquefaction or gasification), extracting high-value chemicals from the resulting liquid, vapour and/or solid phases, and reforming/upgrading biofuels for different applications. Employing a high-value coproduct strategy through the integrated biorefinery approach would significantly enhance the overall cost effectiveness of the production system.

Efficient Photobioreactor Designing (Design of Advanced Photobioreactors)

Choosing an ideal cultivation system is another key aspect that may significantly affect the efficiency and cost-effectiveness of the production process (Lee 2001; Pulz 2001; Carvalho *et al.*, 2006; Chaumont 1993). Carvalho (2006) explained several closed systems in detail. Lee (2001) has discussed a few open systems and compared them with closed systems over different geographical regions. Pulz (2001) stressed more on the process parameters and suggested a number of open systems. Janssen *et al.* (2003) offered useful conceptual diagrams for some of the discussed closed systems and described new systems to be examined, including the use of optical fiber to enhance lighting. Though open pond systems seem to be favoured commercial production systems due to their low capital costs, closed systems offer better control over contamination, mass transfer, and other parameters. A combination of photobioreactor and open pond could be effective at a 2 ha scale (Huntley *et al.*, 2007; Li *et al.*, 2008).

Table 3.6: Some high-value bioproducts extracted from Microalgae.

Product Group	Applications	Products and their Respective Producers
Phycobiliproteins	Pigments,	Phycocyanin- *Spirulina platensis*[a] Phycoerythrin- *Porphyridium cruentu*[b]
Carotenoids	Pro-vitamins, cosmetics, pigmentation	β-carotene- *Dunaliella salina*[c] Astaxanthin - *Haematococcus pluvialis*[d]
Polyunsaturated fatty acids (PUFAs)	Food additive, Nutraceuticals	EPA- *Trachydiscus minutus*[e] DHA- *Chroomonas salina*[f] AA- *Parietochlorisincise*[g]
Vitamins	Nutrition	Biotin- *Euglena gracilis*[h] Vit. E- *Euglena gracilisa*[i] Vit. C- *Prototheca moriformis*[j]

a: Furuki *et al.*, 2003; b: Roman *et al.*, 2002; c: Borowitzka 1991; d: Olaizola 2003; e: Øezanka *et al.*, 2010; f: Henderson *et al.*, 1992; g: Valencia *et al.*, 2007; h: Baker *et al.*, 1981; i: Survase *et al.*, 2006; j: Bremus *et al.*, 2006.

EPA: Eicosapentaenoic acid; DHA: Docosahexaenoic acid; AA: Arachidonic acid.

The lipid depleted algal biomass is a valued resource. It has many alternative applications, including use as a feedstock for plastic additives (glycols from biomass sugars), use in animal nutrition as a feed, and in other fuel producing alternatives (syngas production, methane production by anaerobic digestion, ethanol production *via* fermentation, etc.).

Selection of Cost-Effective Technologies for Biomass Harvesting and Drying

Given the relatively low biomass concentration obtainable in microalgal cultivation systems due to the limit of light penetration (typically in the range of 1–5 g/l) and the small size of microalgal cells (2-20μm dia.), costs and energy consumption for biomass harvesting are significant concerns to be addressed. Technologies including chemical flocculation (Knuckey *et al.*, 2006) biological flocculation (Divakaran *et al.*, 2002), filtration, (Molina *et al.*, 2003) centrifugation, (Olaizola, 2003) and ultrasonic aggregation (Bosma *et al.*, 2003) have been investigated for biomass harvesting. Though chemical and biological flocculation requires only low operating costs, the disadvantages are long processing period and the risk of bioactive product decomposition. Contrarily, filtration, centrifugation and ultrasonic flocculation are more efficient, but the cost factor is a concern. Selecting appropriate harvesting technology depends on the size of target cells, value of the target products and biomass concentration.

Biomass drying and/or thermochemical processing for extraction are steps that need consideration. Sun-drying is probably the cheapest method (Millamena *et al.*, 1990; Prakash *et al.*, 1997). However, this method takes long time, requires large surface, and risks the loss of bioactive products. Low-pressure shelf drying is a low-cost alternative, but is of low efficiency. More efficient but costly drying technologies having been investigated that include drum drying (Prakash *et al.*, 1997), spray drying (Leach *et al.*, 1998; Desmorieux *et al.*, 2006), fluidised-bed drying, freeze-drying, and refractance window dehydration technology (Nindo *et al.*, 2007). It is important to find the balance between the drying efficiency and cost-effectiveness to maximise the net energy output.

Resource and Site Analysis

India, a peninsular country has around 14,500 km of inland navigable waterways (Anon 2011a) and has an 8000 km coastline. There are twelve rivers which are classified as major rivers, with the total catchment area exceeding 2,528,000 km^2 (976,000 mile^2). The contiguous population thrives on capturing (or culturing) the water animals such as fish, crab etc. These water bodies could serve as natural open-water systems for large-scale algal culture, variation in water quality of this water system has big role play on the production and biochemical composition though. As various strains have been reported that produce maximum oilgae at some different conditions, proper strain selection will be a key factor. Patra and coworkers (Patra *et al.*, 2009) have reported algal forms like *Chaetomorpha* sp. and *Phormidium* sp. in brackishwater of Chilika Lake in Odisha.

Environmental and Social Issues

Considering that biodiesel is a credible source of low-carbon energy that delivers greenhouse gas (GHG) savings compared with fossil fuels, many countries strive to set global standards for lowering emissions in the future. Europe aims to cut GHG emission by one-fifth by 2020, partly by biofueling at least one in 10 vehicles. Such efforts will spark a surge in demand for biodiesel. The Federal Government (USA) wishes to reduce its GHG pollution by 28 per cent by 2020. Meanwhile, the Chinese government announced the action to control GHG emissions, by dropping the CO_2 emissions by 40-45 per cent per unit of GDP by 2020 than in 2005, and has also decided to help the African countries to develop clean energy projects. The Japanese government has a GHG emission reduction target of 60–80 per cent by 2050 from its current level (Matsumoto *et al.*, 2009). India, Brazil, South Africa and other countries have also set their GHG reduction target and development programmes of substitute energy in the future. All of these provide biodiesel industry many unprecedented opportunities of development. Right now, due to large-scale deforestation for the purpose of energy crops, the water storage and conservation capability of soil has been very much weakened. Close attention also needed to be paid to the haze caused by deliberate forest fires caused by farmers to clear land for agriculture uses.

Environmental Impact of Large-Scale Operations

Microalgae are advanced biofuels having small ecological footprint – it enables productive use of arid and semi-arid lands and saline water resources unsuitable for agriculture etc. Intensively managed microalgal production facilities are capable of fixing several-fold more CO_2 per unit area than agricultural crops or trees. Although CO_2 will still be released when biofuels derived from algal biomass are combusted, integration of microalgal farms with power plants for flue gas capture can increase the amount of energy produced per unit of CO_2 released by as much as 60 per cent. Materials derived from microalgal biomass also can be used for other long-term uses, serving to sequester CO_2. Flue gas from power plants has the potential to provide sufficient quantities of CO_2 for large-scale microalgae farms. Full life cycle assessment (LCA) with extensive boundaries should continue as production, extraction, conversion, and use technologies evolve to ensure maximum environmental and ecological benefits principally regarding water use and quality. As with any biomass-based technology, the algae-to-fuels concept needs to be analysed from a resource perspective so that critical requirements, such as CO_2, nutrients, sunlight, and water can be aligned with their availability, a significant driver for the development of algal biofuels. Preliminary survey of the resource requirements and availability for large-scale algal cultivation has to be conducted, with special attention on climate, land, water and CO_2 availability. Figure 3.1 suggested a technoeconomically feasible model for value-added algal biofuel production vis-à-vis other utility products.

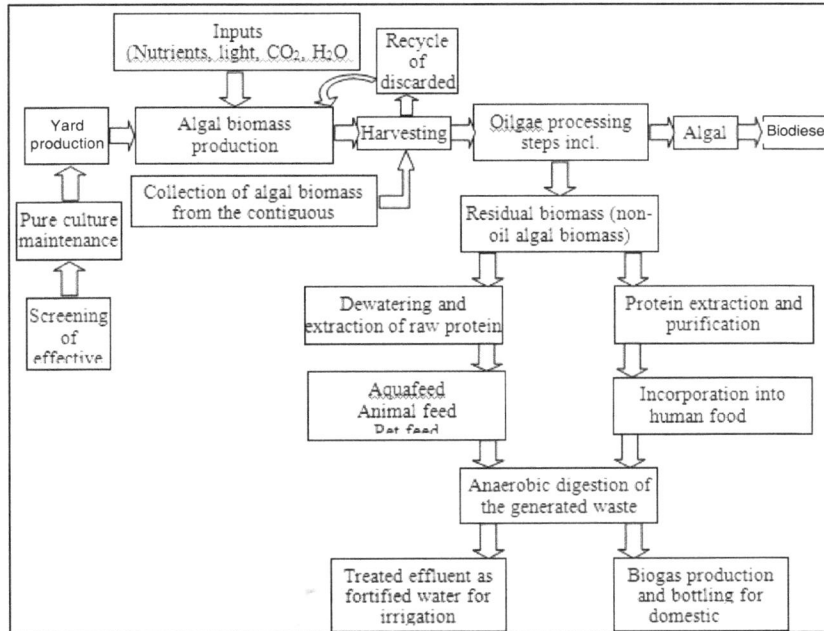

Figure 3.1: A Proposed Complete Utility Model for the Algal Biofuel Production in Combination with other Byproducts of Economic Significance.

Future Prospects

Algae have great potential as a sustainable feedstock for production of diesel-types with the least CO_2 emissions. Currently, there are serious drawbacks and it would be imprudent to overestimate the greenness of this up and coming technology. Algae can be grown in ponds and bioreactors in just a few days, and oil can be extracted directly from the harvested algae. Success in microalgae culture achieved in the US is providing momentum in many other countries. Some companies have just finished R and D on expansion of production areas through location of new farming sites (U.S. Department of Energy, 2006). While some have perfected the culture techniques, others are exploring new ways and are focusing on the protection of existing stocks from over-harvesting through good management practices. Research on such biofuels is still in the inception, and a large-scale operation would require massive investments in production facilities. That may require many years and large revenues, though it might be possible if nations were willing to commit the resources for the purpose. Geographically India, being surrounded by ocean and sea waters on three sides, has a natural advantage. It's India's chance to advance algae-based biofuel technology.

Conclusion

Some microalgae have been exploited for millennia (*Nostoc* in China and *Arthospira* in Chad and Mexico). However, closed system commercialisation has begun in Japan and Israel, and *Chlorella* in Germany. In view of deteriorating effects on the environment due to use of synthetic pigments, researchers are emphasising on the need for natural pigmenting agents as alternative to synthetic chemicals. Algal production system need to be further improved in order to become more competitive and more economically feasible through integrated farming approaches.

Microalgae have the potential to transform the energy industry by supplying cost transformational biofuel production systems, and novel applications of existing technologies to improve the production cost to a point competitive with fossil fuels. It's an opportunity that developing and vast countries like India with a long coastline must explore, standardise the technology, and make it an economically viable proposition so that not only the country gains and saves on the precious foreign exchange but also provide economic benefits far-and-wide cutting across social and economic strata.

References

Ako H, Tamaru CS, Asano L *et al.* (2000). Achieving natural colouration in fish under culture. UJNR Technical Report No-28, 1-4.

Alagappan M, Vijila K, Archana S (2004). Utilization of spirulina algae as a source of carotenoid pigment for blue gouramis (Trichogaster trichopterus Pallas). J *Aquaricult Aquat Sci* 10: 1-11.

Amar EC, Kiron V, Satoh S (2003). Enhancement of innate immunity in rainbow trout (Oncorhynchus mykiss Walbaum) associated with dietary intake of carotenoids from natural products. Fish Shellfish Immunol 16: 527-537.

Anderson S (2000). Salmon color and the consumer. IIFET Proceedings 1-4.

Anon (2010). India Energy Data, Statistics and Analysis - Oil, Gas, Electricity, Coal. http://www.eia.gov/countries/cab.cfm?fips=IN. Accessed on 11 November 2011.

Anon (2011a). Introduction to Inland Water Transport. Government of India. http://iwai.gov.in/introduction.html. Accessed on 29 August 2011.

Anon (2011b). US Energy Information Administration. http://www.eia.gov/countries/country-data.cfm?fips=IN. Accessed on 25 August 2011.

Appler HN, Jauncey K (1983). The utilization of a filamentous green alga [Cladophora glomerata (L. Kutzin)] as a protein source in pelleted feeds for Sarotherodon *Tilapia niloticus* fingerlings. Aquaculture 30: 21-30.

Appler HN (1985). Evaluation of Hydrodictyon reticulatum as a protein source for Oreochromis *Tilapia nilotica* and *Tilapia zillii*. J Fish Biol 27: 327-333.

Aresta M, Dibenedetto A, Barberio G (2005). Utilization of macro-algae for enhanced CO_2 fixation and biofuels production: Development of a computing software for an LCA study. Fuel Proc Technol 86: 1679-1693.

Aslan S, Kapdan IK (2006). Batch kinetics of nitrogen and phosphorus removal from synthetic wastewater by algae. Ecol Eng 28: 64-70.

Avron M, Ben Amotz, A (1992). *Dunaliella*: physiology, Biochemistry and biotechnology.CRC Press, Boca Raton, Florida.

Baker ER, McLaughlin JJA, Hutner SH (1981). Water-soluble vitamins in cells and spent culture supernatants of *Poteriochromonas stipitata, Euglena gracilis*, and *Tetrahymena thermophila*. Arch Microbiol 129: 310-313.

Baker RTM (2001). Canthaxanthin in aquafeed applications: Is there any risk? Trends in Food Science and Technology 7: 240-243.

Banerjee A, Harma RS, Chisti Y *et al.* (2002). *Botryococcus braunii*: A renewable source of hydrocarbons and other chemicals. Critic Rev Biotechnol 22: 245-279.

Basurco B, Abellan E (1999). Finfish species diversification in the context of the Mediterranean marine fish farming development. Cahiers Options Mediterraneennes, Ser. B: Etudes et Recherches, 24: 9-25.

Becker EW (1994). Microalgae. Biotechnology and Microbiology. Cambridge: Cambridge University Press. ISBN 978-0-521-06113.

Becker EW (1994). Biotechnology and Microalgae. Cambridge University Press Cambridge.

Benemann J, Oswald WJ (1996). Systems and economic analysis of microalgae ponds for conversion of CO_2 to biomass. US DOE, Pitburgh Energy Technology Centre.

Benemann JR, Dunahy TG, Roessler PG (1998). A look back at the U.S. department of energy's aquatic species programme biodiesel from algae. Report NREL/TP-580-24190. National Renewable Energy Laboratory, US Department of Energy.

Benemann JR, Koopman BL, Weissman JC *et al.* (1978). An integrated system for the conversion of solar energy with sewage-grown microalgae. Report, Contract D (0-3)-34, U.S. Department of Energy, SAN-003-4-2.

Benemann JR (1992). Microalgae aquaculture feeds. J Appl Phycol 4: 23.

Biendenbach JM, Smith LL, Lawrence AL (1990). Use of a new spray dried algal product in penaeid larval culture. Aquaculture 86: 249-257.

Bjerkeng B, Johnsen G (1995). Frozen storage of rainbow trout (*Oncorhynchus mykiss*) as affected by oxygen, illumination and fillet pigment. J Food Sci 60: 284-288.

Boonyaratpalin M, Lovell RT (1977). Diet preparation for aquarium fishes. Aquaculture 12: 53-62.

Boonyaratpalin M, Unprasert N (1989). Effect of pigments from different sources on colour changes and growth of red *Oreochromis niloticus*. Aquaculture 79: 375-380.

Boonyaratpalin M, Phromkunthong W (1986). Effects of carotenoid pigments from different sources on colour changes of fancy carp, *Cyprinus carpio* Linn. J Sci Technol 8: 11-20.

BioAstin/Naturose™ Technical Bulletin-020, Revision Date: November 9, 2001. Boonyaratpalin M, Lovell RT (1977). Diet preparation for aquarium fishes. Aquaculture 12: 53-62.

Booth M, Warner-Smith R, Allan G *et al.* (2004). Effects of dietary astaxanthin source and light manipulation on the skin colour of Australian snapper *Pagrus auratus* (Bloch and Schneider, 1801). Aquacult Res 35: 458-464.

Borowitzka LJ (1991). Development of Western Biotechnology's algal β-carotene plant. Bioresour Technol 38: 251-252.

Borowitzka MA (1999). Commercial production of microalgae: ponds, tanks, tubes and fermenters . J Biotech 70: 313–321.

Borowitzka MA (1995). Micro algae as a source of pharmaceuticals and other biologically active compounds. J Appl Phycol 7: 3-15.

Bosma R, van Spronsen WA, Tramper J *et al.* (2003). Ultrasound, a new separation technique to harvest microalgae. J Appl Phycol 15: 143-153.

Bosma R, van Zessen E, Reith JH *et al.* (2007). Prediction of volumetric productivity of an outdoor photobioreactor. Biotechnol Bioeng 97: 1108-1120.

Boyd CE (1990). Water quality in ponds for aquaculture. Alabama Agricultural Experiment Station, Auburn University, Alabama.

Bremus C, Herrmann U, Bringer-Meyer S *et al.* (2006). The use of microorganisms in L-ascorbic acid production. J Biotechnol 124: 196-205.

Brown P (2009). Algal Biofuels Research, Development, and Commercialization Priorities: A Commercial Economics Perspective. Energy Overviews. ep Overviews Publishing, Inc, 22 06 2009. http: //epoverviews.com/main_img.jpg. Accessed 23 February 2012.

Burlew JS, ed. (1953). Algal Culture from Laboratory to Pilot Plant; Carnegie Institution, Publication 600: Washington, DC.

Campbell PK, Beer T, Batten D. Greenhouse Gas Sequestration by Algae- Energy and Greenhouse Gas Life Cycle Studies. CSIRO Australia. http: //www.csiro.au/files/files/poit.pdf. Accessed on 31 July 2011.

Carlozzi P (2000). Hydrodynamic aspects and Arthrospira growth in two outdoor tubular undulating row photobioreactors. Appl Microbiol Biotechnol 54: 14-22.

Carlozzi P, Pushparaj B, Degl'Innocenti A *et al.* (2006). Growth characteristics of *Rhodopseudomonas palustris* cultured outdoors, in an underwater tubular photobioreactor, and investigation of photosynthetic efficiency. Appl Microbiol Biotechnol 73: 789-795.

Carlsson AS, van Bilen JB, Möller R *et al.* (2007). Mircro- and macroalgae: utility for industrial applications; 2007. http: //www.epobio.net/pdfs/0709AquaticReport.pdf. Accessed on 24 August 2011.

Carvalho AP, Meireles LA, Malcata FX (2006). Microalgal reactors: A review of enclosed system designs and performances. Biotechnol Prog 22: 1490-1506.

Chae SR, Hwang EJ, Shin HS (2006). Single cell protein production of *Euglena gracilis* and carbon dioxide fixation in an innovative photo-bioreactor. Bioresour Technol 97: 322-329.

Chakraborty RD, Chakabort K, Radhakrishnan EV (2007). Variation in fatty acid composition of Artemia salina nauplii enriched with microalgae and bakers yeast for use in larviculture. J.Agric Food Chem 55: 4043-4051.

Chaumont D (1993). Biotechnology of algal biomass production: a review of systems for outdoor mass culture. J Appl Phycol 5: 593-604.

Chisti Y (2006). Microalgae as sustainable cell factories. Environ Eng Man J 5: 261-274.

Chisti Y (2007). Biodiesel from microalgae. Biotechnol Adv 25: 294-306.

Chou YH, Chien YH (2006). Effects of astaxanthin and vitamin E supplement in Japanese sea bass (*Lateolabrax japonicus*) broodstock diet on their spawning performance and egg quality, J Fish Soc, Taiwan, 33: 157-169.

Choubert G (1979). Tentative utilization of spirulina algae as a source of carotenoid pigments for rainbow trout. Aquaculture 18: 135-143.

Choubert G, Cravedi J, Laurentie M (2005). Pharmacokinetics and bioavailabilities of ^{14}C-keto-carotenoids, astaxanthin and canthaxanthin, in rainbow trout, *Oncorhynchus mykiss*. Aquaculture Research 15: 1526-1534.

Chow CY, Woo NYS (1990). Bioenergetic studies on an omnivorous fish, *Oreochromis mossambicus*: Evaluation of the utilization of Spirulina algae in feeds. In: Hirano R, Hanyu I (ed). Asean Fish Society, Manila, Philippines Second Asian Fisheries Forum, pp. 291-294.

Christiansen R, Torrissen OJ (1996). Growth and survival of Atlantic salmon, Salmo salar L. fed different dietary levels of astaxanthin. Juveniles. Aquacult Nutr 2: 55-62.

Christiansen R, Lie O, Torrissen OJ (1994). Effect of astaxanthin and vitamin A on growth and survival during feeding of Atlantic salmon, Salmo salar L. Aquacult Res 25: 903-914.

Ciferri O, Tiboni O (1985). The biochemistry and industrial potential of *Spirulina*. Annu Rev Microbiol 39: 503-526.

Converti A, Lodi A, Del Borghi A *et al.* (2006). Cultivation of *Spirulina platensis* in a combined airlift-tubular system. Biochem Eng J 32: 13-18.

Craik ICA (1985). Egg quality and egg pigment content in salmonids fishes. Aquaculture 47: 61-88.

Crutzen PJ, Mosier AR, Smith KA (2007). N$_2$O release from agro-biofuel production negates global warming reduction by replacing fossil fuels. Atmos Chem Phys Discuss 7: 11191-11205.

Csogor Z, Herrenbauer M, Schmidt K (2001). Light distribution in a novel photobioreactor-modelling for optimization. J Appl Phycol 13: 325-333.

Danielo O (2005). An algae-based fuel. Biofutur 255.

De Groot,C. (1991). Aquatic Microbial Life, Source of Hope An Expectation, Biotechnology and Development Monitor. University Of Amsterdam, Amsterdam The Netherlands.

de la Noue J, de Pauw N (1988). The potential of microalgal biotechnology: a review of production and uses of microalgae. Biotechnol Adv 6: 725-770.

de Morais MG, Costa JAV (2007). Biofixation if carbon dioxide by *Spirulina* sp. and *Scenedesmus obliquus* cultivated in a three-stage serial tubular photobioreactor. J Biotechnol 129: 439-445.

Degen J, Uebele A, Retze A *et al.* (2001). A novel photobioreactor with baffles for improved light utilization through the flashing light effect. J Biotechnol 92: 89-94.

Del Campo JA, Garcia-Gonzalez M, Guerrero MG (2007). Outdoor cultivation of microalgae for carotenoid production: current state and perspectives. Appl Microbiol Biotechnol 74: 1163-1174.

Demirbas A, Demirbas MF (2011). Energ Convers Manag 52: 163-170.

Demirbas MF (2011). Biofuels from algae for sustainable development. Applied Energy 88: 3472-3480.

Desmorieux H, Decaen N (2006). Convective drying of *Spirulina* in thin layer. J Food Eng 77: 64-70.

Dimitrov K (2007). Green Fuel Technology: A Case Study for Industrial Photosynthetic Energy Capture. http://www.nanostring.net/Algae/CaseStudy.pdf. Accessed 21 November 2011.

Divakaran R, Pillai VNS (2002). Flocculation of algae using chitosan. J Appl Phycol 14: 419-422.

Donovan J, Stowe N. Is the Future of Biofuels in Algae? Renewable Energy World. Renewable Energy World, 12.06.2009. http://www.renewableenergyworld.com/rea/news/article/2009/06/is-the-future-of-biofuels-in-algae. Accessed on 24 August 2011.

Doolan BJ, Allan GL, Booth MA *et al.* (2004). Improving skin colour in farmed snapper (red sea bream, *Pagrus auratus*).School of Ecology and Environment, Deakin University, Warrnambool, Victoria 3280, Australia. www.was.org/documents.

Doucha J, Lývansky K (2006). Productivity, CO_2/O_2 exchange and hydraulics in outdoor open high density microalgal (*Chlorella* sp.) photobioreactors operated in a Middle and Southern European climate. J Appl Phycol 18: 811-826.

Doucha J, Straka F, Lývansky K (2005). Utilization of flue gas for cultivation of microalgae (*Chlorella sp.*) in an outdoor open thin-layer photobioreactor. J Appl Phycol 17: 403-412.

Elnady M, Hassanien HA, Salem MA *et al.* (2010). Algal Abundances and Growth Performances of Nile Tilapia (Oreochromis niloticus) as Affected by Different Fertilizer Sources. J Am Sci 6: 584-593.

Eriksen NT, Riisgard FK, Gunther W *et al.* (2007). On-line estimation of O_2 production, CO_2 uptake, and growth kinetics of microalgal cultures in a gas tight photobioreactor. J Appl Phycol 19: 161-174.

Etheridge DM, Steele LP, Langenfelds RL *et al.* (1996). Natural and anthropogenic changes in atmospheric CO_2 over the last 1000 years from air in Antarctic ice and firn. J Geophys Res 101: 4115-4128.

Fernandez FGA, Hall DO, Guerrero EC *et al.* (2003). Outdoor production of *Phaeodactylum tricornutum* biomass in a helical reactor. J Biotechnol 103: 137-152.

Feuga MA (2004). Microalgae for aquaculture: the current global situation and future trends. In: Richmond A. (ed) Handbook of microalgal culture. Blackwell Science, pp. 352-364.

Floyd RF (2002). Fish nutrition. Fisheries and Aquatic Sciences Department, Florida Cooperative Extension Service, Institute of Food and Agricultural Sciences, University of Florida.VM114.

Furuki T, Maeda S, Imajo S *et al.* (2003). Rapid and selective extraction of phycocyanin from *Spirulina platensis* with ultrasonic cell disruption. J Appl Phycol 15: 319-324.

Galvez-Cloutier R, Leroueil S, Allier D *et al.* (2006). A combined method: precipitation and capping, to attenuate eutrophication in Canadian lakes. J ASTM Int.3.

Gavrilescu M, Chisti Y (2005). Biotechnology - a sustainable alternative for chemical industry. Biotechnol Adv 23: 471-499.

Gilman D (2007). Fueling organ with sustainable biofuels. Portland: Oregon Environmental Council.

Goodwin TW (1984). The Biochemistry of the Carotenoids. Volume II Animals. Chapman and Hall, New York, USA. pp. 224.

Gouveia L, Rema P (2005). Effect of microalgal biomass concentration and temperature on ornamental goldfish (*Carassius auratus*) skin pigmentation. Aquacult Nutr 11: 19-23.

Gouveia L, Ghoubert C, Pereira N (2002). Pigmentation of gilhead seabream, *Sparus aurata* (L.1985), using *Chlorella vulgaris* (Chlorophyta, Volvocales) microalga. Aquacult Res 33: 987–993.

Gouveia L, Gomes E, Empis J (1996). Potential use of microalga (Chlorella vulgaris) in the pigmentation of rainbow trout (*Oncorhynchus mykiss*) muscle. Zertschrift fur Lebensmittel Untersuchung und-Forschung 202: 75-79.

Gouveia L, Rema P, Pereira O (2003). Colouring ornamental fish (*Cyprinus carpio* and *Carassius auratus*) with microalgal biomass. Aquacult Nutr 9: 123–129.

Gray KA, Zhao L, Emptage M (2006). Bioethanol Curr Opin Chem Biol 10: 141-146.

Green BW, El Nagdy Z, Hebicha H (2002). Evaluation of *Nile tilapia* pond management strategies in Egypt. Aquacult Res 33: 1037-1048.

Grima EM, Belarbi EH, Acien Fernandez *et al.* (2003). Recovery of microalgal biomass and metabolites: process options and economics. Biotechnol Adv 20: 491-515.

Grobbelaar JU (2000). Physiological and technological considerations for optimising mass algal cultures. J Appl Phycol 12: 201-206.

Grung M, D´Souza, ML, Borowitzka M *et al.* (1992). Algal carotenoids 51. Secondary carotenoids 2. *Haematococcus pluvialis* aplanospores as a source of (3S, 3´S)-astaxanthin esters. J Appl Phycol 4: 165-171.

Guillou A., Choubert G, Storebakken T *et al.* (1989). Bioconversion pathway of astaxanthin into retinol$_2$ in mature rainbow trout (*Salmo gairdnieri* Rich). Comp Biochem Physiol 94B: 481-485.

Hai T, Ahlers H, Gorenflo V *et al.* (2000). Axenic cultivation of anoxygenic phototrophic bacteria, cyanobacteria, and microalgae in a new closed tubular glass photobioreactor. Appl Microbiol Biotechnol 53: 383-389.

Hall DO, Fernandez FGA, Guerrero EC *et al.* (2003). Outdoor helical tubular photobioreactors for microalgal production: Modelling of fluid-dynamics and mass transfer and assessment of biomass productivity. Biotechnol Bioeng 82: 62-73.

Halten B, Arnmesan A, Jobling M *et al.* (1997). Carotenoid pigmentation in relation to feed intake, growth and social integration in Arctic char, *Salvelinus aipinus* (L.), from two anadromous strains. Aquacult Nutr 3: 189–199.

Hameed MSA (2007). Effect of algal density in bead, bead size and bead concentrations on wastewater nutrient removal. Afr J Biotechnol 6: 1185-1191.

Hanaa H, Abd El-Baky k, baz EL *et al.* (2003). *Spirulina* species as a source of carotenoid and tocopherol and its Anticarcinoma factors. Biotechnology 2: 222-240.

He HZ, Li HB, Chen F (2005). Determination of vitamin B1 in seawater and microalgal fermentation media by high-performance liquid chromatography with fluorescence detection. Anal Bioanal Chem 383: 875-879.

Henderson RJ, Mackinlay EE (1992). Radiolabeling studies of lipids in the marine cryptomonad *Chroomonas salina* in relation to fatty acid desaturation. Plant Cell Physiol 33: 395-40.

Hernandez JP, De-Bashan LE, Bashan Y (2006). Starvation enhances phosphorus removal from wastewater by the microalga *Chlorella spp.* co-immobilized with *Azospirillum brasilense*. Enzyme Microb Technol 38: 190-198.

Higuera-Ciapara I, Felix-Valenzuela L, Goycoolea FM (2006). Astaxanthin: A review of its chemistry and applications. Crit Rev Food Sci Nutr 46: 186-196.

Horton P, Ruban AV, Walters RG (1996). Regulation of light harvesting in green plants. Annu Rev Plant Physiol Plant Mol Biol 47: 655-668.

Hovatta I, Barlow C (2008). Molecular genetics of anxiety in mice and men. Ann Med 40: 92-109.

Hu Q, Kurano N, Kawachi M *et al.* (1998). Ultrahigh-cell-density culture of a marine alga *Chlorococcum littorale* in a flat-plate photobioreactor. Appl Microbiol Biotechnol 49: 655-662.

Huntley ME, Redalje DG (2007). CO_2 mitigation and renewable oil from photosynthetic microbes: a new appraisal. Mitigation Adapt Strat Global Change 12: 573-608.

Ip PF, Chen F (2005). Employment of reactive oxygen species to enhance astaxanthin formation in *Chlorella zofingiensis* in heterotrophic culture. Process Biochem 40: 3491-3496.

Janssen M, de Bresser L, Baijens T *et al.* (2000). Scale-up of photobioreactors: effects of mixing-induced light/dark cycles. J Appl Phycol 12: 225-237.

Janssen M, Tramper J, Mur LR *et al.* (2002). Enclosed outdoor photobioreactors: Light regime, photosynthetic efficiency, scale-up, and future prospects. Biotechnol Bioeng 81: 193-210.

Jensen GS, Ginsberg DI, Drapeau MS (2001). Bluegreen algae as an immuno-enhancer and biomodulator. J Am Nutraceutical Assoc 3: 24–30.

Jiang FC (2000). Algae and Their Biotechnological Potential. Kluwer Academic Publishers, Dordrecht/Boston/London.

Jiang Y, Fan KW, Wong RTY *et al.* (2004). Fatty acid composition and squalene content of the marine microalga *Schizochytrium mangrovei*. J Agric Food Chem 52: 1196-1200.

Johnson EA, Schroeder WA (1995). Microbial carotenoids. In: Fiechter (Eds). Advances in Biochemical Engineering. Berlin: Springer 119-178.

Johnson M, Wen Z (2010). Development of an attached microalgal growth system for biofuel production. Appl Microbiol Biotechnol 85: 525-534.

Kebede-Westhead E, Pizarro C, Mulbry WW (2006). Treatment of swine manure effluent using freshwater algae: Production, nutrient recovery, and elemental composition of algal biomass at four effluent loading rates. J Appl Psychol 18: 41-46.

Khatoon N, Sengupta P, Homechaudhury S *et al.* (2010). Evaluation of algae based feed in Goldfish (*Crassius auratus*) nutrition. Proc Zool Soc 63: 109-114.

Knuckey RM, Brown MR, Robert R *et al.* (2006). Production of microalgal concentrates by flocculation and their assessment as aquaculture feeds. Aquacult Eng 35: 300-313.

Knuckey RM, Semmens GL, Mayer RJ *et al.* (2005). Developement of an optimal micro algal diet for the culture of the calanoid copepod *Acartia sinjiensis*: Effect of algal species and feed concentration on copepod development. Aquacuture 249: 339-351.

Koteng DF (1992). Markedsundersokelse, Norsk laks. Norway: Fis-kerinaeringsens Landsforening (FNL).

Krichnavaruk S, Powtongsook S, Pavasant P (2007). Enhancd productivity of *Chaetoceros calcitrans* in airlift photobioreactors. Biores Technol 98: 2123-2130.

Krishna KB, Mohanty P (1998). Secondary carotenoid production in green algae. J Sci Industr Res 57: 51-63.

Leach G, Oliveira G, Morais R (1998). Spray-drying of *Dunaliella salina* to produce a β-carotene rich powder. J Ind Microbiol Biotechnol 20: 82-85.

Lebeau T, Robert JM (2003). Diatom cultivation and biotechnologically relevant products. II. Current and putative products. Appl Microbiol Biotechnol 60: 624-632.

Lee HS, Seo MW, Kim ZH *et al.* (2006). Determining the best specific light uptake rates for the lumostatic cultures of bubble column photobioreactors. Enzyme Microb Technol 39: 447-452.

Lee YK (2001). Microalgal mass culture systems and methods: their limitation and potential. J Appl Phycol 13: 307–315.

Lee YK (1997). Commercial production of micro algae in the Asia Pacific rim. J App Phycol 9: 403-411.

Lewis NS, Nocera DG (2006). Powering the planet: Chemical challenges in solar energy utilization. Proc. Natl. Acad. Sci USA 103: 15729-15735.

Li J, Shou N, Su WW (2003). Online estimation of stirred-tank microalgal photobioreactor cultures based on dissolved oxygen measurements. Biochem Eng J 14: 51-65.

Li Y, Horsman M, Wu N *et al.* (2008). Biofuels from Microalgae. Biotechnol. Prog 24: 815-820.

Lin MQ, Ushio H, Ohshima T *et al.* (1998). Skin color control of the red sea bream (Pagrus major). LWT Food Sci Tech 31: 27-32.

Liu ZY, Wang GC, Zhou BC (2008). Effect of iron on growth and lipid accumulation in *Chlorella vulgaris*. Bioresour Technol 99: 4717-4722.

Lovell RI (1992). Dietary enhancement of color in ornamental fish. Aquaculture Magazine 18: 77-79.

Ltd ABC (2007). Company news: biodiesel from algae makes debut. Fuels Lubes Int. 13: 28.

Lynd L, Greene N, Dale B *et al.* (2006). Energy returns on ethanol production. Science 312: 1746-1748.

Maeda K, Owada M, Kimura N *et al.* (1995). CO_2 fixation from the flue-gas on coal-fired thermal power-plant by microalgae. Energy Convers Manage 36: 717-720.

Mallick N (2002). Biotechnological potential of immobilized algae for wastewater N, P and metal removal: A review. BioMetals15: 377-390.

Mata TM, Martins AA, Ceatano NS (2010). Microalgae for biodiesel production and Rather applications: A review. Renew. Sustain. Energy Rev 14: 217-232.

Meier RL (1955). Biological cycles in the transformation of solar energy into useful fuels. In: Daniels, F. and Duffie, J.A (ed). Solar Energy Research, Madison, WI: University of Wisconsin Press, pp. 179–183.

Merchuk JC, Gluz M, Mukmenev I (2000). Comparison of photobioreactors for cultivation of the red microalga *Porphyridium sp.* J Chem Technol Biotechnol 75: 1119-1126.

Miki W, Yamaguchi K, Konosu S *et al.* (1985). Origino of tunaxanthin in the integument of yellowtail (Seriola quinqueradiata). Biochem Mol Biol 80: 195-201.

Millamena OM, Aujero EJ, Borlongan IG (1990). Techniques on algae harvesting and preservation for use in culture and as larval food. Aquacult Eng 9: 295-304.

Minowa T, Yokoyama SY, Kishimoto M *et al.* (1995). Oil production from algal cells of *Dunaliella tertiolecta* by direct thermochemical liquefaction, Fuel 74: 1735-1738.

Miron AS, Gomez AC, Camacho FG *et al.* (1999). Comparative evaluation of compact photobioreactors for large-scale monoculture of microalgae. J Biotechnol 70: 249-270.

Mishra S, Ojha SK. Potentials of oilgae: The prospects and challenges. Microbiol Applications (in press).

Mohan D, Pittman CU Jr., Steele PH (2006). Pyrolysis of wood/biomass for biooil: a critical review. Energy Fuels 20: 848-889.

Molina Grima E, Belarbi EH, Acien Fernandez FG *et al.* (2003). Recovery of microalgal biomass and metabolites: process options and economics. Biotechnol Adv 20: 491-515.

Molina E, Fernandez J, Acien FG *et al.* (2001). Tubular photobioreactor design for algal cultures. J Biotechnol 92: 113-131.

Mulbry WW, Wilkie AC (2000). Growth of benthic freshwater algae on dairy manures. J Appl Phycol 13: 301–306.

Munoz R, Guieysse B (2006). Algal-bacterial processes for the treatment of hazardous contaminants: a review. Water Res 40: 2799-2815.

Mussgnug J, Thomas-Hall S, Rupprecht J *et al.* (2007). Engineering photosynthetic light capture: Impacts on improved solar energy to biomass conversion. Plant Biotech J 5: 802–814.

Mustafa MG, Nakagawa H (1995). A review: Dietary benefits of algae as an additive in fish feed. Isr J Aquacult- Bamidgeh 47: 155-162.

Nakagawa H, Kashahara S, Ugiyama T (1987). Effect of Ulva meal supplementation on lipid metabolism of black seabream (*Acanthopagrus schlegeli* Bleeker). Aquaculture 62: 109-121.

Nakano T, Kanmuri T, Sato M *et al.* (1999). Effect of astaxanthin rich red yeast (Phaffia rhodozyma) on oxidative stress in rainbow trout. Biochimica et Biophysica Acta 1426: 119-125.

Nakano T, Tosa M, Takeuchi M (1995). Improvement of biochemical features in fish health by red yeast and synthetic astaxanthin. J Agric Food Chem 43: 1570-1573.

Navarro N, Sarasquete C (1998). Use of freeze dried microalgae for rearing gilhead seabream, *Sparus aurata*, larvae. Growth, histology and water quality. Aquaculture 167: 179-63.

Negoro M, Hamasaki A, Ikuta Y *et al.* (1993). Carbon-dioxide fixation by microalgae photosynthesis using actual flue-gas discharged from a boiler. Appl Biochem Biotechnol 39: 643-653.

Negoro M, Shioji N, Miyamoto K *et al.* (1991). Growth of microalgae in high CO_2 gas and effects of Sox and Nox. Appl Biochem Biotechnol 28: 877- 886.

Nindo CI, Tang J (2007). Refractance window dehydration technology: a novel contact drying method. Drying Technol 25: 37-48.

Ogbonna JC, Tanaka H (2000). Light requirement and photosynthetic cell cultivation Developments of processes for efficient light utilization in photobioreactors. J Appl Phycol 12: 207-218.

Oh HM, Choi A, Mheen TI (2003). High-value materials from microalgae. Korean J Microbiol Biotechnol 31: 95-102.

Olaizola M (2003). Commercial development of microalgal biotechnology: from the test tube to the marketplace. Biomol Eng 20: 459-466.

Oswald WJ (1988). Micro-algae and waste-water treatment. In: Borowitzka MA, Borowitzka LJ (ed) Microalgal Biotechnology, Cambridge University Press, New York, USA, pp. 305–328.

Oswald WJ, Golueke C (1960). Biological transformation of solar energy. Adv. Appl Microbiol 2: 223-262.

Page GI, Russell PM, Davies SJ (2005). Dietary carotenoid pigment supplementation influences hepatic lipid and mucopolysaccharide levels in rainbow trout (*Oncorhynchus mykiss*). Comp Biochem Physiol 142B: 398-402.

Paripatananont T, Tangtrongpairoj J, Sailasuta A *et al.* (1999). Effect of a astaxanthin on pigmentation of goldfish (*Carassius auratus*). J World Aquacult Soc 30: 454-460.

Pascal AA, Liu Z, Broess K *et al.* (2007). Molecular basis of photoprotection and control of photosynthetic light harvesting. Nature 436: 134-137.

Patra JK, Patra AP, Mahapatra NK *et al.* (2009). Biomolecular constituents and antibacterial activity of some marine algae from Chilika Lake (Orissa, India). Int J Algae 11: 222-235.

Perner-Nochta I, Lucumi A, Posten C (2007). Photoautotrophic cell and tissue culture in a tubular photobioreactor. Eng Life Sci 7: 127-135.

Polle JEW, Kanakagiri S, Jin E *et al.* (2002). Truncated chlorophyll antenna size of the photosystems– a practical method to improve microalgal productivity and hydrogen hydrogen production in mass culture. Int J Hydrogen Energy 27: 1257-1264.

Prakash J, Pushparaj B, Carlozzi P *et al.* (1997). Microalgal biomass drying by a simple solar device. Int J Solar Energy 18: 303-311.

Pulz O (2001). Photobioreactors: Production systems for phototrophic microorganisms. Appl Microbiol Biotechnol 57: 287–293.

Raja R (2009). Microalgae [Pourriel probable] a coloumn in the second chapter in un monde invisible. In: Bordenave L (ed) Aubanel- La Martiniere Group, France, pp. 124-126.

Restrom B, Borch G, Skulberg OM *et al.* (1981a). Optical purity of (3S, 3´S)- astaxanthin from Haematococcus pluvialis. Phytochemistry 20: 2561-2564.

Rezanka T, Petrankova M, Cepak V *et al.* (2010). *Trachydiscus minutus*, a new biotechnological source of eicosapentaenoic acid. Folia Microbiologica 55: 265-269.

Richardson JW, Outlaw JL, Allison M (2009). Economics of micro algae oil. In: 13 th ICABR conference on the emerging bio-economy Ravello, Italy June 17–20; 2009.

Richmond A, Cheng-Wu Z, Zarmi Y (2003). Efficient use of strong light for high photosynthetic productivity: interrelationships between the optical path, the optimal population density and cell-growth inhibition. Biomol Eng 20: 229-239.

Roman RB, Pez JM, Fernandez FGA *et al.* (2002). Recovery of pure B-phycoerythrin from the microalga *Porphyridium cruentum*. J Biotechnol 93: 73-85.

Sawayama S, Inoue S, Dote Y *et al.* (1995). CO_2 fixation and oil production through microalga. Energy Convers Manage 36: 729-731.

Saxena A (1994). Health; colouration of fish. International Symposium on Aquatic Animal Health: Program and Abstracts. Univ. of California, School of Veterinary Medicine, Davis, CA, USA, pp. 94.

Schenk PM, Hall SRT, Stephens E *et al.* (2008). Second generation biofuels: high-efciency microalgae for biodiesel production. Bioenergy Res 1: 20–43.

Schiedt K, Leuenberger FJ, Vecchi M et a(1985). Absorption, retention and metabolic transformation of carotenoids in rainbow trout, salmon and chicken. Pure Appl Chem 57: 685-692.

Schluter M, Groeneweg J (1981). Mass production of freshwater rotifers on liquid wastes I. The influence of some environmental factors on population growth of *Brachionus rubens*. Aquacultures 25: 17-24.

Scragg AH, Illman AM, Carden A *et al.* (2002). Growth of microalgae with increased calorific values in a tubular bioreactor. Biomass Bioeng 23: 67-73.

Segner H, Arend P, Von Poeppinghaussen K *et al.* (1989). The effect of feeding astaxanthin to *Oreochromis niloticus* and *Colisa labiosa* on the histology of the liver. Aquaculture 79: 381-390.

Sheehan J, Dunahay T, Benemann J *et al.* (1998). A Look Back at the US Department of Energy's Aquatic Species Program - Biodiesel from Algae. National Renewable Energy Laboratory NREL. National Renewable Energy Laboratory NREL, 1998. http: //www.nrel.gov/docs/legosti/fy98/24190.pdf. NREL/TP-580-24190. Accessed on 5 January 2012.

Shi XM, Jiang Y, Chen F (2002). High-yield production of lutein by the green microalga *Chlorella protothecoides* in heterotrophic fedbatch culture. Biotechnol Prog 18: 723-727.

Shimidzu N, Goto M, Miki W (1996). Carotenoids as singlet oxygen quenchers in marine organisms. Fish Sci 62: 134-137.

Sialve B, Bernet N, Bernard O (2009). Anaerobic digestion of microalgae as a necessary step to make microalgal biodiesel sustainable. Biotechnol Adv 27: 409-416.

Sloth JK, Wiebe MG, Eriksen NT (2006). Accumulation of phycocyanin in heterotrophic and mixotrophic cultures of the acidophilic red alga *Galdieria sulphuraria*. Enzyme Microb Technol 38: 168-175.

Smith RP, Larkin GL, Southwick SM (2008). Trends in U.S. emergency department visits for anxiety-related mental health conditions, 1992-2001. J Clin Psychiatry 69: 286-294.

Sobszuk TM, Camacho FG, Molina Grima E *et al.* (2006). Effects of agitation on the microalgae *Phaeodactylum triconutum* and *Porphyridium cruentum*. Bioprocess Biosyst Eng 28: 243-250.

Sommer TR, Souza FMLD, Morrisssy NM (1992). Pigmentation of adult rainbow trout Oncorhynchus mykiss, using the green alga Haematococcus Pluvialis. Aquaculture 106.

Spolaore P, Joannis-Cassan C, Duran E *et al.* (2006). Commercial applications of microalgae. J Biosci Bioeng 101: 87-96.

Stanley J G, Jonesa J B (1976). Feeding algae to fish. *Aquaculture* 7: 219-223.

Suh IS, Lee CG (2003). Photobioreactor engineering: design and performance. Biotechnol Bioprocess Eng 8: 313-321.

Suh IS, Lee SB (2001). Cultivation of a cyanobacterium in an internally radiating air-lift photobioreactor. J Appl Phycol 13: 381-388.

Survase SA, Bajaj IB, Singhal RS (2006). Biotechnological production of vitamins. Food Technol Biotechnol 44: 381-396.

Torrissen OJ, Hardy RW, Shearer KD (1989). Pigmentation of salmonids: Carotenoid deposition and metabolism. Aquat Sci 1: 209-225.

Torrissen OJ (1995). Strategies for salmonid pigmentation. J Appl Ichthyol 11: 276–281.

Torrissen OJ (1989). Pigmentation of salmonids: interaction of astaxanthin and cantaxanthin on pigment deposition in rainbow trout. Aquaculture 79: 363-374.

Torrissen KR, Torrissen OJ (1985). Protease activities and carotenoid levels during the sexual maturation of Atlantic salmon (*Salmo salar*). Aquaculture 50: 113-122.

Torrissen KR (1984). Characterization of proteases in the digestive tract of Atlantic salmon (*Salmo salar*). in comparison with rainbow trout (*Salmo gairdneri*). Comp Biochem Physiol 77B: 669-674.

Torzillo G, Pushparaj B, Masojidek J *et al.* (2003). Biological constraints in algal biotechnology. Biotechnol Bioprocess Eng 8: 338-348.

Travieso L, Hall DO, Rao KK *et al.* (2001). A helical tubular photobioreactor producing *Spirulina* in a semicontinuous mode. Int Biodeterior Biodegradation 47: 151-155.

Tredici MR (2004). Mass production of microalgae: photobioreactors. In: Richmond A (ed) Handbook of Microalgal Culture: Biotechnology and Applied Phycology. Oxford: Blackwell Science pp. 178-214.

Tsukahara K, Sawayama S (2005). Liquid fuel production using microalgae. J Jpn Petrol Inst 48: 251-259.

Trinadha B, Prabhakara R, Madhavi R (2003). Potential benefits of algae in shrimp disease management. Fishing Chimes 23 (1).

Um, B.H., Kim, Y.S. (2009). Review: A chance for Korea to advance algal-biodiesel technology. J Ind Eng Chem 15: 1-7.

Valencia I, Ansorena D, Astiasaran I (2007). Development of dry fermented sausages rich in docosahexaenoic acid with oil from the microalgae *Schizochytrium* sp.: Influence on nutritional properties, sensorial quality and oxidation stability. Food Chem 104: 1087-1096.

Vassallo-Agius R, Imaizumi H, Watanabe T *et al.* (2001). The influence of astaxanthin supplemented dry pellets on spawning of striped jack. Fisheries Sci 67: 260-270.

Venkataraman LV (1980). Algae as food/feed: A critical appraisal based on Indian experience. In: Seshadri CV,Thomas S, Jeegibai N (ed) Proceedings National Workshop on Algal Systems. Indian Society of Biotechnology: New Delhi pp. 83-134.

Verakunpiriya V, Watanabe K, Mushiake K (1997). Effect of krill meal supplementation in soft dry pellets on spawning and quality of egg of yellowtail. Fisheries Sci 63: 433-439.

Vunjak-Novakovic G, Kim Y, Wu X *et al.* (2005). Air-lift bioreactors for algal growth on flue gas: mathematical modelling and pilot-plant studies. Ind Eng Chem Res 44: 6154-6163.

Wang JK (2003). Conceptual design of a microalgae based recirculating oyster and shrimp system. Aquacult Eng 28: 37-46.

Wen ZY, Chen F (2003). Heterotrophic production of eicosapentaenoic acid by microalgae. Biotechnol Adv 21: 273-294.

White DA, Ornsrud R, Davies SJ (2003). Determination of carotenoid and vitamin A concentrations in everted salmonids intestine following exposure to solutions of carotenoid *in vitro*. Comp Biochem Physiol 136: 683-692.

Wilkie AC, Mulbry WW (2002). Recovery of dairy manure nutrients by benthic freshwater algae. Bioresour Technol 84: 81-91.

Williams PJ, le B, Laurens LML (2010). Microalgae as biodiesel and biomass feedstocks: Review and analysis of the biochemistry, energetics, and economics. Energy Environ Sci 3: 554-590.

Yamaguchi K (1997). Recent advances in micro algal bioscience in Japan, with special reference to utilization of biomass and metabolites: A review. J Appl Phycol 8: 227-223.

Zatkova I, Sergejevova M, Urban J *et al.* (2010). Carotenoid-enriched microalgal biomass as feed supplement for freshwater ornamentals: albinic form of wels catfish (*Silurus glanis*). Aquacult Nutr 17: 278–286.

Zitelli GC, Rodolfi L, Biondi N (2006). Productivity and photosynthetic efficiency of outdoor cultures of *Tetraselmis suecica* in annular columns. Aquaculture 261: 932-943.

2014, Advances in Biochemistry and Biotechnology Volume 2   *Pages 57-66*
Edited by: Dr. Biplab Sarkar and Dr. Chiranjib Chakraborty
Published by: DAYA PUBLISHING HOUSE

4

Pattern Recognition Receptors and Innate Immunity

*Mrinal Samanta**

*Fish Health Management Division, Central Institute of Freshwater Aquaculture,
Kausalyaganga, Bhubaneswar – 751 002, Orissa*

ABSTRACT

The innate immune response is the first line of defense against invading pathogens and is the most universal, rapidly acting, and by some appraisals, the most important type of immunity. It exists in plants and animals, well conserved from invertebrates to higher mammals and mostly relies on germline-encoded pattern recognition receptors (PRRs) that recognize conserved components of microorganisms called microbes/pathogen-associated molecular patterns (PAMPs or MAMPs) (Akira, 2009). Among these, the key PRRs are toll-like receptors (TLRs), nucleotide binding and oligomerization domain (NOD) receptors, retinoic acid inducible gene-I (RIG-I) receptors and melanoma differentiation associated gene-5 (MDA5). These PRRs recognize PAMPs and trigger the activation of overlapping signaling cascades involving protein-protein interactions and phosphorylations. These culminate in activation of transcription proteins that control the expression of a vast array of antimicrobial effector molecules like inflammatory cytokines,

* *Corresponding author.* E-mail: msamanta1969@yahoo.com

interferons, chemokines, reactive nitrogen and oxygen radicals and antimicrobial peptides that attack microorganisms at many different levels and provide protection to host against a diverse range of pathogens or their products. The innate immune system appeared early in evolution, and the basic mechanisms of pathogen recognition and protection against diseases are much conserved throughout the animal kingdom.

Keywords: PAMPS, TLR, NOD, RIG-I, MDA5, Innate immunity.

Innate Immunity

We encounter an astronomical number of pathogens daily yet in most cases we are able to avoid infections and survive. How is this possible? It is possible because organisms are able to discriminate between self and non-self, enabling them to detect, defend and protect against invading pathogens, which are recognized as non-self. Host immune system discriminates between self and non-self by its two arms: innate immunity and acquired immunity and triggers immune responses against invading pathogens (non-self) to eliminate them. Between these two arms of immunity, innate immunity is regarded as antigen-nonspecific first line of defense mechanisms that a host uses immediately or within several hours of infection and is regarded as the primeval and hence the universal form of host defense (Beutler, 2004). It exists in plants as well as in animals (vertebrates and invertebrates) and initiates immediate defense mechanisms on the basis of non-clonal recognition of microbial components. While higher vertebrates like birds and mammals show presence of higher level of immune defense mechanism like adaptive immunity, which is a slower process, insects and other lower vertebrates like fish and amphibian predominantly depend upon innate immune system, a more faster one but less specific than adaptive immunity (Mushegian *et al.*, 2001). Innate immune system recognizes pathogens or conserved pathogen derived structures like flagellin, lipopolysaccharides (LPS), lipoproteins, peptidoglycan (PGN), lipoteichoic acid (LTA), zymosan, heat shock protein (hsp), CpG-DNA and nucleic acids (DNA or RNA) of the micro-organisms (pathogen- associated molecular patterns, PAMPs or microbes associated molecular patterns, MAMPs) by germ-line-encoded pattern recognition receptors (PRRs) that are distributed in cell surface, in intracellular compartments, or secreted into the blood stream and tissue fluids (Akira *et al.*, 2006). Three major classes of PRRs have been identified: Toll-like receptors (TLRs) that recognize ligand on either the extracellular surface or within the endosome, NOD receptors that function as cytoplasmic sensors and Rig-I-like receptors (RLRs): retinoic acid inducible gene-I (RIG-I), melanoma differentiation-associated gene-5 (MDA-5) that recognize viruses (Opitz *et al.*, 2009).

Toll like Receptors

The story of toll-like receptor (TLR) started in 1985, when proteins inducing dorsal- ventral polarity in fruit fly (*Drosophila melanogaster*) embryos were discovered by Christiane Nusslein-Volhard *et al.*, and was termed as "Toll" means "weird" in German. Flies lacking "Toll" develop in weird away and thus the term "Toll" was coined. Christiane Nusslein-Volhard and her collaborators later rewarded with the Nobel Prize for their cutting edge discovery of "Toll" signaling pathway and other components of Drosophila embryogenesis (The story Toll'd 2010). It was the late Charles Janeway who first hypothesized that there might be a family of pattern-recognition receptors (PRRs) that are expressed by cells of the innate immune system that are capable of recognizing specific pathogen-associated molecular patterns (PAMPs) to initiate antimicrobial immune responses. The extraordinary insight and accuracy of Janeway's predictions was later validated with the identification of the human toll-like receptor (TLR) and RIG-like helicase (RLH) families. The first family of molecules which fit Janeway's PRR model was the TLRs. Toll-like receptors (TLRs) are a family of PRR that are evolutionarily conserved from the worm *Caenorhabditis elegans* to mammals and sense a diverse range of PAMPs to initiate a well coordinated immune response to limit or eradicate invading microbes (Akira and Takeda, 2004). TLRs vary in their types and at present, 13 TLR types are known in mammals and 17 in lower vertebrates.

Structure of TLR

TLRs are type-I integral membrane glycoproteins characterized by the extracellular domains containing varying number of scattered leucine-rich repeat (LRR) motifs involved in recognition of PAMPs, a trans-membrane domain, and a cytoplasmic signal transducing domain known as Toll/IL-1 receptor (TIR) domain. While the LRR domains specifically recognize and discriminate between a broad spectrum of PAMPs, the intracellular TIR domain interact with downstream signaling molecules, activating overlapping but distinct signal pathways and ultimately resulting in different biological effects. The extracellular, N-terminal ligand recognizing ectodomains of TLRs consists of a variable number of leucine-rich repeats (LRR), bent into a horseshoe-shaped solenoid and a 60 amino acids domain rich in cysteines (Bell *et al.*, 2003). The LRR domains are composed of 19-25 tandem LRR motifs (LXXLXLXXNXL; L = leucine/isoleucine/valine/phenylalanine; N = asparagine/threonine/serine/cysteine; X = any amino acids), each of which is 24-29 amino acids in length. LRR motifs are sandwiched between the LRRNT (cysteine rich cluster at N-terminal end) and LRRCT (cysteine rich cluster at C-terminal end). Each LRR consists of a β-strand and α-helix connected by loops (Kobe *et al.*, 2001). Transmembrane domain exists in between the extracellular and intracellular domain. The C-terminal intracellular globular cytoplasmic signaling domain is homologous to that of interleukin-1 receptor (IL-1R), termed as Toll/IL-1R homology (TIR) domain. The TIR domain contains ~200 amino acids that include three conserved domains: boxes1-3 and are essential in signal transduction (Gay *et al.*, 2006).

TLR Types and their Localization in Cells

TLRs are classified into various types depending upon their primary sequence and types of ligands (PAMPs) recognition. In mammals, 13 members (TLR1-13) of the TLR family are known, 10 of which are present in humans. In lower vertebrates like fish, 17 TLRs (TLR1-5, TLR5S, TLR7-9, TLR13-14, and TLR18-23) have been identified in more than a dozen of teleost species (Aoki *et al.*, 2008; Basu *et al.*, 2012; Samanta *et al.*, 2012). TLRs are mostly expressed on various immune cells, including macrophages, dendritic cells (DCs), neutrophils, B-cells, specific types of T-cells, and in non-immune cells such as fibroblast, epithelial cells and dermal endothelial cells. The localization of TLRs in the cell varied greatly among the TLR types and they are also classified into two subfamilies according to their cellular localization; TLR1, TLR2, TLR4, TLR5, TLR6 and TLR10 are expressed on the cell surface while TLR3, TLR7, TLR8 and TLR9 are found on intracellular compartments, such as endosomes and endoplasmic reticulum (Takeda *et al.*, 2005). The localization of TLRs is not static and may vary between cell types and physiological conditions.

TLR-Ligands

TLR1 mostly remain associated with TLR2, and therefore, they also recognize TLR2 ligands. Some of the TLR1 ligands are glycosylphosphatidylinositol (GPI)-anchored protein, lipoarabinomannan, Pam3CSK4, tryacylated lipopeptides. TLR2 recognizes lipoproteins of various pathogens, peptidoglycan(PGN) and lipoteichoic acid (LTA) from Gram-positive bacteria (Samanta *et al.*, 2012), lipoarabinomannan from mycobacteria, glycosylphosphatidylinositol of *Trypanosoma cruzi*, modulin from *Staphylococcus epidermis*, zymosan from fungi and glycolipids from *Treponema maltophilum*.TLR3 recognizes dsRNA, ssRNA and poly I:C ; TLR4: LPS, fusion protein, lipoteichoic acid, mannuronic acid polymers, heat shock proteins 60,70; TLR5: flagellin (Basu *et al.*, 2012) ; TLR6: diacetylated lipopeptides, LTA, modulin, zymosin; TLR7 :imidazoquinolines, ssRNA, GC-rich ssRNA oligonucleotides; TLR8: ssRNA, resiquimod; TLR9: unmethylated CpG oligodeoxynucleotides, viral/ bacterial genomic DNA; TLR11: uropathogenic bacteria, profilin. Ligands for TLR10, 12 and TLR13 are unknown.

TLR Signaling Pathway

TLR activation is a sequential process. Recognition of PAMPs by their respective TLRs trigger the activation of signaling cascades leading to the activation of genes involved in antimicrobial host defense. Once TLRs recognize their ligand by LRRs, usually they form homo/hetero dimer and undergo conformational changes at the C-terminal region of the ECD, this induces stability in TLR-TLR interaction resulting into conformational changes in the TLR transmembrane helices of the receptor dimer, and is critical in transmitting the signal from the cell surface to the cytoplasm and interaction with downstream adaptor molecules utilizing TIR domains. There are four well known adaptor molecules namely MyD88 (myeloid differentiation primary response protein 88), TIR-associated protein (TIRAP), TRIF/TICAM1, and TRIF related adaptor molecule (TRAM). Among all the adaptor protein, MyD88 is the key and crucial adaptor for all TLRs except TLR3. With the selective usage of MyD88 and TRIF adaptor protein, TLR signaling pathway is broadly divided into MyD88-dependent and MyD88-independent (TRIF-dependent) pathways leading to the production of pro-inflammatory cytokines and type-I interferon (IFN) respectively (Akira *et al.*, 2006; Zhang *et al.*, 2010). TRIF is the only adapter used by TLR3. TLR that activates signal through MyD88-dependent as well as independent pathway is TLR4. In MyD88 independent pathway, TLR4 uses TRIF coupled to TRAM, and in MyD88-dependent pathway, it uses TIRAP. In MyD88-dependent signaling pathway, TIRAP is essential for TLR1, 2, 6 but non for TLR5, 7, and TLR9. In addition to these adaptor molecules, some accessory molecules like CD14, CD36, RP105, MD-1, MD-2, gp96, LL37, PRAT4A, HMGB1 and Unc93B etc. are required for microbial recognition, signaling and modulation of TLR responses.

In MyD88-dependent signaling, a MyD88 TIR domain binds TLR TIR alone or with TIRAP and recruits members of the IRAK (interleukin-1 receptor-associated kinase) family, notably IRAK4, which once activated phosphorylates IRAK1 and activates it. Activated IRAK1 then binds to TRAF domain of TRAF6 (TNF receptor associated factor 6), which acts as an ubiquitin protein ligase (E3). The association of IRAK4/IRAK1/TRAF6 induces conformational changes and this complex disengages itself from the receptor complex. IRAK1/TRAF6 complex are then transferred to a preformed membrane complex consisting of TAK1 (TGF-β-activated kinase-1) and TAK1 binding proteins, TAB1, TAB2/3. Formation of IRAK1/TRAF6/TAK/TAB complex engages itself to phosphorylation by a local kinase. TRAF6/TAK/TAB complex then dissociates from IRAK1 and translocate to cytosol to form another complex with E2 ligases consisting of Ubc13 and Uev1A. Subsequently, TRAF6 along with E2 catalyzes the synthesis of lysine 63-linked polyubiquitin chains on TRAF6 itself and on IKK-γ/NF-κB (nuclear factor κB) essential modulator (NEMO). The next step is the autophosphorylation of TAK1 which induces IKKα and β and thus activate IKK complex (IKKα, β and γ). This activation leads to the phosphorylation of IκB and MAP (mitogen-activated protein) kinase. Phosphorylation of IκB results in degradation of IκB, enabling the release and translocation of NF-κB from the cytoplasm to nucleus and thus induces the expression of inflammatory cytokines. Activation of MAP kinase cascades leads

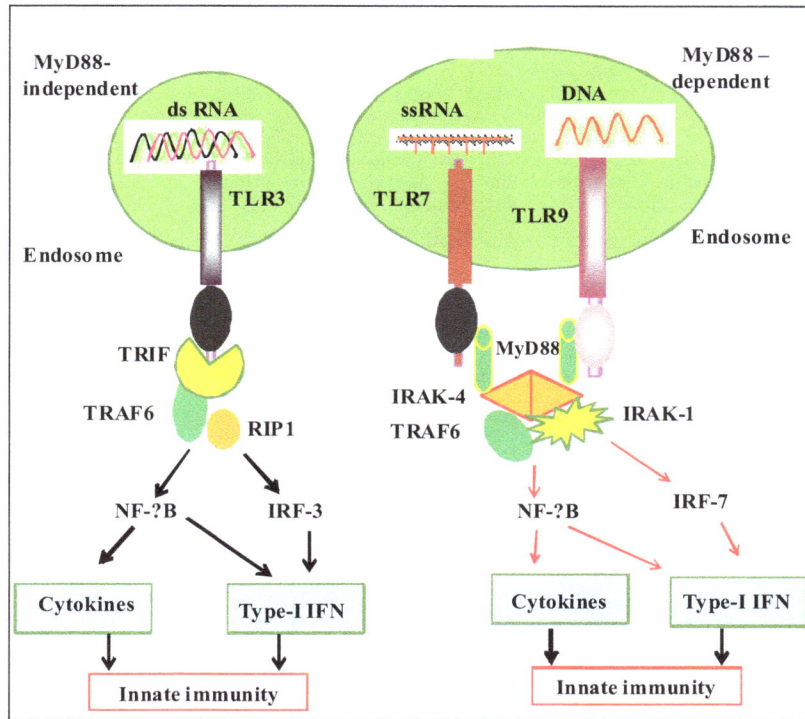

Figure 4.1:T LR Signaling Pathway.

to the activation of AP-1, which is also crucial for the induction of immune and inflammatory cytokines (Akira *et al.,* 2004; Akira *et al.,* 2006).

MyD88-independent and TRIF-dependent pathway occurs in TLR3. Ligand binding to TLR3 results in TRIF recruitment at TLR TIR domain. In one hand, TRIF interacts with RIP1 (receptor-interacting protein1) and activates NF-κB to induce pro-inflammatory cytokines. On the other hand, TRIF activates TANK (TRAF-family member associated NF-κB activator) binding kinase-1 (TBK1 also known as NAK or T2K) through TRAF3. TBK1 activation leads to phosphorylation of IRF3 and IRF7 enabling the formation of their homodimer, translocation into the nucleus and binding to the respective motifs on the DNA to induce the expression of type-I IFNs.

TLR as Therapeutic Targets

TLRs are implicated as novel therapeutic targets and an increasing numbers of immunotherapeutic approaches have been developed based on both activation and inhibition of TLR signaling. TLR agonists as vaccine adjuvants are immensely promising (Zhu *et al.,* 2010). Some TLR agonists have been approved as drug and numerous TLR agonists are under different phase of clinical trials (Gomariz *et al.,* 2010). Approved drugs include TLR4 agonists: fendrix in HPV vaccine; TLR7 agonists: aldara (imidazoquinoline) in actinic keratosis, HPV warts, melanoma and basal cell carcinoma. Drugs under phase III trial include TLR4 agonists: stimuvax in lung cancer, eritoran in septic shock; TLR9 agonists: MAGE-A3 and Vaximmune in lung cancer (Imgenex, 2010).

Nucleotide Binding and Oligomerization Domain (NOD) Receptor

NOD receptors are one of the members in the intracellular PRR family and are implicated in the recognition of bacterial components in the cytoplasm and are structurally related to the nucleotide

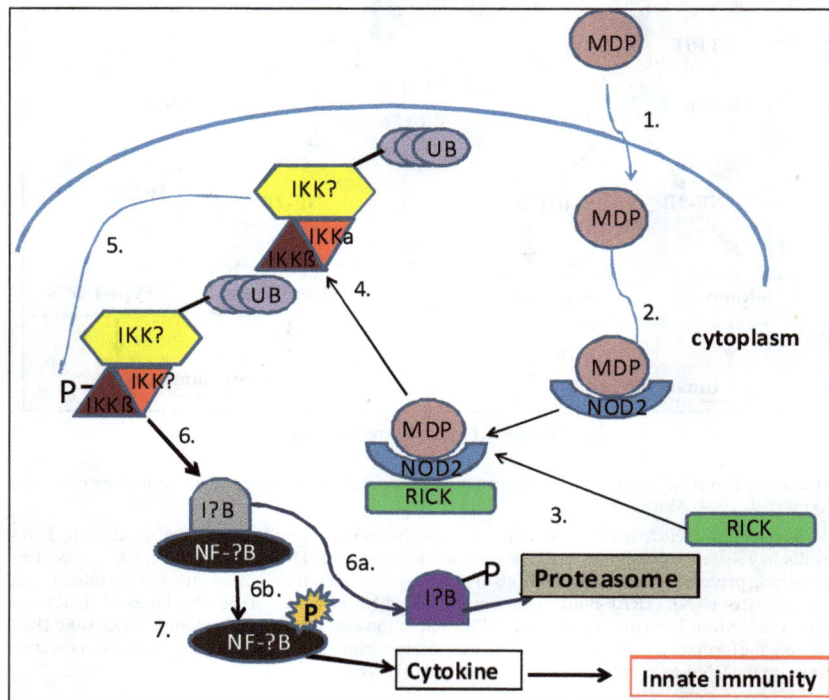

Figure 4.2: NOD2-Signaling Pathway.

binding site (NBS)-leucine-rich repeats (LRR) proteins class of plant R gene products that mediate disease resistance against pathogens in plants (Proell *et al.*, 2008).

Structure and Classification

This family of receptors is characterized with presence of three domains. At C-terminal, a leucin-rich repeat (LRR) domain, at the center a nucleotide oligomerization (NACHT) domain, and a protein-protein interaction domain at the N-terminal end (Rafika *et al.*, 2004). The C-terminal LRR domain recognizes specific ligand to which the NLR is to be associated, the NACHT domain mediates self-regulation and oligomerization and the N-terminal domain generates downstream signals (Fritz *et al.*, 2006). Based on various N-terminal domains, like pyrin domain (PYD), caspase recruitment domain (CARD) or baculovirus inhibitor of apoptosis repeat domain (BIR), NLR is subdivided into three classes *viz.*, NALP (NACHT, LRR and PYD containing proteins), NOD (NACHT, LRR and CARD containing proteins) and NAIP (for neuronal apoptosis inhibitor protein). NOD sub-family consists of five members NOD1, NOD2, NOD3, NOD4 and NOD5 (Ting *et al.*, 2008). Among the large number of NOD family members NOD1 and NOD2 are well characterized. NOD-2 differs from NOD-1 having two amino terminal caspase recruitment domains (CARD1 and CARD2) that trigger down-stream signaling (Wilmanski *et al.*, 2008).

NOD-Ligands

NOD1 (CARD4 :caspase-activating and recruitment domain-4) recognizes peptidoglycan containing the muramyl dipeptide NAG-NAM- γ-D-glutamyl-meso-diaminopimelic acid, part of the peptidoglycan monomer in common gram-negative bacteria and just a few gram-positive bacteria, but NOD-2 detects muramyl dipeptide (MurNAc-L-Ala-D-iso Gln) found in both Gram positive and negative bacterial peptidoglycan (Chen *et al.*, 2009).

NOD-Signaling

Prior to the activation by ligand, NOD protein remains in an inactive form due to folding of LRR region and it's binding to NACHT, and on the arrival of ligand the LRR region unfolds and mediates signal transduction. Following ligand binding, oligomerization of the NACHT domains initiates the recruitment of interacting proteins, the RIP2 or RICK (receptor interacting serine-threonine protein kinase-2) via CARD-CARD-interaction. Recruitment of RICK causes activation of I$\kappa\kappa$ complex and stimulates NF-κB activation by ubiquitinylation of I$\kappa\kappa$-γ subunit of I$\kappa\kappa$ complex. NOD signaling also activates MAPK (mitogen-activated protein kinase) pathway that results in activation of specific transcription factors like AP-1, and induces the expression of pro-inflammatory cytokines and chemokines like IL-1β, IL-6, IL-8, TNF and IFN-γ (Athman *et al.*, 2004 ; Sabbah *et al.*, 2009; Monie *et al.*, 2009).

RIG-I and MDA5

Retinoic acid-inducible gene-I (RIG-I, also known as DDX58) and MDA5 (melanoma-differentiation-associated gene 5, also known as Ifih1 or Helicard) are virus sensors (dsRNA), and are expressed ubiquitously in the cytoplasm. RIG-I and MDA5 contain two caspase-recruitment domains (CARDs) at N-terminal and a DExD/H-box helicase domain at C-terminal and share ~25 per cent homology within the CARD domain regions and 40 per cent within the helicase domains. The helicase domain binds dsRNA (including short RNAs, ~25-bp) and 52-ppp RNA and the CARD domains relay the down-stream signal (Barral *et al.*, 2009).

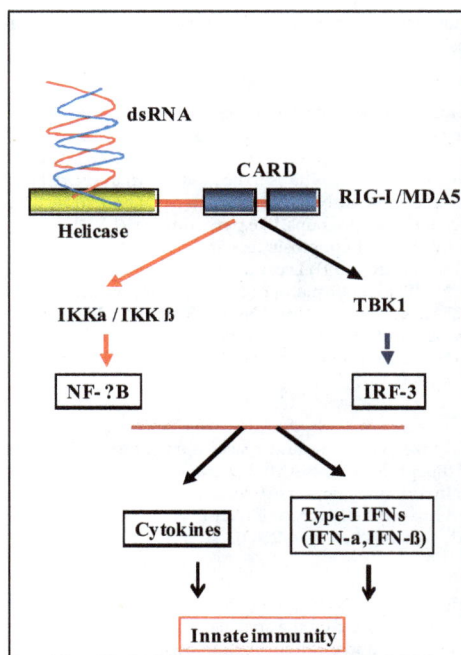

Figure 4.3: RIG-1 and MDA5 Signaling Pathway.

RIG-I localizes to membrane ruffles in non-polarized epithelial cells where it associates with the F-actin cytoskeleton and the actin depolymerization results in cellular migration of RIG-I. It is also localized in the apical junction complexes in polarized epithelial and endothelial cells.

MDA-5 remains localized in the cytoplasm and do not associate with F-actin.

Signaling Pathway

In the absence of its ligand, RIG-I remain in an inactivated form and upon binding of ligands (dsRNA or 52-ppp RNA) to the helicase domain it recruits a CARD-containing adaptor, IPS-1 (also known as MAVS, VISA or Cardif). MDA5 recognizes short sequence of RNA through its helicase domain and also recruits IPS-1. In this way both RIG-I and MDA5 signaling converge at IPS-1. Then IPS-1 relays the signal to the kinases TBK1 and IKK-i, which phosphorylate interferon-regulatory factor-3 (IRF-3) and IRF-7 and upon phosphorylation, IRF3 and IRF7 translocate to nucleus and bind to the respective nuclear motifs to induce the expression of cytokine and type-I IFNs (IFN-α and β) (Kato *et al.*, 2006; Samanta *et al.*, 2006).

Conclusion

The innate immune system is primeval and diverse. It rapidly detects invading pathogens as non-self, and eliminates them by expressing a battery of antimicrobial peptides. Pattern recognition receptors (PRR) which are germ line encoded are the key components of innate immune system. Three major classes of PRRs: TLR, NLR and RIG-I/MDA5 play essentially very important role in host defense. A wide variety of bacterial pathogens are being detected and defended by several members of the TLR and NOD-like receptors (NLRs) family. They are the first to detect the bacterial infections and to induce innate immunity by activating respective signaling cascades that results into the expression of several inflammatory cytokines and protection of host against diseases.

Two signaling pathways activate the host innate immunity against viral infection. One of the pathways utilizes members of the Toll-like receptor (TLR) family to detect viruses that enter the endosome through endocytosis. The other antiviral pathway is RNA helicase RIG-I or MDA5 signaling. RIG-I or MDA5 acts as the receptor of intracellular viral double-stranded RNA, the genetic components of some viruses or is produced as replicative intermediate during virus multiplication. Both TLR and RIG-I/MDA5 signaling triggers the expression of several innate immune cytokines and type I interferon (IFN) that inactivate the virus and protect the host against diseases.

References

Akira S, Takeda K (2004). Toll-like receptor signaling. Nat Rev Immunol 4: 499-511.

Akira S (2009). Pathogen recognition by innate immunity and its signaling. Proc Jpn Acad Ser 85: 143-156.

Akira S, Uematsu S, Takeuchi O (2006). Pathogen recognition and innate immunity. Cell 124: 783–801.

Barral PM, Sarkar D, Zao-zhong S et al. (2009). Functions of the cytoplasmic RNA sensors RIG-I and MDA-5: Key regulators of innate immunity. Pharmacol and Therap 124: 219–234.

Beckmann BU, Heine H, Wiesmuller KH et al. (2006). TLR1- and TLR6-independent recognition of bacterial lipopeptides. J Biol Chem 281: 9049–9057.

Bell JK, Mullen GE, Leifer CA et al. (2003). Leucine-rich repeats and pathogen recognition in Toll-like receptors. Trends Immunol 24: 528–533.

Beutler B (2004). Innate immunity: an overview. Curr Opin Microbiol 7: 25–32.

J Zhu, Mohan C (2010). Toll-Like Receptor Signaling Pathways-Therapeutic Opportunities. Mediators Inflamm. doi: 10.1155/2010/781235.

McDonald C, Inohara N, Nunez G (2005). Peptidoglycan Signaling in Innate Immunity and Inflammatory Disease. J Biol Chem 280: 20177-20180.

Mushegian A, Medzhitov R (2001). Evolutionary perspective on innate immune recognition. Mol Immunol 40: 845–859.

Opitz B, Eitel J, Meixenberger K et al. (2009). Roll of Toll-like receptors, NOD-like receptors and RIG-like receptors in endothelial cells and systemic infections. J Thromb Haemost 102: 1103-1109.

Rafika A, Philpott D (2004). Innate immunity via Toll-like receptors and Nod proteins. Curr Opin Microbiol 7: 25-32.

Sabbah A, Chang TH, Harnack R et al. (2009). Activation of innate immune antiviral responses by Nod2. Nature Immunol 10: 1073-1080.

Toll-like receptors, IMgenex and Innate Immunity: The story Toll'd (2010).

Voss E, Wehkamp J, Wehkamp K *et al*. (2006). NOD2/CARD 15 Mediates Induction of the Antimicrobial Peptide Human Beta-defensin-2. J Biol Chem 281: 2005-2011.

Wilmanski JM, Ocwieja TP, Kobayashi KS (2008). NLR proteins: integral members of innate immunity and mediators of inflammatory diseases. J Leukoc Biol 83: 13–30.

Zhang AN, Cheng Q, XueTao CAO (2010). Regulation of Toll-like receptor signaling in theinnate immunity. Sci China Life Sci 53: 34–43.

2014, Advances in Biochemistry and Biotechnology Volume 2
Edited by: Dr. Biplab Sarkar and Dr. Chiranjib Chakraborty
Published by: DAYA PUBLISHING HOUSE

Pages 67-79

5

Deciphering Nanotoxicity on Zebrafish Model

Indarchand Gupta[1]*, Mahendra Rai[1] and Biplab Sarkar[2]
[1]*Department of Biotechnology, SGB Amravati University, Amravati – 444 602, Maharashtra, India*
[2]*KIIT School of Biotechnology, KIIT University, Patia, Bhubaneswar – 751 024, Orissa, India*

ABSTRACT

Nanotechnology deals with the construction of new materials, devices, and different technological systems. It holds promise for several biomedical and life science applications. As a consequence of their use these nanomaterials are released into the environment intentionally or unintentionally. Therefore, nanotoxicology has become the subject of concern in nanotechnology as it is necessary to determine the hazardous effects of those nanomaterials on the environment, particularly the aquatic environment. To understand the potential toxicological impacts of nanoparticulates released to aquatic environments, the zebrafish is the best model organism.

The present chapter outlines the toxic effect of nanoparticles on zebrafish highlighting different reports and evaluating the potential eco-toxicity of manufactured nanomaterials.

* *Corresponding author.* E-mail: indarchandgupta@gmail.com

Introduction

Nanotechnology has appeared as new zone in science and engineering, leading to the advanced structures, devices and systems that have new functional properties with size ranging between 1 and 100 nm (Roco, 1999). In the last few years, nanolevel substances with dimensions became unique. Owing to exclusive physical, chemical, electrical, optical, thermal, biological and magnetic properties, nanomaterials have great potential for industrial development.There has been a spectacular increase in the use of nanoparticles (NPs) in research in food packaging, medical devices, pharmaceuticals, cosmetics, odor-resistant textiles and household appliances. As a result the environment is exposed to particles of variable origin in the air, water and soil. The overuse of these nanoparticles has raised many questions such as: what is the potential toxicity of such materials after their release from these sources? (Lewinski *et al.,* 2008 and Meng *et al.,* 2009), what happens at the end-of-life stage of these products? When they gets disposed or recycled? Therefore, there is great demand to find the toxic potential of nanomaterials in order to ease public concern and to contribute regulators in defining environmental and health risks of engineered nanomaterials (Hoet *et al.,* 2004, Guzman *et al.,* 2006 and Hurt *et al.,* 2006). This is an area of nanotechnology where risk associated with the use of nanomaterials remains mainly unexplored. Thus the field of nanotoxicology was born which now become critical segment in safety assessments of nanomaterials in foods, drugs, medical devices, cosmetics etc.

Although various applications of different nanoparticles (NPs) are rising in industry and consumer products, there are still little knowledge about their potential toxicity. For such a purpose there is also an utmost need for low-cost, high-throughput animal models in some fields of biomedical research such as drug screening and toxicity assessment of various materials (Lieschke and Currie,2007; Bull and Levin 2000).Thus regarding nanomaterials, it is quite easy and cheap method to screen initially the nanotoxicity by utilizing the *in vitro* cell culture. But on the other hand it not possible to replicate the *in vitro* results in *in vivo* condition. Therefore small animal models are commonly used to evaluate the possible risk associated with them. To address such issues the fishes like Zebrafish (*Danio rerio*), fathead minnow, rainbow trout (*Oncorhynchus mykiss*) etc are routinely used for the study. Now Zebrafish is firmly accepted as a general research model for many areas of biology and medicine (Lieschke and Currie,2007, Hsu *et al.,* 2007; Chakraborty *et al.,* 2009). It is mainly valuable during the earlier stages of research as it is a better model organism to reveal efficacy and toxicity of new treatment prior to use of costlier mammalian models. To meet these challenge Zebrafish model is being employed worldwide to determine nanomaterial toxicity.In the present chapter, we describe the toxic effects of various types of nanomaterials causing either deformities or death of adult and embryonic zebrafish. The chapter also highlights different reports comparing effect of the nanoparticle versus ion on zebrafish.

Ideal Aquatic Model: Zebrafish

Zebrafish are a small (about 3cm in length) cyprinids which are native to the Indian subcontinent. They were firstly described by Hamilton (1822) during his survey of fishes of the river Ganga. Its domestication began a century ago and later gained popularity in the 1930s as a valuable experimental and tachin organism (Creaser, 1934). Subsequently it was then widely accepted for vertebrate research in developmental genetics, toxicological and environmental monitoring, cancer, aging, behavioural and disease studies (Kishi 2004; Trede *et al.,* 2004; Parng 2005; Wright *et al.,* 2006; Beckman 2007; Scholz and Mayer 2008; Hsu *et al.,* 2007; Chakraborty *et al.,* 2009; Chakraborty and Agoramoorthy, 2010; Chakraborty *et al.,* 2011).

The use of Zebrafish as a model is advantageous over other aquatic organism. Their embryo is permeable to small molecules and their transparent chorion facilitates the easy observation of development. Lee *et al.* (2007) studied the effect of silver nanoparticles on early embryonic development in zebrafish. For this study they made use of highly purified and stable silver nanoparticles. Their study revealed that a single silver nanoparticle get transported in and out of embryos through chorion-pore canals (CPC). Different silver nanoparticles were seen inside embryos at each developmental stage. Moreover, the genome organization, cellular and physiological processes appear to be highly conserved between zebrafish and humans having 40 to >80 per cent similarity, depending upon gene examined (Barbazuk *et al.*, 2000) and therefore zebrafish may be used for modeling of human diseases. Additionally, several cellular and molecular pathways involved in response to chemical or stress are conserved among zebrafish and the mammals (Voelker *et al.*, 2007).Also, some features of brain patterning, their structure, function, anatomical and physiological characteristics and genomic sequence are extensively homologous between zebrafish and other vertebrates including humans (Guo, 2004; Tropepe, 2003; Veldman and Lin, 2008; Postlethwait *et al.*, 2000). Neuronal plate formation in zebrafish embryo occurs at 10 hours, subsequently organogenesis occurs at 24 hours as compared to rat which takes 9.5 days and 5-6 days respectively. Similarly the first heartbeat occurs at 30 hours for the zebrafish and 10.2 days for rats. Furthermore, zebrafish embryos develop visible red blood cells by 24 hours post fertilization (hpf), organogenesis of major organs is completed in 5 days post fertilization (dpf) and complete immune system in 30days (Rubinstein, 2003). Certainly, zebrafish embryos might be an appropriate replacement for some of the adult fish toxicity tests, thus offering more technical advantages (Lammer *et al.*, 2009).

The Zebrafish embryo is also proposed as a link among *in vitro* assays and assays of biological validation in whole animals like rodents (Lieschke and Currie,2007). According to a study conducted by Parng *et al.* (2002) the toxicity of 18 toxic compounds in zebrafish was well correlated with response reported in the rodents. Therefore, zebrafish cannot replace rodent models but is similar to them, being mainly useful for fast, high-throughput and low-cost assays (Redfern *et al.*, 2008).

Adult zebrafish and zebrafish embryo are being utilised for determining acute toxicity of several compounds by determining LC50 (the concentration that is lethal to 50 per cent of the test fishes) value of test compounds. For this purpose a range of standard toxicity tests has been recommended by the International Standardization Organisation (ISO) (ISO, 1996), the U.S. Environmental Protection Agency (USEPA), the Organisation for Economic Cooperation and Development (OCED) (OCED, 1992), the American Society for Testing and Materials (ASTM). These recommendations have been established for toxicity testing on both adult zebrafish and zebrafish embryo (Braunbeck *et al.*, 2005). Therefore, hereafter we are discussing various researches reporting the toxicity of nanoparticles on zebrafish.

In vivo Aquatic Models for Nanotoxicity Testing

Zebrafish, a small aquatic vertebrate species, can be rapidly and successfully bred and easily maintained in laboratory. Size of the Zebrafish eggs ranges in 1.0–1.2 mm in diameter. Generally they are transparent and develop rapidly and synchronously, which facilitate direct optical examination of the toxic effects on their internal organs (Hallare *et al.*, 2006, Samson and Shenker, 2000). The developing fish embryo or larvae is usually believed to be the highly sensitive stage in the life cycle of a teleost which is specifically sensitive to low level environmental pollutant (Westernhagen, 1988). These embryos are use to be transparent. Additionally they offer an economically feasible, high-throughput screening platform for noninvasive real-time assessments of toxicity.

Nanotoxicity on Early Life Stages of Zebrafish

The embryonic stage of zebrafish has been utilized many times for assessing wide variety of chemical classes. In spite of additional challenges, the zebrafish embryo is being useful for determining toxic potential and potential mechanisms of action of different nanomaterials. One of those studied nanomaterial is fluorescent core-shell silica nanoparticle. In a study, uptake and toxicity of fluorescent core-shell silica nanoparticles (FSNP) was assessed in early life stages of zebrafish (Fent *et al.*, 2010). The finding suggests that Ru@SiO$_2$ nanoparticles with average size of 200 nm encapsulating [Ru(bpy)3](2+)Cl$_2$ dye and Cy5.5@SiO$_2$ with average size of 60 nm, at concentration between 0.0025 and 200mg/L, get accumulated on the chorion of embryo without their uptake and translocation in embryo. Furthermore, these nanoparticles didn't affected hatching time and hatching success with no mortality and deformities in the embryo, indicating the non embryotoxic nature of the said nanoparticles.

Cheng *et al.* (2007) examined the impact of single and double walled carbon nanotubes on Zebrafish embryo. They reported the delay in embryo hatching by both type of the nanotubes. In particular, the Double-walled CNTs (DWCNT) delayed hatching at a concentration greater than 240mg/L as compared to Single-walled CNTs (SWCNT) which delayed the hatching at concentration more than 120 mg/L. The delayed hatching was likely induced by the Co and Ni catalyst used during the production of SWCNT, suggesting that the raw materials associated with their synthesis have the potential to affect the aquatic life when released in aquatic environment.

Copper nanoparticles are also reported to have toxicity, especially in water and therefore assessment of their toxicity in the aquatic systems is very important. In this concern Bai *et al.* (2010a) studied the effect of copper nanoparticles suspension to zerbrafish embryos. Their study concluded that nano-Cu suspension retard the hatching of zebafish embryos and also caused morphological changes in larvae whereas at concentrated nano-Cu *i.e.* more than 0.1 mg/L killed the gastrula-stage zebrafish embryos. They have also performed similar experiment on zebrafish embryo by exposing then with Zinc Oxide (ZnO) nanoparticles.

This study revealed that nano-ZnO killed zebrafish embryos at 50 and 100mg/L and further retarded the embryo hatching at in concentration between 1-25mg/L. The embryo toxicity test revealed that nano-ZnO killed zebrafish embryos (50 and 100 mg/L), retarded the embryo hatching (1–25 mg/L), reduced the body length of larvae, and caused tail malformation after the 96 hpf exposure. Zn$_{(dis)}$ only partially contributed to the toxicity of nano-ZnO. This research highlights the need to further investigate the ecotoxicity of nano-ZnO in the water environment. Several recent studies has been summarized in Table 5.1.

To know the potential ecotoxicological impacts of metal oxide nanoparticles released in the aquatic environments, Zhu *et al.* (2008) assessed toxicities of aqueous suspensions of nanoscale zinc oxide (nZnO), titanium dioxide (nTiO$_2$) and alumina (nAl$_2$O$_3$) on the zebrafish embryo larvae. nZnO particles were found to be more toxic as compared to nAl$_2$O$_3$ aqueous suspensions. While in contrast nTiO$_2$ was not found to be toxic under same experimental conditions. Similarly, Asharani *et al.* (2008) also studied the toxicity of silver nanoparticles on zebrafish. In their study they found that silver nanoparticle causes the concentration dependent toxicity by obstructing the normal development resulting in abnormal body axes, twisted notochord, slow blood flow, pericardial edema and cardiac arrhythmia with increased apoptosis in zebrafish embryos.Likewise colloidal silver (cAg) and colloidal gold (cAu) nanoparticles also found to have size dependent toxicity at certain concentrations. The most important point is that the colloidal gold induces more toxic effects as compared to colloidal silver of equivalent sizes. This indicates that the nanoparticle chemistry defines their toxicity. Toxicity and types of abnormalities in the embryo were highly dose dependent. Later, similar results were obtained by Bar-Ilan *et al.* (2009). They also reported size-dependent mortality and malformations in zebrafish embryos exposed to silver nanoparticles.

Table 5.1: Different Report Showing Toxicity Evaluation of Various Nanoparticles on Zebrafish.

Nanoparticle	Embryo/Adult Zebrafish	Concentration	Result	References
C60, C60(OH)16–18	Embryo	C60 : 1.5 mg/mL C60(OH)16–18: 50mg/mL	C60(OH)16–18: no toxicity C60 : embryo and larval development delayed, Free radical-induced toxicity	Zhu (2007)
C60, C60(OH)16–18	Embryo	0-300 ppb	Mortality and the incidence of fin malformations and pericardial edema increased>200 ppb in dark. Light activated toxicity.	Usenko (2008)
AgNP, AuNP, PtNP	Embryo		Both Ag-NP and Pt-NP induced hatching delays, caused concentration dependant drop in heart rate, touch response and axis curvatures. Au-NP did not show any indication of toxicity.	Asharani *et al.*, 2011
AuNP	Adult Zebrafish	36–106 ng gold/fish/day	Dysfunctions at the sub cellular scale, Mitochondrial dysfunctions, modulation of expression of genes involved in DNA repair, detoxification processes, apoptosis, mitochondrial metabolism and oxidative stress,	Geffroy *et al.*, 2011
CuNP	Zebrafish embryo	0.01 and 0.05 mg/L>0.1 mg/L	Retarded hatching of zebrafish embryos, caused morphological malformation of the larvaekilled the gastrula-stage zebrafish embryos	Bai, *et al.*, 2010b
nZnObulk ZnO	Adult Zebrafish	3.969 mg L^{-1} 2.525 mg L^{-1}	Dissolved Zn^{2+}, from nZnO and bulk ZnO in suspensions, were toxic to zebrafish	Yu *et al.*, 2011
CdSe/ZnS quantum dots	Adult Zebrafish			Lewinski *et al.*, 2011 (QDs)
ZnO NP	Zebrafish embryo	50 and 100 mg/L 1–25 mg/L	Killed embryos Retarded the embryo hatching	Bai *et al.*, 2010b
ZnO NP	Zebrafish embryo	2 µg/mL	Interferes hatching	Xia *et al.*, 2011
TiO₂ NPs	Larval Zebrafish	0.1 to 10 mg/L	Affected fish locomotor parameters without causing mortality and deformity	Chen *et al.*, 2011
Ag NP	Liver of Adult Zebrafish		Oxidative stress and apoptosis	Choi *et al.*, 2010
TiO₂ NPs			Accumulation and distribution in gill, liver, heart, brain	Chen *et al.*, 2010
TiO₂ NPs	Zebrafish	0.1 mg/L	Impairs reproduction	Wang *et al.*, 2011

Nanotoxicity on Late Stages of Zebrafish

One of the most commercialized nanoparticles is TiO_2 nanoparticles, having vast industrial applications. Therefore risk associated with the use of this nanoparticle is also required to be assessed.

In an interesting study, Palaniappan and Pramod (2011a) attempted to compare effect of bulk and nano TiO_2 on Zebrafish brain by using FT-IR technique. Their reports are extremely opposite to Zhu *et al.* (2008), as mentioned in the previous section. They have analyzed the response of brain by measuring the differences in absorbance intensities between control and TiO_2 exposed tissue. The observations reflected alterations on major biochemical constituents such as proteins, lipids and nucleic acids in the zebrafish brain tissues. These biochemical changes could be due to the overproduction of ROS as a result of nano TiO_2 exposure Furthermore, the nano TiO_2 shown to be more toxic as compared to its bulk counterpart. Similar results were obtained by them while investigating the effect of nano and bulk TiO_2 on zebrafish by FT-Raman Spectroscopy, a useful tool for rapid assessment of nanoparticles interaction with living system (Palaniappan and Pramod, 2011b). Progress in different instrumentation are making Raman spectroscopy the tool of choice for an increasing number of (bio) chemical applications. This technique is greatly advantageous as it can provide the information on the concentration, structure and interaction of biochemical molecules in their microenvironments within intact cells and tissues without destructing them. The results of this study suggested that the microenvironment of zebrafish liver significantly altered due to nano TiO_2 as compared to bulk TiO_2. The basis of result is a shift to a higher wavenumber and an increase in the intensity of the band.

In another study Chae *et al.* (2009) suggested that the Ag-NPs led to cellular and DNA damage. Additionally carcinogenic and oxidative stresses, genes related with metal detoxification/metabolism regulation and radical scavenging action were also reported to induced. In contrast, the ionic silver lead to an induction of inflammatory response and metallic detoxification processes in the liver of the exposed fish, but caused a lower overall stress response as compared with the Ag-NPs. The toxic effects of silver nanoparticles on liver of adult zebrafish has been also studied by Choi *et al.* (2010). They reported the alterations like disruption of hepatic and apoptotic changes in silver nanoparticles exposed zebrafish. Further, the induction of DNA damage with reduction in mRNA levels of the enzyme catalase and glutathione reductase and upregulation of p-53 related propoapoptotic genes like Bax, Noxa and p21 were also reported.

Metallic nanoparticles like nickel are used in catalytic, sensing, and electronic applications, but health and environmental affects have not been fully investigated. As per earlier reports it is imperative that metal nanoparticles are toxic at certain concentration. In addition it is also important to determine whether nanoparticles of the same metal but of different size and shape affect toxicity. In this respect Ispas *et al.* (2009) studied the toxic effects of Nickel nanoparticles (Ni NPs) on zebrafish. The range of nanoparticles studied was 30 nm, 60 nm, 100nm and larger particle clusters of aggregated 60nm entities with a dendritic structure. As a result it has been reported that 30, 60 and 100nm Ni NPs are equally or less toxic as compared to soluble nickel salts. Each of these nanoparticle exposures initially resulted in thinning of intestinal epithelium while further exposure resulted in separation of skeletal muscle fiber. These results indicates that configuration of nanoparticles may affect toxicity more than size. This report also suggests that the defects from exposure by Ni NPs occur by different mechanism than soluble nickel.

Likewise nanocopper is acutely toxic to Zebrafish at the concentration of 1.5 mg/L. Like other nanoparticles the gill is found to be the primary target of nanocopper. Furthermore, the nanocopper is reported to give different morphological effects and different global gene expression patterns in the gill that the soluble copper (Griffitt *et al.*, 2007). This study clearly suggests that the effects of nanocopper on gill are independent of dissolved copper.

The systemic effects of zinc oxide nanoparticles and titanium dioxide nanoparticles on zebrafish shown the damage induced through oxidative stress. The oxidative stress affected mostly the liver as compared to guts (Xiong *et al.,* 2011). The higher damage in liver may be due to the well-known fact that liver is more active metabolically as compared to the other organs. In a different study Jovanovic *et al.* (2011) performed the gene microarray analysis of zebrafish embryos exposed by sublethal dose of engineered TiO_2 and hydroxylated fullerenes (C60 (OH) 24). This study firstly reported that these nanoparticles cause circadian rhythm gene regulation in aquatic animals, which signifies the potential for broad physiological and behavioral effects controlled by the circadian system.

In another study it has been reported that exposure to silver nanoparticles results into the impairment of neurodevelopment in zebrafish. Moreover, silver nanoparticles treated cells shown distinct effects in comparison to the Ag^+ ions alone. If the coating solely affected the dissolution of Ag+, then all the comparative effects would have been alike. By the same time, the bigger nanoparticles had superior effects than the smaller nanoparticles on most of the results. Studies with gold nanoparticles demonstrated that particles of the size ≤ 50 nm are actively get entry into cells, however smaller particles do not (Johnston *et al.,* 2010), therefore providing a probable explanation for the generally greater effects seen for the larger coated nanoparticles like PVP coated AgNP. The results differ according to the size and coating of silver nanoparticles where PVP- coated AgNPs showing the greater effect as compared to Citrate coated AgNPs (Powers *et al.,* 2011).

The research of Chen *et al.* (2010) revealed that TiO_2 NPs causes the adverse effects to zebrafish. The chronic toxicity of these nanoparticles is time and concentration dependent. As mentioned earlier these nanoparticles also accumulate and distributes in gill as well as liver, heart and brain. In addition to these findings, Chen *et al.* (2010) also the reported translocation of TiO_2 NPs among organs and passes through the blood-brain and the blood-heart barrier after prolonged exposure.

Nanoparticle against Ion Effects

Precise characterization of exposure circumstances and suitable dosimetry is an important concern for nanotoxicologists (Teeguarden *et al.,* 2007), predominantly in aquatic exposures. It is mostly reported that metallic nanoparticles when added to water have a tendency to aggregate to form larger particles or it can get dissolved to release soluble metal ions. Every one of these will change exposure conditions which signify that the real situations to which organisms are exposed may have little or no relation to the initial added dose. Growing use of metallic nanoparticles probably results in release of dissolved metal species into aqueous environments. It is however unclear if these materials are harmful to aquatic animals. Conversely, it is not clear that whether the nanoparticles itself or the ions released by them causes the hazard to aquatic organisms. The question is raised since some dissolution of metal particles will occur and thus it is important to differentiate effects of nanoparticles from dissolved metals.

By various researches across the globe it has been already demonstrated that metallic nanoparticles produce toxicity in aquatic organisms largely due to effects of particles as opposed to release of dissolved ions. For example both copper and silver nanoparticles after exposing to zebrafish found to increase metal content associated with gill tissue of the fish. Here silver concentrations were found to be much higher suggesting that intact silver nanoparticles are associated with the gill. Copper nanoparticles increased mean gill filament width by three to four times while nanosilver did not altered gill filament width. These different responses amongst the exposures points shows that every particle is having a discrete biological effect that does seems to be driven exclusively by the released soluble metal ions into the water column. Based on these results, care should be taken when inferring toxicity of nanomaterials from data on a different material (Griffitt *et al.*, 2008).

Later, Griffitt *et al.* (2009) examined the interplay of nanoparticle composition and dissolution on response of the zebrafish gill following exposure to toxic nanometals like nanocopper, nanosilver and nontoxic (nano-TiO_2) nanometals. The exposure resulted in the association of intact silver nanoparticles with zebrafish gill. It indicates that each of these nanoparticles induces the distinct biological response, which is not solely driven by release of soluble metal ions into the water column.

According to Griffitt *et al.* (2009) it is apparent that there is development of relatively insoluble metal oxide/hydroxide layers on the surface of the particles after suspension in water that confines consequent dissolution. After release, some metal ions gets complexed by organic matter in water followed by their removal from the water. This complex formation thus reduces the release of the soluble ions back into the water and decreases the effect of dissolution in nanotoxicity to aquatic organisms. This study therefore highlights need of understanding the mechanisms of nanoparticle toxicity in aquatic organisms as dissolution and the presence of nanoparticle alone.

Conclusion

With the fast development of nanotechnology and its applications, a broad array of nanostructured materials are now available with various applications in pharmaceutics, cosmetics, biomedical products and industries. It is well known fact that nanomaterials have novel and unique physicochemical properties as compared to their bulk counterparts. Thus the importance of nanoparticles has grown rapidly. It is therefore crucial to obtain upto-date information about the likely risk associated with their use as they also have hazardous impact on the human health and environment. Therefore it is always a question of concern that what happens with nanomaterials when they enter and interact with an organism. This scientific curiosity is drawing a great attention towards concern for the human and environment.

In the last decade, different technologies have been increasingly used in fish biology research to investigate the physiology, development biology and the impact of contaminants in fish model organisms, such as zebrafish (*Danio rerio*), with some commercially available species produced in aquaculture. The biological impact of engineered nanoparticles released into the aquatic environment is a major concern. However, the lack of previous genetic information on most fish species has been a major drawback for getting the complete detailed knowledge about the risk associated with the different kinds of nanoparticles. Also, the toxic effects of nanoparticles on the organism with unique physiological characteristics cannot be directly related from the study of small laboratory fish models. Thus in future it is needed to perform such study on diverse types of aquatic organisms to get detailed idea about toxicity of nanoparticles in aquatic environment.

In conclusion, it can be suggested that in any study or application of nanoparticles, their toxicological aspects should be understood critically using different preparations, different dosing regimens and/or other bioassays to better assess their mechanisms of toxicity and their determinants. Eventually such assessments using the aquatic model organisms like zebrafish will lead to the identification of nanomaterial characteristics that comes up with negligible or no toxicity and help to get more balanced designs of materials on the nanoscale.Ultimately such assessments using the zebrafish embryo model should lead to the identification of nanomaterial characteristics that afford minimal or no toxicity and guide more rational designs of materials on the nanoscale.

References

Asharani,P.V., Wu, Y. L., Gong, Z. and Valiyaveettil, S. (2008).Toxicity of silver nanoparticles in zebrafish models, *Nanotechnology*, 19(25), Article ID 255102.

Asharani PV, lianwu Y, Gong Z, Valiyaveettil S (2011). Comparison of the toxicity of silver, gold and platinum nanoparticles in developing zebrafish embryos. Nanotoxicology 5(1): 43-54. (doi: 10.3109/17435390.2010.489207).

Bai, W, Tian, W, Zhang, Z, He, X, Ma, Y, Liu, N, Chai, Z (2010a). Effects of Copper Nanoparticles on the Development of Zebrafish Embryos. Journal of Nanoscience and Nanotechnology, 10(12): 8670-8676(7).

Bai, W, Zhang, Z, Tian, W, He, X,Ma, Y, Zhao, Y, Chai, Z (2010b). Toxicity of zinc oxide nanoparticles to zebrafish embryo: a physico-chemical study of toxicity mechanism. J Nanopart Res 12(5): 1645–1654.

Bar-Ilan O, Albrecht RM, Fako VE, Furgeson DY.(2009). Toxicity assessments of multisized gold and silver nanoparticles in zebrafish embryos. Small. 5(16): 1897-1910.

Beckman, M., 2007. Zebrafish take the stage in cancer research. J. Natl. Cancer Inst. 99, 500-501.

Beliaeva NF, Kashirtseva VN, Medvedeva NV, Khudoklinova IuIu, Ipatova OM, Archakov AI. (2010). Zebrafish as a model organism for biomedical studies. Biomed Khim. 56(1): 120-31.

Bull J, Levin B (2000). Perspectives: microbiology. Mice are not furry petri dishes. Science 287: 1409–1410.

Chakraborty, C., Agoramoorthy, G. (2010). Why zebrafish? Riv. Bio., 103(1): 25-7.

Chakraborty, C., Hsu, C.H. Wen, Z.H., Lin, C.S., Agoramoorthy, G. (2011). Effect of caffeine, norfloxacin and nimesulide on heartbeat and VEGF expression zebrafish larvae. J. Environ. Biol., 32(2): 179-83.

Chae, Y. J., Pham,C.H., Lee, J., Bae,E., Yi, J., and Gu,M.B. (2009). Evaluation of the toxic impact of silver nanoparticles on Japanese medaka (*Oryzias latipes*). Aquatic Toxicology Volume 94, Issue 4, 4 October 2009, 320-327.

Chen J, Dong X, Xin Y and Zhao M. (2010). Effects of titanium dioxide nanoparticles on growth and some histological parameters of zebrafish (*Danio rerio*) after a long term exposure. Aquatic Toxicology 101(3-4), 493-499.

Chen, TH, Lin, CY, Tseng, M-C (2011). Behavioral effects of titanium dioxide nanoparticles on larval zebrafish (*Danio rerio*). Marine Pollution Bulletin. Article in Press, Corrected Proof - doi: 10.1016/j.marpolbul.2011.04.017.

Cheng J, Flahaut E, Cheng SH. (2007). Effect of carbon nanotubes on developing zebrafish (*Danio rerio*) embryos. Environ Toxicol Chem 26(4): 708-716.

Choi JE, Kim S, Ahn, JH, Youn,P, Kang, JS, Park, K, Yi, J, Ryu, D-Y. (2010). Induction of oxidative stress and apoptosis by silver nanoparticles in the liver of adult zebrafish. Aquatic Toxicology, 100(2): 151-159. doi: 10.1016/j.aquatox.2009.12.012.

Chakraborty C, Hsu CH, Wen ZH, Lin CS, Agoramoorthy G. (2009). Zebrafish: A complete animal model for *in vitro* drug discovery and development. Current Drug Metabolism. 10(2): 116-24.

Creaser C.W. 1934. The technic of handling the zebra fish (*Brachydanio rerio*) for the production of eggs which are favorable for embryological research and are available at any specified time throughout the year. Copeia 1934: 159-161.

Environmental Protection Agency (2007). Science Policy Council, Nanotechnology Workgroup Nanotechnology White Paper. Available http: //www.epa.gov/osa/nanotech.htm.

Fent K, Weisbrod CJ, Wirth-Heller A, Pieles U.(2010). Assessment of uptake and toxicity of fluorescent silica nanoparticles in zebrafish (*Danio rerio*) early life stages. Aquat Toxicol. 2010 Oct 15; 100(2): 218-28.

Geffroy B, Ladhar C, Cambier S, Treguer-Delapierre M, Brèthes D, Bourdineaud, J-P. (2011). Impact of dietary gold nanoparticles in zebrafish at very low contamination pressure: The role of size, concentration and exposure time. Nanotoxicology doi: 10.3109/17435390.2011.562328.

Griffitt RJ, Hyndman K, Denslllow ND and Barber DS (2008). Comparison of Molecular and Histological Changes in Zebrafish Gills Exposed to Metallic Nanoparticles. Toxicological Sciences 107(2), 404-415.

Griffitt RJ, Hyndman K, Denslow ND, Barber DS.(2009). Comparison of molecular and histological changes in zebrafish gills exposed to metallic nanoparticles. Toxicol Sci. 107(2): 404-415.

Griffitt RJ, Weil R, Hyndman KA, Denslow ND, Powers K, Taylor D, Barber DS. (2007). Exposure to copper nanoparticles causes gill injury and acute lethality in zebrafish (*Danio rerio*). Environ Sci Technol. 41(23): 8178-86.

Guo S (2004). Linking genes to brain, behavior and neurological diseases: what can we learn from zebrafish? Genes Brain Behav 3: 63–74.

Guzman, K.A.D., M.R. Taylor, and J.F. Banfield, (2006). Environmental risks of nanotechnology: National nanotechnology initiative funding, 2000-2004. Environmental Science and Technology, 40(5): 1401-1407.

Hallare A, Nagel K, Kohler HR, Triebskorn R (2006). Comparative embryotoxicity and proteotoxicity of three carrier solvents to zebrafish (*Danio rerio*) embryos. Ecotoxicol Environ Saf 63: 378–388.

Hamilton F. 1822. An account of the fishes found in the River Ganges and its branches.Archibald Constable and Company, Edinburgh.

Hoet, P., I. Bruske-Hohlfeld, and O. Salata (2004). Nanoparticles- known and unknown health risks. Journal of Nanobiotechnology. 2: 12-37.

Hsu CH, Wen ZH, Lin CS, Chakraborty C (2007). Zebrafish model: use in studying cellular mechanisms for a spectrum of clinical disease entities. Current Neurovascular Research, 4: 111-120.

Hurt, R.H., M. Monthioux, and A. Kane. (2006). Toxicology of carbon nanomaterials: status, trends, and perspectives on the special issue. Carbon44: 1028-1033.

Ispas C, Andreescu D, Patel A, Goia DV, Andreescu S and Wallace KN. (2009). Toxicity and Developmental Defects of Different Sizes and Shape Nickel Nanoparticles in Zebrafish. Environ. Sci. Technol. 43 (16), 6349–6356.

Jovanovic, B., Ji, T. Palic, D. (2011). Gene expression of zebrafish embryos exposed to titanium dioxide nanoparticles and hydroxylated fulerenes. Ecotoxicolgy and Environmental safety. 74(0147): 1518-1525.

King-heiden, TC, Wiecinski, PN, Mangham, AN, Metz, KM, Nesbit, D, Pedersen, JA, Hamers, R J, Heideman, W, Peterson, RE (2009). Quantum Dot Nanotoxicity Assessment Using the Zebrafish Embryo. Environ. Sci. Technol. 43: 1605–1611.

Kim Y.S., Song M.Y., Park J.D., Song K.S., Ryu H.R., Chung, Y.H., Chang H.K., Lee J.H., Oh K.H., Kelman, B.J., Hwang, I.K., and Yu I J. 2010. Subchronic oral toxicity of silver nanoparticles. Particle and Fibre Toxicology 7: 20 from http: //www.particleandfibretoxicology.com/content/7/1/20.

Kishi S. 2004. Functional senescence and gradual aging in zebrafish. Annals of the New York Academy of Science 1019: 521-526.

Kreyling, W. G., Semmler, M., Erbe, F., Mayer, P., Takenaka, S., Schulz, H.,Oberdö rster, G., and Ziesenis, A. (2002). Translocation of ultrafine insoluble iridium particles from lung epithelium to extrapulmonary organs is size dependent but very low. J. Toxicol. Environ. Health A 65, 1513–1530.

Lammer E, Carr GJ, Wendler K, Rawlings JM, Belanger SE, et al. (2009). Is the fish embryo toxicity test (FET) with the zebrafish (Danio rerio) a potential alternative for the fish acute toxicity test? Comp Biochem Physiol C Toxicol Pharmacol 149: 196–209.

Lee, K. J., Nallathamby, P. D., Browning, L. M., Osgood, C. J. and Xu, X. H. (2007).In vivo imaging of transport and biocompatibility of single silver nanoparticles in early development of zebrafish embryos, ACS Nano, 1(2): 133–143,.

Lewinski, N.; Colvin, V.; Drezek, R. (2008). Cytotoxicity of Nanoparticles. Small, 4, 26–49.

Lewinski,NA, Zhu,H, Ouyang,CR, Conner,GP, Wagner,DS, Colvin, VL, Drezek, RA (2011). Trophic transfer of amphiphilic polymer coated CdSe/ZnS quantum dots to Danio rerio. Nanoscale, Advance Article DOI: 10.1039/C1NR10319A.

Li T, Albee B, Alemayehu M, Diaz R, Ingham L, Kamal S, Rodriguez M, Bishnoi SW. (2010). Comparative toxicity study of Ag, Au, and Ag–Au bimetallic nanoparticles on Daphnia magna. Anal Bioanal Chem 398: 689–700.

Lieschke GJ, Currie PD (2007). Animal models of human disease: zebrafish swim into view. Nat Rev Genet 8: 353–367.

Lynch, I., and Dawson, K. A. (2008). Protein-nanoparticle interactions. NanoToday 3, 40–47.

MacNee, W., Li, X., Gilmour, P., and Donaldson, K. (2000). Systemic effect of particulate air pollution. Inhal. Toxicol. 12, 233–244.

Meng, H.; Xia, T.; George, S.; Nel, A. E. (2009). A Predictive Toxicological Paradigm for the Safety Assessment of Nanomaterials. ACS Nano, 3, 1620–1627.

Muller J, Delos M, Panin N, Rabolli V, Huaux F, Lison D (2009). Absence of Carcinogenic Response to Multiwall Carbon Nanotubes in a 2-Year Bioassay in the Peritoneal Cavity of the Rat. Toxicological Sciences 110(2), 442–448.

Oberdorster, G., Sharp, Z., Atudorei, V., Elder, A., Gelein, R., Lunts, A.,Kreyling, W., and Cox, C. (2002). Extrapulmonary translocation of ultrafinecarbon particles following whole-body inhalation exposure of rats. J Toxicol.Environ. Health A 65, 1531–1543.

Palaniappan, PL. RM., Pramod, K.S. (2011a). The effect of titanium dioxide on the biochemical constituents of the brain of Zebrafish (Danio rerio): An FT-IR study. Spectrochimica Acta Part A: Molecular and Biomolecular Spectroscopy. 79(1): 206-212.

Palaniappan, PL.RM., Pramod, K.S. (2011b). Raman spectroscopic investigation on the microenvironment of the liver tissues of Zebrafish (*Danio rerio*) due to titanium dioxide exposure. Vibrational Spectroscopy, 56(2): 146-153.

Parng C, Seng WL, Semino C, McGrath P (2002). Zebrafish: A preclinical model for drug screening. Assay Drug Dev Technol 1: 41–48.

Parng C. (2005). *In vivo* zebrafish assays for toxicity testing. Current Opinions in Drug Discovery and Development 8: 100-106.

Postlethwait JH, Woods IG, Ngo-Hazelett P, Yan YL, Kelly PD, Chu F, Huang H, Hill-Force1 A. and Talbot, W.S. (2000). Zebrafish comparative genomics and the origins of vertebrate chromosomes. Genome Research 10: 1890–1902.

Powers,C.M., Badireddy, A. R., Ryde,I. T., Seidler,F.J., and Slotkin, T. A. (2011). Silver Nanoparticles Compromise Neurodevelopment in PC12 Cells: Critical Contributions of Silver Ion, Particle Size, Coating, and Composition. Environ Health Perspect. 119(1): 37–44.

Redfern WS, Waldron G, Winter MJ, Butler P, Holbrook M, *et al.* (2008). Zebrafish assays as early safety pharmacology screens: paradigm shift or red herring? J Pharmacol Toxicol Methods 58: 110–117.

Roco, M C (1999). Nanoparticles and nanotechnology research. J Nanopart Res 1: 1-6.

Rubinstein AL (2003). Zebrafish: from disease modeling to drug discovery. Curr Opin Drug Discov Devel 6: 218–223.

Samson JC, Shenker J (2000). The teratogenic effects of methylmercury on early development of the zebrafish, Danio rerio. Aquat Toxicol 48: 343–354.

Scholz S, Mayer I (2008). Molecular biomarkers of endocrine disruption in small model fish Molecul Cell Endocrinol 293: 57–70.

Scown T M, Santos E M, Johnston BD, Gaiser B, Baalousha M, Mltov S, Lead JR, Stone V, Fernandes TF, Jepson M, van Aerlllle R, Tyler CR.(2010). Effects of Aqueous Exposure to Silver Nanoparticles of Different Sizes in Rainbow Trout. Toxicological Sciences 115 (2) 521-534.

Teeguarden JG, Hinderliter PM, Orr G, Thrall BD, Pounds JG (2007). Particokinetics *in vitro*: Dosimetry considerations for *in vitro* nanoparticle toxicity assessments. Toxicol. Sci. 95: 300-312.

Trede, N.S., Langenau, D.M., Traver, D., Look, A.T., Zon, L.I., 2004. The use of zebrafish to understand immunity. Immunity 20, 367-379.

Tropepe V, Sive HL (2003). Can zebrafish be used as a model to study the neurodevelopmental causes of autism? Genes Brain Behav 2: 268–281.

Usenko CY, Harper SL, Tanguay RL (2008). Fullerene C60 exposure elicits an oxidative stress response in embryonic zebrafish. Toxicol Appl Pharmacol 229: 44-55.

Veldman MB, Lin S (2008). Zebrafish as a developmental model organism for pediatric research. Pediatr Res 64: 470–476.

Voelker D, Vess C, Tillmann M, Nagel R, Otto GW, *et al.* (2007). Differential gene expression as a toxicant-sensitive endpoint in zebrafish embryos and larvae. Aquat Toxicol 81: 355–364.

von Westernhagen H (1988). Sublethal effects of pollutants on fish eggs and larvae. In: oar W, Randall DJ (eds) The physiology of developing fish. Fish physiology II. Academic Press, New York, 253–346.

Wang B, Feng WY, Wang M, Wang TC, Gu YQ, Zhu MT, Ouyang H, Shi JW, Zhang F, Zhao YL, Chai ZF, Wang HF, Wang J (2008). Acute toxicological impact of nanoand submicro-scaled zinc oxide powder on healthy adult mice. J Nanopart Res 10(2): 263–276.

Wang ZL (2004). Zinc oxide nanostructures: growth, properties and applications. J Phys Condens Matter 16: 829–858.

Wang, J, Zhu, X, Zhang, X, Zhao,Z, Liu, H, George,R, Wilson-Rawls,J, Chang, Y, Chen, Y (2011). Disruption of zebrafish (*Danio rerio*) reproduction upon chronic exposure to TiO_2 nanoparticles. Chemosphere,83(4): 461-467.

WB Barbazuk, I Korf, C Kadavi, *et al.* (2000). Genome Research 10: 1351.

Wright, D., Nakamichi, R., Krause, J., Butlin, R.K. (2006). QTL analysis of behavioural and morphological differentiation between wild and laboratory zebrafish (*Danio rerio*). Behav. Genet. 36, 271-284.

Xiong, D., Fang, T., Yu, L., Sima, X. and Zhu, W. (2011). Effects of nano-scale TiO_2, ZnO and tgeir bulk counterparts on zebrafish: Acute toxicity, oxidative stress and oxidative damage.Science of the Total Environment 409: 8, 1444-1452.

Yu,L-P, Fang,T, Xiong,D-W, Zhu, W-T, Sima, X-F. (2011). Comparative toxicity of nano-ZnO and bulk ZnO suspensions to zebrafish and the effects of sedimentation, ÿOH production and particle dissolution in distilled water. J. Environ. Monit., 13: 1975-1982. DOI: 10.1039/C1EM10197H.

Zhang Y, Chen W, Zhang J, Liu J, Chen G, Pope C. (2007). *In vitro* and *in vivo* toxicity of CdTe nanoparticles J Nanosci Nanotechnol. 2007 Feb; 7(2): 497-503.

Zhu X, Zhu L, Duan Z, Qi R, Li Y, Lang Y. (2008). Comparative toxicity of several metal oxide nanoparticle aqueous suspensions to Zebrafish (*Danio rerio*) early developmental stage. Journal of Environmental Science and Health Part A, 43 (3), 278 – 284.

Zhu X, Zhu L, Li Y, Duan Z, Chen W, Alvarez PJJ (2007). Developmental toxicity in Zebrafish (*Danio rerio*) embryos after exposure to manufactured nanomaterials: Buckminsterfullerene aggregates (nC60) and fullerol. Environ Toxicol Chem 26: 976-979.

Zhu, X, b, Wang, J, Zhang,X, Chang, Y (2010). Trophic transfer of TiO_2 nanoparticles from daphnia to zebrafish in a simplified freshwater food chain. Chemosphere 79(9): 928-933.

2014, Advances in Biochemistry and Biotechnology Volume 2   *Pages 81-97*

Edited by: Dr. Biplab Sarkar and Dr. Chiranjib Chakraborty

Published by: DAYA PUBLISHING HOUSE

6

Innate and Adaptive Components of Immune System in Fish

Jaya Kumari[1]* and Trilochan Swain[2]**

[1]*Norwegian College of Fishery Science, Faculty of Biosciences, Fisheries and Economics,*
University of Tromsø, N-9037 Tromsø, Norway
[2]*Shree-Kshetramohan Biocomplex, Jagatsinghpur, Orissa, India*

ABSTRACT

Innate immune response is a primitive form of defense mechanism existent in plants and animals. It is a complex system which, in vertebrates, is composed of cellular and humoral responses. The vertebrate teleost fish, which diverged from the tetrapod lineage about 450 million years ago, has an innate immune component that shows considerable conservation with higher vertebrates particularly in mammals highlighted by the presence of orthologous pattern recognition receptors (PRRs) and stimulated cytokines. However, there is also increasing evidence of teleost fish components and functions that are not observed in mammals suggesting complexity

Corresponding E-mail: *jaya_kumari2005@rediffmail.com; jaya.kumari@uit.no; **tjay1975@gmail.com and diversity in teleost fish innate immune function. The innate system also plays an instructive role in the acquired immune response and homeostasis and is therefore equally important in higher vertebrates. The innate immune system is divided into physical barriers, cellular and humoral components. The adaptive system is divided into two main branches. In the humoral branch, the effector molecules are the antibodies (Ab) which all belong to proteins called immunoglobulins (Ig), whereas, T-cells are a key component in the cell-mediated response, the specific immune response that utilizes T-cells to neutralize cells that have been infected with viruses and certain bacteria. Knowledge about the network and function of these immune-related molecules and also the crossroads between the innate and adaptive immune responses in model and/or economically important fish is therefore important and new molecular biological tools will help elucidate such information and thus can contribute to the control of fish disease and thereby improve aquaculture.

Keywords: Innate immunity, Adaptive immunity, Vertebrates, Fish.

Introduction

Fish, as the first vertebrate group appearing in evolution after adaptive radiation from the Devonic period, still represents the most successful and diverse group of vertebrates. Teleost fish represent a transition point on the phylogenetic spectrum between invertebrates that depend only on innate immunity and mammals that heavily depend on adaptive immunity. However, an increasing body of evidence, both from fish and mammalian immunology, shows that these are combinational systems. Innate immune response generally precedes the adaptive response, activates and determines the nature of the adaptive response and co-operates in the maintenance of homeostasis (Fearon 1997; Fearon *et al.*, 1996). Importantly, immune organs homologues to those of mammalian immune system are present in fish. However, their structural complexity is less, potentially limiting the capability to generate fully functionally adaptive immune response against pathogen invasion.

This chapter will provide to outline the function of innate and acquired immune defences in bonyfish, describing both humoral and cellular components. Emphasis is given to particularities present in fish but not in mammals, whose defensive mechanisms are known in greater details (Janeway 2005). In-depth immune studies have been primarily carried out on teleost fish species of commercial importance. Thus, a considerable body of work exists on the immunology of zebrafish *Danio rerio*, carp *Cyprinus carpio*, tilapia *Oreochromis mossambicus*, sea bream *Dicentrarchus labrax*, sea bass *Sparus aurata*, turbot *Scophthalmus maximus*, Atlantic salmon *Salmo salar*, rainbow trout *Oncorhynchus mykiss*, Channel catfish *Ictalurus punctatus*, and eel *Anguilla anguilla* (Buchmann *et al.*, 2001; Iwama 1996; Manning 1998; Nielsen *et al.*, 2006; Simon 2001; Stein *et al.*, 2007).

The Innate Immune System

The innate immune system is the earliest or primeval immune mechanism and hence universal form of host defense. It is characterized by being non-specific and therefore not depending upon previous recognition of the surface structures of the invader. Innate immunity is generally subdivided into two parts, the cellular and humoral defense responses. As in all vertebrates, fish have cellular and humoral immune responses, and central organs whose the main function is involved in immune system.

Immune System Morphology in Teleosts

Fish and mammals show some similarities and some differences regarding immune function (Table 6.1). Most of the generative and secondary lymphoid organs present in mammals are also found in fish, except the lymphatic nodules and the bone marrow (Press *et al.*, 1999). Instead, the head kidney, aglomerular, assumes hemopoietic functions (Meseguer 1995) (Zapata *et al.*, 1997), and unlike higher vertebrates is the principal immune organ responsible for phagocytosis (Dannevig *et al.*, 1994), antigen processing (Brattgjerd *et al.*, 1996; Kaattari *et al.*, 1985) and formation of IgM and immune memory through melanomacrophagic centres (Herraez 1986; Tsujii *et al.*, 1990). Thus, the head kidney in teleost is a major lymphoid organ, in addition to the thymus and spleen (Press *et al.*). The HK of fish exhibits similarity to red bone marrow in terms of morphology and its functional role in haematopoiesis. Thymus and HK are the primary T cell and B cell organs, respectively. The HK serves as a secondary

Table 7.1: Relevant Immune differences between Jawed Fishes and Mammals (Tort *et al.*, 2003)

	Jawed Fishes	Mammals
Biotic constrictions		
Temperature range	−2 to 35°C	36.5 to 37.5°C
Primary environment	Water	Air
Metabolism	Poikilothermia, Endothermia (eg. Bluefin tuna and some pelagic fishes)	Homeothermia
External interfaces	Mucous skin, gills	Respiratory tree
Humoral diversity		
Igisotypes	IgM, IgD, IgT, IgM, IgX/IgR, IgW, NAR(C) (*Chondrichthyes*), IgM redox forms	IgM, IgA, IgD, IgE, IgG
Ig gene arrangement	Multicluster (*Chondrichthyes* and some *Teleostei*)	Translocon
Non-specific diversity	Several C3 isoforms (*Teleostei*)	No C3 isoforms
Overall performance		
Antibody affinity	Low	High
Antibody response	Slow	Fast
Memory response	Weak	Strong
Affinity maturation	Low or absent	High
Low temperatures	High dependence, immunosuppressive response (only in poikilothermic fish)	Low dependence
Lymphoid organs		
Haematopoietic tissue	Head kidney (Teleostei), Epigonal and Leydig organs, meningeal tissue,orbital and subcranial hematopoietic tissue (Chondrichthyes)	Bone marrow
Thymus	Involution species-dependent, influenced by seasonal changes and hormonal cycles	Involution with age
Lymphoid nodes	Absent	Present
Gut-associated lymphoid tissues	Not organized, lymphoid aggregates, Leydig organ and spiral valve *(Chondrichthyes)*	Organized, Peyerpathes
Germinal centres	Absent (melanomacrophagecentres?),dendritic cells probably present	Present

lymphoid organ in the clearance of soluble and particulate antigens from the circulation and it is a major site of antibody production (Workenhe *et al.*, 2010). The spleen of teleosts has also been implicated in the clearance of blood-borne antigens and immune complexes in splenic ellipsoids, and also has a role in the antigen presentation and the initiation of the adaptive immune response (Workenhe *et al.*, 2010).Gut associated lymphoid tissues are also known lymphoid organs, and have been shown to function in eliciting immune responses in carp (Joosten *et al.*, 1996). Some teleosts, such as plaice, have been shown to possess a lymphatic system that is differentiated from the blood vascular system (Wardle, 1971), though the existence of such a system has been challenged in other species. Mucosa associated lymphoid tissues in fish include the gut, skin and gills and form an initial barrier to invasion by pathogens (Dalmo *et al.*, 1997).

Non-Specific Humoral Immunity

The skin of fish forms the first line of defence against pathogens, as do the mucosal membranes covering the gills and the gastrointestinal (GI) tract. Apart from any scales, spines or secreted toxic substances that may be present on skin, mucus covering the skin, the gills and the GI tract is also involved in defensive mechanisms, as it contains several antimicrobial and antiparasitic compounds: lysozyme and proteases, complement factors, C-reactive protein, lectins, interferons, eicosanoids, transferring, peptides such as piscidins, somatostanin and ACTH, and various carbohydrates (Buchmann *et al.*, 2001; Woo 2007; Magnadottir 2006; Manning 1998). Several of the products found in fish mucus are also present in serum, from where they can be transported to the fish surface. Alternatively, they can be synthesized by epithelial or mucous cells (Buchmann, 1999).

The complement system appears to be one of the central immune response in fish. Complement is a series of serum proteins responsible for three primary immune functions: (a) to cover pathogens and foreign particles to facilitate their recognition and destruction by phagocytic cells (opsonization); (b) to initiate inflammatory reactions by stimulating the contraction of smooth muscle, vasodilation and chemo attraction of leucocytes; and (c) to lyse pathogens through the perforation of their membranes. The classical, alternative and possibly also the lectin pathways have been described in several teleost groups (Endo *et al.*, 1998; Nonaka *et al.*, 2000; Zarkadis *et al.*, 2001). Moreover, it has been suggested that the lectin-mediated pathway may have preceded the immunoglobulin mediated pathway (Quesenberry *et al.*, 2003). The third component of the complement series (C3) is present in all vertebrates and is the key element in the activation of the system. Here, there are some relevant differences compared with mammals. The first is that fish possess multiple active isoforms of the key activation molecule C3. Mammals have one isoform of the C3 molecule whereas fish express several functionally active C3 isoforms, three in trout (*Oncorhynchus mykiss*) and medaka (*Oryzias latipes*), five in seabream (*Sparus aurata*) and carp (*Cyprinus carpio*), and three loci coding for three isoforms in zebrafish (*Danio rerio*) (Gongora *et al.*, 1998; Kuroda *et al.*, 2000; Nakao *et al.*, 1997; Sunyer *et al.*, 1997; Sunyer *et al.*, 1996). Teleost C3 share the two-chain structure although showing variations in the catalytic residues of the protein, they maintain a differential affinity for several substrates and they probably are products of several polymorphic genes (Sahu *et al.*, 2001; Slierendrecht *et al.*, 1993). The biological meaning of the variability may be the specialization to bind specific surfaces and to increase efficiency to eliminate immunogens. This specialization remains, however, to be fully demonstrated. Similar to mammals in which Ig variability gives more efficiency in binding immunogens, the same variability process may have occurred in fish regarding the complement response (Sunyer *et al.*, 1996). Furthermore bacteriolytic and haemolytic activity of these C3 isoforms has been demonstrated to be higher than in mammals. This also would justify the preference for the alternative pathway response in fish (Sunyer *et al.*, 1995).

Lysozyme is one of the most studied innate responses in fish (Saurabh *et al.*, 2008). It is a lytic enzyme acting on the peptidoglycan component of the bacterial cell wall, especially of gram positive bacteria; it can also act as an opsonin (Magnadottir 2006). In Gram negative bacteria, lysozyme may become effective after complement and other factors have disrupted the outer cell wall, exposing the inner peptidoglycan layer. Lysozyme has been found in mucus and ova, and serum lysozyme, probably coming from peritoneal macrophages and blood neutrophils, has been used as an indicator of non-specific immune response. It appears that the lysozyme response in fish may be induced very rapidly and not only related to bacterial presence but also to other alarm situations such as after stress (Tort *et al.*, 2003). Thus, lysozyme in fish would be involved in the overall alarm response, acting as an acute-phase protein.

Lectins are important immune mediators in lower vertebrates and invertebrates. Mucosal or serum agglutinins and precipitins are lectins like C-type lectins and pentraxins. C-type lectins show binding specificity for different carbohydrates like mannose, N-acetyl glucosamine or fucose in the presence of Ca ions. The interaction of these carbohydrate binding proteins and carbohydrate leads to opsonization, phagocytosis and activation of the complement system (Arason 1996). Most widely studied is the mannose binding lectin (MBL), which shows specificity for mannose, N-acetyl glucosamine, fucose and glucose. Lectins, with various carbohydrate specificities, have been isolated from the serum of several fish species (Ewart *et al.*, 2001). Some show similar carbohydrate affinity, molecular structure and function to mammalian MBL, while others, also implicated in innate immune defence, have different carbohydrate binding specificity or heterologous sequence structure (Magnadottir, 2006). Calcium dependent LPS binding protein had been isolated from some fish sera (Fenton and Golenbock 1998; Hoover *et al.*, 1998). A lectin with binding affinity for N-acetyl-glucosamine and mannose has recently been isolated from cod serum. Proteomic analysis of this lectin showed homology with ficolin. Ficolin is believed to play a role in host defence through opsonization and complement activation in a similar manner to MBL (Magnadottir 2006). Transferrin is an iron binding lectin, which inhibits bacterial growth by limiting the availability of this essential nutrient (Manning 1998).

Pentraxins (C-reactive protein, CRP and serum amyloid protein, SAP) are lectins, which are present in the body fluids of both invertebrates and vertebrates and are commonly associated with the acute phase response (Magnadottir 2006). As well as showing significantly increased serum levels following tissue injury, trauma or infection (acute phase response), the pentraxins take part in innate immune defence through their lectin type binding role (PRR), activate the complement pathways and play a role in the recognition and clearance of apoptotic cells (Magnadottir, 2006). By definition CRP binds to the phosphorylcholine moiety of the bacterial cell wall in the presence of Ca ions whereas SAP shows affinity for phosphoryl-ethanolamine and is also known to bind LPS of Gram negative bacteria. Some fish species appear to have either the CRP pentraxin (like cod and channel catfish) or the SAP pentraxin (like salmon, wolffish and halibut) whereas others (like plaice and rainbow trout) have both types like higher vertebrates. The level of pentraxin is normally high in fish compared to mammals and may or may not be elevated during an acute phase response (Magnadottir, 2006).

The integument and integumental secretions of fish, such as the multifunctional skin mucus, have been shown to play a significant role in host defence against bacteria and viruses. Antimicrobial polypeptides have been identified as a component of the innate immune response and are widespread, both in the plant and the animal kingdom. Piscidins are antimicrobial peptides of 22 amino acids forming an alpha helix, are located in mucous tissues and immune cells, and have been identified in several fish species *viz.* tilapia, seabream and seabass (Silphaduang *et al.*, 2006).

Interferons (IFN) are a heterologous family of proteins that confer resistance to viral infections (Secombes C.J 1997). They are categorized in three groups: IFNα and IFNβ are produced by cells infected by viruses, and it is thought that any cellular type can produce them. IFNγ is a cytokine produced by T-cells and recently it is shown that it also plays important role in viral immunity together with IFNα (Sun *et al.*, 2011). The gene structure, protein structure and functional properties of fish interferons show great similarity to those of mammalian interferons (Robertsen 2006; Zou *et al.*, 2011).

Eicosanoids include prostaglandins, thromboxanes and leukotrienes, and are potent proinflammatory mediators. They participate in several physiological processes, including haemostasis, immune regulation and inflammation, and can increase phagocytosis and act as chemoattractants for neutrophils (Manning 1998; Secombes 1997).

Although antibodies (immunoglobulins) are an acquired immune parameter, natural antibodies can also be classified as components of the innate system. Natural antibodies are produced in the absence of gene-rearrangement and without any apparent specific antigen stimulation. Natural antibodies are a well known phenomenon in fish and have been shown to play an important role in their innate/acquired immune defence. Natural antibodies of rainbow trout and goldfish take part in both viral and bacterial defence and high non-specific antibody activity in the serum of goldfish inhibited the specific antibody response (Magnadottir 2006). Variation in the natural antibody specificity repertoire between different fish species have been reported, activity against haptenated (TNP/DNP) proteins being relatively strongest (Gonzalez *et al.*, 1988).

Food additives like vitamins, lipids or high carbohydrate content may or may not enhance innate parameters but can still be of general benefit as regards growth and survival (Kumari *et al.*, 2005; Lygren *et al.*, 1999). There is considerable interest in upregulating the innate immune system with the help of various immunostimulants. The immunostimulants that are commonly used are components that activate the pattern recognition mechanism of the innate system like fungal b-1,3 glucans, peptidoglycans of Gram negative and positive bacteria, LPS, common to all Gram negative bacteria and various carbohydrates like levamisol, lactoferrin, polymannuronic acid, chitosan, also bacterial or synthetic oligo-dexanucleotides (CpG motives), and herbal remedies (Kumari and Sahoo 2006; Zhang *et al.*, 2009). Immunostimulation studies with the aid of extensive gene expression profiling like ESTs, cDNA microarray and Serial Analysis of Gene Expression (SAGE) generated information on various proinflammatory cytokines that are potential for vaccine/adjuvant development.

Non-Specific Cellular Immunity

The cellular component of non-specific immune defenses includes the mobile phagocytic cells (macrophages and granulocytes) recruited from the blood and lymphoid tissues; the less motile eosinophilic granular cells (EGC), which occur at mucosal sites such as the gut or the gills and are considered analogous to mammalian mast cells; and the non-specific cytotoxic cells of fish (NCC) which are considered to be equivalent functionally to the mammalian natural killer (NK) cells (Manning 1998; Secombes 1997). To recognize antigens and initiate immune responses, the cell types mentioned above possess diverse receptors. Toll-like receptors are a type of pattern recognition receptor (PRR), and now one of the most studied biological molecules, are transmembrane proteins present in cells mediating innate immunity which enable recognition of non-self repetitive patterns called pathogen associated molecular pattern (PAMPS). Although toll-like receptors have been shown to be involved in non-specific immune responses in fish, these are found in all animals. So far, a total of 13 TLRs have been identified in mammals (Meylan *et al.*, 2006), and several more have been found in fish. TLRs are highly specific, as each respond to different agonists (Table 6.2) (Holvold, 2007). There are receptors from the immunoglobulin (Ig) superfamily regulating innate immunity which up to date have only been detected in fish: the novel immune-type receptors (NITR) (Ostergaard *et al.*, 2009). Although structurally analogous to lymphocyte B immunoglobulin, NITR are not rearranged like antibodies.

Table 6.2: A Selection of Toll-like Receptors and their Agonists.
Toll-like receptors 3, 7, 8 and 9 all recognize PAMPs in endosomal/lyzosomal compartments, while the rest are expressed on the cell surface (Linn 2007).

	Properties of the Receptor	*Agonists*
TLR2	The TLR2 receptor is dependent on the formation ofDimmers with TLR1 or TLR6. Due to this heterodimerization, the TLR2 is able to recognize a great variety of ligands.	Microbial lipopeptide β-glucan (Laminaran) Atypical lipopolysaccharide (LPS) Bacterial lipoprotein Heat shock protein (HSP)
TLR3	Binding of agonists to the receptor will induce synthesisof type-I interferons (IFNα and IFNβ), which then exert antiviral and immuno-stimulatory activities.	Double stranded RNA Polyinosinicpoly- cytidylic acid (polyI:C)
TLR4	TLR4 is unique in the TLR family in that it requires the molecule MD-2 in addition to LPS in order to initiate signaling. This molecule is indispensable for TLR4 but will not affect the response to other bacterial components such as peptidoglycans or CpGDNA.	LPS
TLR5	The TLR5 receptor recognizes bacterial flagellin (Hayashi *et al.*, 2001). The receptor is expressed on the basolateral surface of intestinal epithelia, and will there for reactivate pro-inflammatory gene expression only if flagellin crosses the epithelium.	Flagellin
TLR7/8	Alongwith TLR3 and 9, TLR7 and 8 recognize PAMPs in endosomal/lysozomal compartments, though the natural ligand for the receptors is still not known.	Single stranded RNA Imidazoquinoline compounds – Imiquimod – Resiquimod
TLR9	Despite a variety of effects concerning this receptor, they are all dependent on the TLR9-MyD88-mediated pathway.	Bacterial and viral CpG (pDNA)

Non-specific cellular immunity comprises three main defensive mechanisms, which are outlined in the following section: inflammation, phagocytosis and non-specific cytotoxicity. Inflammation is a response involving granulocytes, monocytes/macrophages and lymphocytes which follows exposure to an antigenic insult. Upon contact with the antigen, which can be of chemical, bacterial, mycotic, or parasitic origin, the affected area receives an increased supply of blood, followed by increased capillary permeability and migration of leucocytes from the bloodstream into the tissue. A variety of host-derived and pathogen-derived factors stimulate this migration. Host chemoattractants include the complement fragment C5a, leukotrienes and some cytokines, which are secreted by granulocytes, the first cellular types to accumulate around the antigenic insult. Additionally, fish leucocytes may be responding to soluble factors secreted by the pathogen; for instance, fish leucocytes have been shown to exhibit chemokinetic responses to bacterial, nematode, acanthocephalan and cestode products. Inflammatory reactions start rapidly, within an hour of exposure to the insult, and reach their peak after about 2 d. However, if the insult persists, inflammation can become chronic and lead to the formation of granulomas or the encapsulation of the antigenic source (Rubio-Godoy, 2010).

A cascade of pro-inflammatory cytokines is released as part of the non-specific innate immune response. In the last few years, much interest has been generated in the study of fish chemokines and cytokines and significant progress has been made in isolating these molecules from fish. Most of the progress has been attributed mainly to the enormous advances in genome projects for the Fugu (*Takifugu rubripes*) and zebrafish genome, and the large increase of fish expressed sequence tag entries in the GenBank.

The process of phagocytosis in teleosts is very similar to that observed in higher vertebrates: it includes the stages of antigen recognition, attachment, engulfment, killing and digestion. Both neutrophils and macrophages are the effector cells; macrophages in addition cooperate with lymphocytes through antigen presentation and cytokine secretion. Phagocytes possess a variety of killing mechanisms, both non-oxidative and oxidative; the most important one is the oxygen-dependent respiratory burst, which results in the formation of reactive oxygen species (ROS), including superoxide anion, hydrogen peroxide and hypochlorous acid. Phagocytosis is enhanced by opsonization; thus, lectins, C-reactive protein, complement and antibodies facilitate phagocytosis. The killing abilities of phagocytes are modulated by host-derived factors, such as IFN-γ and macrophage-activating factor (MAF), which enhance the cells' respiratory burst and their ability to kill microorganisms (Manning 1998; Rubio-Godoy 2010; Sakai 1992). Recent evidence suggests that distinct fish phagocytes, such as acidophilic granulocytes and macrophages, differ in their ability to recognize and eliminate pathogens and in their capacity to regulate adaptive immune responses (Sepulcre *et al.*, 2007).

Eosinophilic granular cells (EGC) are thought to be functionally equivalent to the mast cells of higher vertebrates, since they can be degranulated experimentally (Reite and Evensen 2006). EGC are uncommon in the blood, but are found in high numbers in the connective tissue of skin, gill and gut; they have been shown to degranulate after exposure to bacterial antigens and this is followed by an increase of histamine levels in blood (Reite *et al.*, 2006). EGC also release piscidins upon degranulation (Silphaduang and Noga, 2001).

Non-specific cytotoxic cells (NCC) have been detected in peripheral blood, peritoneal fluid, thymus, spleen and kidney, and have been shown to be cytotoxic to a range of normal and transformed cell lines of both mammalian and fish origins, and to virus-infected cells and parasitic protozoa (Manning 1998; Utke *et al.*, 2007).

The Acquired Immune System

In fish all the prerequisites to mount a specific immune response are present, but the main differences from the mammalian system are that the secondary response is relatively minor and IgG is not present. Acquired immunity in fish includes both humoral and cell mediated responses. A characteristic feature of both cell-mediated and antibody mediated immune responses in fish is their dependence upon environmental temperature. There is also evidence that, in some species at least, nutritional factors and behavior patterns may also influence the immune response.

Specific Humoral Immunity

The morphological and functional characterization of fish immune cells reveals cells that are equivalent to mammalian macrophages, neutrophils, monocytes, thrombocytes, B-cells, plasma cells, T-cells, natural killer cells and eosinophils (Workenhe *et al.*, 2010). The adaptive immune system of fish utilizes cellular components more or less similar to mammals. B-cells of fish produce antibody when stimulated. Teleost fish produce IgM as a primary antibody response and lack isotype switching to mount virus-specific antibodies during the infection process. The immunoglobulin (Ig) of fish is restricted to tetrameric IgM with a heavy chain quite similar to the mammalian M-chain (Swain *et al.,* 2004). However, further two heavy chain isotypes have been identified, IgD (Ohta *et al.,* 2006) and IgZ (immunoglobulin-zebrafish)/IgT (immunoglobulin-trout or immunoglobulin–teleost) (Danilova *et al.,* 2005). IgD is thought to be located in the cell membrane of B-cells, where it might act as receptor. The exploration of IgD and IgT functions has recently been initiated (Chen *et al.,* 2009). Whereas, IgT is a mucosal-epithelial immunoglobulin preferentially expressed in the gut, bound to resident bacteria and induced specifically by a mucosal pathogen. In contrast to tetrameric IgM, IgT existed as monomer in serum. Notably, in the gut mucus, IgT is present as a polymer, a situation analogous to that of human IgA, which is found in polymeric form in the gut mucus and as a monomer in the serum (Woof 2006). Much like IgA, IgT (and mucosal IgM) is transported by means of the fish polymeric immunoglobulin receptor (pIgR) and maintains a portion of pIgR as an associated secretory piece (Zhang *et al.,* 2010).

Immunoglobulin produced against an antigen may result in protective responses against it. The most direct protective mechanism is the neutralization of small molecular weight molecules, such as bacterial toxins. The multivalent binding capacity of immunoglobulin enables it to agglutinate and/ or precipitate soluble antigens. Antibodies also act as opsonins, by coating antigens and promoting phagocytosis. Additionally, antigen binding elicits conformational changes in the Fc region, which enable it to activate the complement system via the classical pathway (Manning 1998).

An important aspect of the specific immune response is that of immunological memory, which results in more rapid and pronounced production of antibodies upon a secondary exposure to the same antigen; this of course is a prerequisite for successful vaccination. Research suggests that immunological memory exists in fish similar to the anamnestic response in higher vertebrates. Fish mount a greater immune response to antigens with successive exposures. Specific Ig in fish functions in opsonization of bacteria, neutralization of toxins or viruses and is a potent activator of complement.

Effective fish vaccines against several bacterial pathogens are available, and are crucial to large scale fish aquaculture. For instance, there are formulations protecting fish against 17 common bacterial infections, including vibriosis (caused by *Listonella anguillarum* and *Vibrio* spp.), furunculosis (*Aeromonas salmonicida*), yersiniosis (*Yersinia ruckeri*), enteric septicemia of catfish (*Edwardsiella ictaluri*) and bacterial kidney disease (*Renibacterium salmoninarum*). In contrast, there are five commercial vaccines available against viruses (Sommerset *et al.,* 2005), and only experimental ones against parasites (Kim *et al.,* 2000; Rubio-Godoy *et al.,* 2003).

The first appearance of IgM in lymphocytes varies considerably among fish species (Magnadottir *et al.,* 2005). Generally, the first appearance of B-lymphocytes harboring superficial Ig is later in marine species compared to fresh water species. Rainbow trout and channel catfish show IgM positive lymphocytes at about 1 wk after hatching. Marine species like sea bass, spotted wolffish and cod show the first appearances of surface IgM 1-10 wk after hatching. Transfer of maternal antibody to eggs, embryos and hatchlings has been demonstrated in several species; examples include plaice, tilapia, carp, asian catfish, sea bass and salmon, but not cod (Magnadottir *et al.,* 2005; Swain *et al.,* 2006).

Mucosal surfaces are extensive in fishes: mucus covers external surfaces as well as internal ones. For this reason, the relationships between the mucosal and the systemic components of the immune system are interesting. That they are related is apparent from the fact that fish do develop detectable antibody levels after immersion in solutions of soluble and suspensions of particulate antigens; and these immunoglobulins can be detected in the gut, the bile, the gill mucus and the skin (Moore *et al.,* 1998; Nakanishi 1997). As described earlier, the antibodies found in mucus are slightly different structurally to serum immunoglobulins. Zhang *et al.*, (Zhang *et al.*, 2010), elegantly demonstrated the pressure to sustain essentially two adaptive immune systems-one systemic, scanning for pathogens infecting tissue and blood, and a second, perhaps more sublime system that is highly regulated and specific to mucosal surfaces.

Specific Cellular Immunity

Intracellular pathogens are controlled by cell-mediated immunity. The cell-mediated response in fish is similar to that in mammals and relies on the presence of accessory cells (macrophages) to present antigen to T-cells. The correct presentation of antigen results in a cascade of events that includes cytokine production that regulates or enhances the cellular response.

Specific cell-mediated immune responses have been demonstrated in both elasmobranches (sharks and rays) and teleost fishes. In both fish types, phenomena suggesting the presence of cytotoxic T-cells have been characterized: allograft rejection, graft-versus-host reaction (GVHR), delayed hypersensitivity reaction, and cell-mediated cytotoxicity against allogeneic target cells (Nakanishi *et al.*, 1999). Specific cellular immunity depends on cells bearing MHC class I receptors presenting antigens to CD8+ve T-lymphocytes. Most information on *in-vivo* cell-mediated immunity has come from transplantation experiments demonstrating host responses characterized by specificity and memory. For example, GVHR were demonstrated to follow the injection of allogenic triploid cells into tetraploid hosts, which were killed by the graft within a month (Nakanishi *et al.*, 1999; Nakanishi *et al.*, 1999). Delayed (type-IV) hypersensitivity reactions are also a cell-mediated immune phenomenon, which has been shown to take place after exposing fish to bacterial antigens (Iwama 1996) and to the protozoan parasites *Cryptobia salmositica* and *Ichthyophthirius multifiliis* (Thomas *et al.*, 1990). Since specific cell-mediated immune responses are restricted to MHC class I molecules, they may play a role in the recognition of viral antigens presented by infected cells (Nakanishi *et al.*, 1999). Recently, viral DNA vaccination was demonstrated to induce cytotoxic responses to virus-infected MHC class I matched targets (Utke *et al.*, 2007). Interactions between immune cells are mediated not only by direct cell-to-cell contact, but also through the release of soluble factors (cytokines).

Specific cell-mediated immunity in fish is to date a relatively poorly studied area in fish immunology. Despite breakthroughs in the cloning of the fish TcR and major histocompatibility (MHC) molecules, and more recently the CD3 and CD8 marker molecules, assays to measure specific T-cell responses are still in their infancy. The classical division of T-cells into cytotoxic (Tc) and helper (Th) subpopulations is probably relevant to fish, based on the presence of these functional activities and MHC class I and II molecules, but as yet even this is not definitively proved (Secombes *et al.*, 2005). Most CD4+ T-cells in the periphery are naive T-cells which produce mainly interleukin (IL)-2 and small amounts of IL-3 and granulocyte–macrophage colony-stimulating factor (GM-CSF). T-helper (Th) lymphocytes secrete a panel of cytokines which determine their functional role in immune regulation. The classic division of T helper subsets, Th1 and Th2, has recently been challenged as four lineages of naïve CD4+ T-cells have been recognized. Th cells are known to be divided into at least four subsets based on their cytokine production profile (Mosmann *et al.*, 1996). These are Th1, Th2, Th17 and Treg, each of which will produce a subset of cytokines.

The cells, which are at an intermediate stage of CD4+ T-cell development between naive and Th1/Th2/Th17/Treg cells, have the pattern of cytokine production of Th1/Th2/Th17/Treg cells. Generally, Th1 cytokines interleukin-2 (IL-2), interferon gamma (IFN-γ) and tumor necrosis factors alpha (TNF-α) and beta (TNF-β) induce defenses against intracellular pathogens by activating macrophages, enhancing antigen presentation and inducing T-cell differentiation and are also responsible for delayed-type hypersensitivity responses (Janeway CA 2005). In contrast, Th2 cytokines (IL-4, IL-5, IL-6, IL-10 and IL-13) activate B-cells and thus coordinate immunity against extracellular pathogens through antibody production and allergic responses (Janeway *et al.*, 2005; Mosmann *et al.*, 1996; Paul *et al.*, 1994). Similarly, Th17 cells are biased towards secretion of IL-17, IL-22, IL-21, and are involved in mucosal immunity and pathogenesis of autoimmune diseases (Kumari *et al.*, 2009b; Stockinger and Veldhoen 2007) and Treg cells secretes IL-10, and TGF-β and play crucial roles in the induction of peripheral tolerance to self and foreign antigens (Wu *et al.*, 2007). A number of ILs may still remain to be discovered in sh, many of which act on T and B-cells and are involved in the adaptive immune response. However, recently, Th1 responses mediated by IFN-γ have been shown functionally in rainbow trout *O. mykiss* (Zou *et al.*, 2005) and Atlantic salmon (Sun *et al.*, 2011) and Th2 responses mediated by IL-4 in pufferfish Tetraodon (Li *et al.*, 2007) and salmonids (Takizawa *et al.*, 2011). There is also evidence suggesting that infection by monogeneans of the genus *Gyrodactylus* induces Th1 responses in salmonids fishes (Buchmann K., 2004).

Besides these, transcription factors also play a crucial role in the T-cell differentiation. Studies in mammals have shown GATA-3 as the master regulator of Th2 differentiation inducing this differentiation even in absence of STAT6 (Ouyang *et al.*, 2000; Zheng *et al.*, 1997). Similarly, T-bet is the master regulator of Th1 differentiation (Mullen *et al.*, 2001; Szabo *et al.*, 2000). T-bet is required for type-1 helper immune response and may skew the development of naive CD4+ T-cells into Th1 cells by increasing the production of IFN-γ (Glimcher, 2007). ROR γt is required for Th17 differentiation and FoxP3 for Treg differentiation. In teleosts, the role of transcription factors have been reported for hematopoiesis in zebrafish (Hsia *et al.*, 2005) and for B-cell function in catfish (Hikima *et al.*, 2005) and torafugu (Ohtani *et al.*, 2006). However, little is known about transcription factors involved in T-cell function and the differentiation and maturation of T-cell subsets. Recently, important role of GATA-3, T-bet and FoxP3 in T-cell immune response has been elucidated in salmonids (Kumari *et al.*, 2009a; Wang *et al.*, 2010a; Wang *et al.*, 2010b), ginbuna carp (Takizawa *et al.*, 2008a; Takizawa *et al.*, 2008b) and cod (Chi et al., 2012), but further functional studies has to be done. Moreover, some recombinant proteins for T-cell associated cytokines and antibodies for T-cell surface receptors have been generated that will facilitate studying the functional roles of teleost T-cell during immune responses. Although there is still a long way to go, major advances have occurred in recent years for investigating T-cell responses, thus phenotypic and functional characterization is on the near horizon.

Conclusions

Innate immunity provides fish with pre-existing, fast-acting defense mechanisms which are relatively independent of temperature. These defenses are fundamental for poikilothermic organisms, and are effective against various types of pathogens. Teleosts can also mount acquired, immune responses, characterized by their specificity although these are slower than innate responses and late appearance of acquired parameters and are temperature-dependent.

Knowledge of the immune system of teleost fishes, apart from providing basic scientific information on the origin of defensive systems of higher vertebrates, has enables the development of methods to stimulate defenses of commercially-important fishes, reducing mortality and increasing productivity of fish farms. Vaccination is crucial for intensive aquaculture and has been essential to the success of salmon and trout farming. Apart from the vaccines available to protect salmonids there are reparations to immunize catfish, seabream, seabass, amberjack/yellowatil, tilapia and cod. In general, available vaccines have been developed empirically based on inactivated bacterial pathogens. Nonetheless, there are only a few commercial vaccines against viruses and there is none that protects against parasites. Increasing the knowledge of bony fish immunology will enable improvements to immune stimulation and vaccination regimes, which would significantly benefit aquaculture, an activity that will presumably become increasingly more relevant. The availability of 6 fish genomic databases (for zebrafish, fugu, green spotted pufferfish, stickleback, medaka and recently cod) will certainly fast tract the study of these fish-specific phenomenon. This will allow for a better understanding of overall fish immunity as well as how this relate to the evolution of innate and acquired immunity in vertebrates and their crosstalks. Knowledge of fish immunology would also enable a reduction of the environmental impact of fish farms, by decreasing the use of chemicals to prevent and control infections.

References

Arason GJ (1996). Lectins as defence molecules in vertebrates and invertebrates. Fish Shellfish Immunol 6: 277-289.

Brattgjerd S, Evensen O (1996). A sequential light microscopic and ultrastructural study on the uptake and handling of *Vibrio salmonicida* in phagocytes of the head kidney in experimentally infected Atlantic salmon (*Salmo salar* L). Vet Pathol 33: 55-65.

Buchmann K (1999). Immune mechanisms in fish skin against monogeneans - a model. Folia Parasitol 46: 1-9.

Buchmann K, Lindenstrom T, Bresciani J (2001). Defence mechanisms against parasites in fish and the prospect for vaccines. Acta Parasitologica 46: 71-81.

Buchmann K Lindenstrom T, Bresciani J (2004). Interactive associations between fish hosts and monogeneans. Symp Soc Exp Biol 55: 161-184.

Chen K, Xu W, Wilson M, *et al.* (2009). Immunoglobulin D enhances immune surveillance by activating antimicrobial, proinflammatory and B cell-stimulating programs in basophils. Nat Immunol 10: 889-898.

Chi H, Zhang Z, Inami M *et al.* (2012). Molecular characterizations and functional assessments of GATA-3 and its splice variant in Atlantic cod (*Gadus morhua* L.). Dev Comp Immunol 36: 491-501.

Dalmo RA, Ingebrigtsen K, Bogwald J (1997). Non-specific defence mechanisms in fish, with particular reference to the reticuloendothelial system (RES). J Fish Diseases 20: 241-273.

Danilova N, Bussmann J, Jekosch K *et al.* (2005). The immunoglobulin heavy-chain locus in zebrafish: identification and expression of a previously unknown isotype, immunoglobulin Z. Nature Immunology 6(3): 295-302.

Dannevig BH, Lauve A, Press CM *et al.* (1994). Receptor-mediated endocytosis and phagocytosis by rainbow-trout head kidney sinusoidal cells. Fish Shellfish Immunol 4: 3-18.

Endo Y, Takahashi M, Nakao M *et al.* (1998). Two lineages of mannose-binding lectin-associated serine protease (MASP). in vertebrates. Journal of Immunology 161: 4924-4930.

Ewart KV, Johnson SC, Ross NW (2001). Lectins of the innate immune system and their relevance to fish health. ICES J Mar Sci 58: 380-385.

Fearon DT (1997). Seeking wisdom in innate immunity. Nature 388: 323-324.

Fearon DT, Locksley RM (1996). Elements of immunity - The instructive role of innate immunity in the acquired immune response. Science 272: 50-54.

Fenton M, Golenbock D (1998). LPS-binding proteins and receptors. J Leukoc Biol 64: 25-32.

Glimcher LH (2007). Trawling for treasure: tales of T-bet. Nature immunology 8: 448-450.

Gongora R, Figueroa F, Klein J (1998). Independent duplications of Bf and C3 complement genes in the zebrafish. Scand J Immunol 48: 651-658.

Gonzalez R, Charlemagne J, Mahana W *et al.* (1988). Specificity of natural serum antibodies present in phylogenetically distinct fish species. Immunology 63: 31-36.

Herraez MP Zapata AG (1986). Structure and function of the melano-macrophage centres of the goldfish Carassius auratus. Vet Immunol Immunopathol 12: 117-126.

Hikima J, Middleton DL, Wilson MR *et al.* (2005). Regulation of immunoglobulin gene transcription in a teleost fish: identification, expression and functional properties of E2A in the channel catfish. Immunogenetics 57: 273-282.

Holvold LB (2007). Immunostimulants connecting innate and adaptive immunity in Atlantic salmon (*Salmo salar*). University of Tromso. http://www.ub.uit.no/munin/bitstream/handle/10037/1268/thesis.pdf?sequence=3.

Accessed 1 February 2012.

Hoover GJ, El-Mowafi A, Simko E *et al.* (1998). Plasma proteins of rainbow trout (*Oncorhynchus mykiss*) isolated by binding to lipopolysaccharide from *Aeromonas salmonicida*. Comp Biochem Physiol-Part B: Biochem Mol Biol 120: 559-569.

Hsia N, Zon LI (2005). Transcriptional regulation of hematopoietic stem cell development in zebrafish. Exp Hematol 33: 1007-1014.

Iwama G NT (1996). The Fish Immune System: Organism, Pathogen, and Environment Academic Press Limited, London.

Janeway CA, Travers P, Walport M *et al.* (2005). Immunobiology; the Immune System in Health and Disease. Garland Science Publishing, New York.

Joosten PHM, Kruijer WJ, Rombout JHWM (1996). Anal immunisation of carp and rainbow trout with different fractions of a *Vibrio anguillarumbacterin*. Fish Shellfish Immunol 6: 541-551.

Kaattari SL, Irwin MJ (1985). Salmonid spleen and anterior kidney harbor populations of lymphocytes with different B cell repertoires. Dev Comp Immunol 9: 433-444.

Kim KH, Whang YJ, Cho JB *et al.* (2000). Immunization of cultured juvenile rockfish Sebastes schlegeli against *Microcotyle sebastis* (Monogenea). Dis Aquat Organ 40: 29-32.

Kumari J, Bogwald J, Dalmo RA (2009a). Transcription factor GATA-3 in Atlantic salmon (Salmo salar): Molecular characterization, promoter activity and expression analysis. Mol Immunol 46: 3099-3107.

Kumari J, Larsen AN, Bogwald J *et al.* (2009b). Interleukin-17D in Atlantic salmon (*Salmo salar*): Molecular characterization, 3D modelling and promoter analysis. Fish Shellfish Immunol 27: 647-659.

Kumari J, Sahoo P (2005). High dietary vitamin C affects growth, non-specific immune responses and disease resistance in Asian catfish, Clarias batrachus. Mol Cell Biochem 280: 25-33.

Kumari J, Sahoo PK (2006). Non-specific immune response of healthy and immunocompromised Asian catfish (*Clarias batrachus*) to several immunostimulants. Aquaculture 255: 133-141.

Kuroda N, Naruse K, Shima A *et al.* (2000). Molecular cloning and linkage analysis of complement C3 and C4 genes of the Japanese medaka fish. Immunogenetics 51: 117-128.

Li JH, Shao JZ, Xiang LX *et al.* (2007). Cloning, characterization and expression analysis of pufferfish interleukin-4 cDNA: The first evidence of Th2-type cytokine in fish. Mol Immunol 44: 2078-2086.

Lygren B, Sveier H, Hjeltnes B *et al.* (1999). Examination of the immunomodulatory properties and the effect on disease resistance of dietary bovine lactoferrin and vitamin C fed to Atlantic salmon (Salmo salar). for a short-term period. Fish Shellfish Immunol 9: 95-107.

Magnadottir B (2006). Innate immunity of fish (overview). Fish Shellfish Immunol 20: 137-151.

Magnadottir B, Lange S, Gudmundsdottir S *et al.* (2005). Ontogeny of humoral immune parameters in fish. Fish Shellfish Immunol 19: 429-439.

Manning M (1998). Immune defence systems. Sheffield Academic Press, Sheffield.

Meseguer J, Lopez-Ruiz A, Garcia-Ayala A. (1995). Reticulo-endothelial stroma of the head-kidney from the seawater teleost gilthead seabream (Sparus aurata L.): an ultrastructural and cytochemical study. Anat Rec 241: 303-309.

Meylan E, Tschopp J (2006). Toll-Like Receptors and RNA Helicases: Two Parallel Ways to Trigger Antiviral Responses. Mol cell 22: 561-569.

Moore JD, Ototake M, Nakanishi T (1998). Particulate antigen uptake during immersion immunisation of fish: The effectiveness of prolonged exposure and the roles of skin and gill. Fish Shellfish Immunol 8: 393-407.

Mosmann TR, Sad S (1996). The expanding universe of T-cell subsets: Th1, Th2 and more. Immunol Today 17: 138-146.

Mullen AC, High FA, Hutchins AS *et al.* (2001). Role of T-bet in commitment of TH1 cells before IL-12-dependent selection. Science 292: 1907-1910.

Nakanishi T, Aoyagi K, Xia C *et al.* (1999). Specific cell-mediated immunity in fish. Veterinary Immunology and Immunopathology 72: 101-109.

Nakanishi T, Ototake M (1997). Antigen uptake and immune responses after immersion vaccination. Dev Biol Stand 90: 59-68.

Nakanishi T, Ototake M (1999). The graft-versus-host reaction (GVHR). in the ginbuna crucian carp, *Carassius auratus* langsdorfii. Dev Comp Immunol 23: 15-26.

Nakao M, Obo R, Mutsuro Ji, Yano T (1997). Sequence diversity of cDNA encoding the third component (C3) of carp (*Cyprinus carpio*) complement. Dev Comp Immunol 21: 144-144.

Nielsen ME, Esteve-Gassent MD (2006). The eel immune system: present knowledge and the need for research. J Fish Diseases 29: 65-78.

Nonaka M, Smith SL (2000). Complement system of bony and cartilaginous fish. Fish Shellfish Immunol 10: 215-228.

Ohta Y, Flajnik M (2006). IgD, like IgM, is a primordial immunoglobulin class perpetuated in most jawed vertebrates. Proceedings of the National Academy of Sciences 103: 10723-10728.

Ohtani M, Miyadai T, Hiroishi S (2006). Molecular cloning of the BCL-6 gene, a transcriptional repressor for B-cell differentiation, in torafugu (Takifugu rubripes). Mol Immunol 43: 1047-1053.

Ostergaard AE, Martin SAM, Wang T *et al.* (2009). Rainbow trout (Oncorhynchus mykiss) possess multiple novel immunoglobulin-like transcripts containing either an ITAM or ITIMs. Developmental and Comparative Immunology 33: 525-532.

Ouyang W, Lohning M, Gao Z, *et al.* (2000). Stat6-independent GATA-3 autoactivation directs IL-4-independent Th2 development and commitment. Immunity 12: 27-37.

Paul WE, Seder RA (1994). Lymphocyte responses and cytokines. Cell (Cambridge) 76: 241-251.

Press CM, Evensen O (1999). The morphology of the immune system in teleost fishes. Fish Shellfish Immunol 9: 309-318.

Press CML, Evensen O (1999). The morphology of the immune system in teleost fishes. Fish Shellfish Immunol 9: 309-318.

Quesenberry MS, Ahmed H, Elola MT *et al.* (2003). Diverse lectin repertoires in tunicates mediate broad recognition and effector innate immune responses. Integr Comp Biol 43: 323-330.

Reite OB, Evensen O (2006). Inflammatory cells of teleostean fish: a review focusing on mast cells/eosinophilic granule cells and rodlet cells. Fish Shellfish Immunol 20: 192-208.

Robertsen B (2006). The interferon system of teleost fish. Fish Shellfish Immunol 20: 172-91.

Rubio-Godoy M (2010). Teleost fish immunology. Review. Tec Pecu Mex 48: 47-57.

Rubio-Godoy M Sigh J, Buchmann K *et al.* (2003). Immunization of rainbow trout Oncorhynchus mykiss against Discocotyle sagiffata (Monogenea). Dis Aquat Organ 55: 23-30.

Sahu A, Lambris JD (2001). Structure and biology of complement protein C3, a connecting link between innate and acquired immunity. Immunological Reviews 180: 35-48.

Sakai DK (1992). Repertoire of complement in immunological defense mechanisms of fish. Annu Rev Fish Dis 2: 223-247.

Saurabh S, Sahoo PK (2008). Lysozyme: an important defence molecule of fish innate immune system. Aquacult Res 39: 223-239.

Secombes CJ (1997). 2 The Nonspecific Immune System: Cellular Defenses. Fish Physiol 15: 63-103.

Secombes CJ, Bird S, Zou J (2005). Adaptive immunity in teleosts: cellular immunity. Dev Biol (Basel) 121: 25-32.

Sepulcre MP, Lopez-Castejon G, Meseguer J *et al.* (2007). The activation of gilthead seabream professional phagocytes by different PAMPs underlines the behavioural diversity of the main innate immune cells of bony fish. Molecular Immunology 44: 2009-2016.

Silphaduang U, Colorni A, Noga EJ (2006). Evidence for widespread distribution of piscidin antimicrobial peptides in teleost fish. Dis Aquat Organ 72: 241-252.

Silphaduang U, Noga EJ (2001). Antimicrobials: Peptide antibiotics in mast cells of fish. Nature 414: 268-269.

Jones SR (2001). The occurrence and mechanisms of innate immunity against parasites in fish. Developmental and Comparative Immunology 25: 841-852.

Slierendrecht WJ, Jensen LB, Horlyck V *et al.* (1993). Genetic polymorphism of complement component C3 in rainbow trout (*Oncorhynchus mykiss*) and resistance to viral haemorrhagic septicaemia. Fish Shellfish Immunol 3: 199-206.

Sommerset I, Krossoy B, Biering E *et al.* (2005). Vaccines for fish in aquaculture. Expert Review of Vaccines 4: 89-101.

Stein C, Caccamo M, Laird G *et al.* (2007). Conservation and divergence of gene families encoding components of innate immune response systems in zebrafish. Genome Biol 8: R251.

Stockinger B, Veldhoen M (2007). Differentiation and function of Th17 T cells. Curr Opin Immunol 19: 281-286.

Sun BJ, Skjaeveland I, Svingerud T *et al.* (2011). Antiviral Activity of Salmonid Gamma Interferon against Infectious Pancreatic Necrosis Virus and Salmonid Alphavirus and Its Dependency on Type I Interferon. Journal of Virology 85: 9188-9198.

Sunyer JO, Tort L (1995). Natural hemolytic and bactericidal activities of sea bream Sparus aurata serum are effected by the alternative complement pathway. Veterinary Immunology and Immunopathology 45: 333-345.

Sunyer JO, Tort L, Lambris JD (1997). Diversity of the third form of complement, C3, in fish: Functional characterization of five forms of C3 in the diploid fish *Sparus aurata*. Biochem J 326: 877-881.

Sunyer JO, Zarkadis IK, Sahu A *et al.* (1996). Multiple forms of complement C3 in trout that differ in binding to complement activators. Proc Natl Acad Sci USA 93: 8546-8551.

Swain P, Dash S, Bal J, *et al.* (2006). Passive transfer of maternal antibodies and their existence in eggs, larvae and fry of Indian major carp, *Labeo rohita* (Ham.). Fish Shellfish Immunol 20: 519-527.

Swain T, Mohanty J, Sahu AK (2004). One step purification and partial characterisation of serum immunoglobulin from Asiatic catfish (*Clarias batrachus* L.). Fish Shellfish Immunol 17: 397-401.

Szabo SJ, Kim ST, Costa GL *et al.* (2000). A novel transcription factor, T-bet, directs Th1 lineage commitment. Cell 100: 655-669.

Takizawa F, Araki K, Kobayashi I *et al.* (2008a). Molecular cloning and expression analysis of T-bet in ginbuna crucian carp (*Carassius auratus* Langsdorfii). Mol Immunol 45: 127-136.

Takizawa F, Koppang EO, Ohtani M, *et al.* (2011). Constitutive high expression of interleukin-4/13A and GATA-3 in gill and skin of salmonid fishes suggests that these tissues form Th2-skewed immune environments. Mol Immunol 48: 1360-1368.

Takizawa F, Mizunaga Y, Araki K *et al.* (2008b). GATA3 mRNA in ginbuna crucian carp (*Carassius auratus* Langsdorfii): cDNA cloning, splice variants and expression analysis. Developmental and Comparative Immunology 32: 898-907.

Thomas PT, Woo PTK (1990). *In vivo* and *in vitro* cell-mediated immune responses of rainbow trout, *Oncorhynchus mykiss* (Walbaum), against *Cryptobia salmositica* Katz, 1951 (Sarcomastigophora: Kinetoplastida). J Fish Dis 13: 423-433.

Tort L, Balasch JC, Mackenzie S (2003). Fish immune system. A crossroads between innate and adaptive responses. Immunologia 22: 277-286.

Tsujii T, Seno S (1990). Melano-macrophage centers in the aglomerular kidney of the sea horse (teleosts) - morphologic studies on its formation and possible function. Anat Rec 226: 460-470.

Utke K, Bergmann S, Lorenzen N *et al.* (2007). Cell-mediated cytotoxicity in rainbow trout, *Oncorhynchus mykiss*, infected with viral haemorrhagic septicaemia virus. Fish Shellfish Immunol 22: 182-196.

Wang T, Holland JW, Martin SAM *et al.* (2010a). Sequence and expression analysis of two T helper master transcription factors, T-bet and GATA3, in rainbow trout Oncorhynchus mykiss and analysis of their expression during bacterial and parasitic infection. Fish Shellfish Immunol 29: 705-715.

Wang T, Monte MM, Huang W, Boudinot P, Martin SAM, Secombes CJ (2010b). Identification of two FoxP3 genes in rainbow trout (*Oncorhynchus mykiss*) with differential induction patterns. Molecular Immunology 47: 2563-2574.

Wardle CS (1971). New Observations on the Lymph System of the Plaice Pleuronectes Platessa and other Teleosts. J Mar Biol Assoc UK 51: 977-990.

Woo PTK (2007). Protective immunity in fish against protozoan diseases. Parassitologia 49: 185-191.

Woof JM, Kerr M (2006). The function of immunoglobulin A in immunity. J Pathol 208: 270-282.

Workenhe ST, Rise ML, Kibenge MJT *et al.* (2010). The fight between the teleost fish immune response and aquatic viruses. Mol Immunol 47: 2525-2536.

Wu K, Bi YT, Sun K *et al.* (2007). IL-10-Producing Type 1 regulatory T cells and allergy. Cellular and Molecular Immunology 4: 269-275.

Zapata AG, Chiba A, Varas A (1997). 1 Cells and Tissues of the Immune System of Fish. 15: 1-62.

Zarkadis IK, Mastellos D, Lambris JD (2001). Phylogenetic aspects of the complement system. Dev Comp Immunol 25: 745-762.

Zhang YA, Salinas I, Li J, *et al.* (2010). IgT, a primitive immunoglobulin class specialized in mucosal immunity. Nature Immunology 11: 827-835.

Zhang Z, Swain T, Bogwald J *et al.* (2009). Bath immunostimulation of rainbow trout (*Oncorhynchus mykiss*) fry induces enhancement of inflammatory cytokine transcripts, while repeated bath induce no changes. Fish Shellfish Immunol 26: 677-684.

Zheng W, Flavell RA (1997). The transcription factor GATA-3 is necessary and sufficient for Th2 cytokine gene expression in CD4 T cells. Cell 89: 587-596.

Zou J, Carrington A, Collet B *et al.* (2005). Identification and bioactivities of IFN-gamma in rainbow trout *Oncorhynchus mykiss*: The first Th1-type cytokine characterized functionally in fish. Journal of Immunology 175: 2484-2494.

Zou J, Secombes CJ (2011). Teleost fish interferons and their role in immunity. Dev Comp Immunol 35: 1376-1387.

2014, Advances in Biochemistry and Biotechnology Volume 2   *Pages 99-120*

Edited by: Dr. Biplab Sarkar and Dr. Chiranjib Chakraborty

Published by: DAYA PUBLISHING HOUSE

7

Anticancer Drugs Designed by Mother Nature: An Old Lock Needs a New Key

Chanakya Nath Kundu*, Purusottam Mohapatra, Ranjan Preet,
Dipon Das and Shakti Ranjan Satapathy

KIIT School of Biotechnology, KIIT University, Campus-11, Patia,
Bhubaneswar – 751 024, Orissa, India

ABSTRACT

Carcinogenesis is a multistage process consisting of initiation, promotion and progression phases involving sequential generations of cells that exhibit continuous disturbance of cellular and molecular signalling cascades. Agents that can suppress these multiple pathways have great potential as chemoprevention. In recent years, natural products which have been traditionally used for treatment of multiple ailments or other purposes, received a great attention for cancer prevention owing to their various health benefits, noticeable lack of toxicity and side effects, and the limitations of chemotherapeutic agents. A variety of grains, cereals, nuts, soy products,

* *Corresponding author.* E-mail: cnkundu@gmail.com

olives, beverages such as tea and coffee, and spices including turmeric, garlic, ginger, black pepper, cumin, caraway and several medicinal plant derived products consists of a wide variety of biologically active phytochemicals including phenolics, flavonoids, carotenoids, alkaloids, nitrogen containing as well as organosulfur compounds and small molecule, which have been shown to suppress early and late stages of carcinogenesis. In this present review, we have given an overview about cancer and anti cancer potentiality of natural products including fruits, vegetables, spices, and medicinal plants derived agents. We have cited a comparison between synthetic and plant derived anti cancer drugs. In addition, we have provided evidence that cancer is a preventable disease that requires major lifestyle changes.

Keywords: Synthetic drugs, Natural anti cancer agents, Medicinal plants.

Introduction

Cancer is a frightful disease and is one of the chief killers now-a-days. It is a class of diseases in which a group of cells display uncontrolled growth, invasion and destruction of adjacent tissues. Cancer may affect people at all ages, even foetuses, but the risk for most varieties increases with age. Cancer causes about 13 per cent of all human deaths. According to the American Cancer Society, 7.6 million people died from cancer in the world during 2007.

Mainly cancerous cells have two properties, (1) reproduce in defiance of the normal restrains on cell division and (2) invade and colonize territories normally reserved for other cells. Combination of these actions makes cancers peculiarly dangerous. An isolated abnormal cell whose proliferation is out of control, will give rise to a *tumor* or *neoplasm*–a relentlessly growing mass of abnormal cells. As long as the neoplastic cells remain clustered together in a single mass, the tumor is said to be benign and when its cells have acquired the ability to invade surrounding tissue, considered as malignant. The property of invasiveness usually implies an ability to break, loose, enter the bloodstream or lymphatic vessels and form secondary tumors called metastasis at other sites of the body. Today, the Greek term *carcinoma* is the medical term for a malignant tumour derived from epithelial cells. It is Celsus who translated *carcinos* into the Latin *cancer*, also meaning crab. Galen used "*oncos*" to describe *all* tumours, the root for the modern word oncology. Hippocrates described several kinds of cancers. He called benign tumours *oncos*, Greek for swelling, and malignant tumours *carcinos*, Greek for crab or crayfish. This name comes from the appearance of the cut surface of a solid malignant tumour, with "the veins stretched on all sides as the animal the crab has its feet, whence it derives its name". He later added the suffix -*oma*, Greek for swelling, giving the name *carcinoma*. Since it was against Greek tradition to open the body, Hippocrates only described and made drawings of outwardly visible tumours on the skin, nose, and breasts.

Cancer is a multistage process consisting of initiation, promotion and progression phases involving sequential generations of cells that exhibit continuous disturbance of cellular and molecular signal cascades. Agents that can suppress these multiple pathways have great potential for chemoprevention. An ideal chemopreventive agent should have (i) little or no toxicity, (ii) high efficacy in multiple sites, (iii) capability of oral consumption, (iv) known mechanisms of action, (v) low cost, and (vi) human acceptance. Natural products have great attention for cancer prevention owing to their various health benefits, noticeable lack of toxicity and side effects, and the limitations of chemotherapeutic agents. Overall, natural products have been used worldwide as traditional medicines for thousands of years to treat various forms of diseases including cancer. Several studies have revealed that natural products exhibit an extensive spectrum of biological activities such as, stimulation of the immune system, antibacterial, antiviral, anti-hepatotoxic, anti-ulcer, anti-inflammatory, antioxidant, anti-mutagenic, and anti-cancer effects. Very recently, scientists are checking the anticancer potentiality of natural products which were earlier used for treatment of other ailment. A variety of grains, cereals, nuts, soy products, olives, beverages such as tea and coffee, and spices including turmeric, garlic, ginger, black pepper, cumin and caraway confer a protective effect against cancer. Several studies have also documented the relationship between decreased cancer risk and high consumption of vegetables, including cabbage, cauliflower, broccoli, brussels sprout, tomatoes, and fruits such as, apples, grapes, and berries. In addition, a number of medicinal plants and herbs such as milk thistle have also been reported to reduce the risk of cancer in multiple sites. In particular, natural products consist of a wide variety of biologically active phytochemicals including phenolics, flavonoids, carotenoids, alkaloids and nitrogen containing as well as organosulfur compounds, which have been shown to suppress early and late stages of carcinogenesis. Several epidemiological studies have validated the inverse relation between the consumption of natural products and the risk of wide range of human cancers including colon, breast, prostate, etc. Cancer is the preventable diseases for prevention little of lifestyle changes is needed.

Types of Cancer

Cancers are classified according to the tissue and cell type from which they arise. Examples of general categories include:

☆ *Carcinoma*: Malignant tumours derived from epithelial cells. This group represents the most common cancers, including the common forms of breast, prostate, lung and colon cancer.

☆ *Sarcoma*: Malignant tumours arise from the tissues derived from mesoderm such as connective tissues (bones, cartilages, tendons, and adipose tissue), lymphoid tissue and muscles.

☆ *Osteoma*: It is the cancer of bones.

☆ *Lymphoma and leukaemia*: Malignancies derived from hematopoietic (blood-forming) cells

☆ *Germ cell tumour*: Tumours derived from totipotent cells. In adults most often found in the testicle and ovary; in foetuses, babies, and young children most often found on the body midline, particularly at the tip of the tailbone; in horses most often found at the poll (base of the skull).

☆ *Blastic tumour or blastoma*: A tumour (usually malignant) which resembles an immature or embryonic tissue. Many of these tumours are most common in children.

☆ *Myeloma (multiple myeloma or Kahler's disease)*: It is a type of cancer of plasma cells (B-lymphocytes) which are immune system cells in bone marrow that produces antibodies.

☆ *Melanoma*: It is the cancer of the pigment producing cells present especially in the skin (melanocytes).

About 90 per cent of human cancers are carcinomas, perhaps because most of the cell proliferation in the body occurs in epithelia, or because epithelial tissues are most frequently exposed to the various forms of physical and chemical damage that favour the development of cancer.

Causes of Cancer

Cancer is neither hereditary nor a contagious disease. It can be caused by countless unknown reasons. Chemical and physical agents that can cause cancer are called carcinogens. Examples of such carcinogens are coal tar, N-nitrosodimehylene present in cigarette smoke, cadmium oxide, mustard gas, asbestos, caffeine, nicotine, UV rays, X-rays etc. Cancer of large intestine is linked to with diet rich in animal protein or low in cereals. Dye workers have a high rate of bladder cancer and chimney sweepers tend to develop scrotum cancer. Sedentary life style and food habits are the major cause of cancer in developed countries.

Many biological agents such as bacteria and viruses can also cause cancer. Viruses that are involved with cancer include the human papilloma virus, which causes cervical cancer, the human T-cells lymphocytic virus, and hepatitis B virus. Known bacterial agents related to various cancers are *Helicobacter pylori*, *Helicobacter hepaticus*, *Enterococcus faecalis* and *Citrobacter rodentium* etc. (Pagano *et al.*, 2004).

Signs and Symptoms

Symptoms of cancer metastasis depend on the location of the tumour. Roughly, cancer symptoms can be divided into three groups:

☆ *Local symptoms*: Unusual lumps or swelling (tumour), haemorrhage (bleeding), pain and ulceration. Compression of surrounding tissues may cause symptoms such as jaundice (yellowing of the eyes and skin).

☆ *Symptoms of metastasis*: Enlarged lymph nodes, cough, hepatomegaly *i.e.* enlarged liver, bone pain, fracture of affected bones and neurological symptoms. Although advanced cancer may cause pain, it is often not the first symptoms.

☆ *Systemic symptoms*: Weight loss, poor appetite, fatigue and cachexia (wasting), excessive sweating (night sweats), anaemia and specific paraneoplastic phenomena, i.e. specific conditions that are due to an active cancer, such as thrombosis or hormonal changes.

Diagnosis and Treatments

Early detection of cancer can greatly improve the odds of successful treatment and survival. Physicians use information from symptoms and several other procedures to diagnose cancer. Imaging techniques such as X-rays, CT scans, endoscopy, MRI scans, PET scans, and ultrasound scans are used regularly in order to detect where a tumour is located and what organs may be affected by it. Recently DNA based techniques also available for early detection of cancer.

Surgical Treatment

At benign stage, a complete cure can usually be achieved by removing the mass surgically but in case of malignant tumor, it becomes difficult to eradicate due to its metastasis.

Radiotherapy

X-rays are used to destroy the cancer cells with radiotherapy. X-rays can be administered by a variety of machines and devices to many sites of the body. Two types of radiotherapies internal and external are used to treat the various types of cancer. Radiotherapy has many side effects which includes fatigue, nausea, vomiting, hair loss, mouth ulcers, skin changes, abdominal or chest problems.

Chemotherapy

Synthetic Drugs

Chemotherapy drugs are sometimes feared because of a patient's concern about toxic effects. Their role is too slow and hopefully halts the growth and spread of a cancer. There are three goals associated with the use of the most commonly-used anticancer agents.

1. Damages the DNA of the affected cancer cells.
2. Inhibits the synthesis of new DNA strands to stop the cell from replicating.
3. Stops mitosis or the cell division (replication) of the original cell into two new cells.

The majority of drugs currently on the market are not specific, which leads to the many common side effects associated with cancer chemotherapy. Because the common approach of all chemotherapy is to decrease the growth rate (cell division) of the cancer cells, the side effects are seen in bodily systems that naturally have a rapid turnover of cells including skin, hair, gastrointestinal, and bone marrow. These healthy, normal cells also end up damaged by the chemotherapy programme. In general, chemotherapy agents can be divided into three main categories based on their mechanism of action.

Directly Damages the DNA in the Nucleus of the Cell

These agents chemically damage DNA and RNA. They disrupt replication of the DNA and either totally halts replication or cause the manufacture of nonsense DNA or RNA (*i.e.* the new DNA or RNA does not code for anything useful). Examples of drugs in this class include cisplatin (Platinol), antibiotics - daunorubicin (Cerubidine), doxorubicin (Adriamycin), and etoposide (VePesid).

Stops the Synthesis of Pre-DNA Molecule Building Blocks

These agents work in a number of different ways. DNA building blocks are folic acid, heterocyclic bases, and nucleotides, which are made naturally within cells. All of these agents work to block some step in the formation of nucleotides or deoxyribonucleotides (necessary for making DNA). When these steps are blocked, the nucleotides, which are the building blocks of DNA and RNA, cannot be synthesized. Thus the cells cannot replicate because they cannot make DNA without the nucleotides. Examples of drugs in this class include (1) methotrexate (Abitrexate), (2) fluorouracil (Adrucil), (3) hydroxyurea (Hydrea), and (4) mercaptopurine (Purinethol).

Effects the Synthesis or Breakdown of the Mitotic Spindles

Mitotic spindles serve as molecular railroads with "North and South Poles" in the cell when a cell starts to divide itself into two new cells. These spindles are very important because they help to split the newly copied DNA such that a copy goes to each of the two new cells during cell division. These drugs disrupt the formation of these spindles and therefore interrupt cell division. Examples of drugs in this class of 8) mitotic disrupters include: Vinblastine (Velban), Vincristine (Oncovin) and Pacitaxel (Taxol).

The various chemotherapy drugs and their mechanism of actions are described below.

1. *Methotrexate*: Methotrexate inhibits folic acid reductase which is responsible for the conversion of folic acid to tetrahydrofolic acid. At two stages in the biosynthesis of purines (adenine and guanine) and at one stage in the synthesis of pyrimidines (thymine, cytosine, and uracil), one-carbon transfer reactions occur which require specific coenzymes synthesized in the cell from Tetrahydrofolic acid itself is synthesized in the cell from folic acid with the help of an enzyme, folic acid reductase. Methotrexate looks a lot like folic acid to the enzyme, so it binds to it thinking that it is folic acid. In fact, methotrexate looks so good to the enzyme that it binds to it quite strongly and inhibits the enzyme. Thus, DNA synthesis cannot proceed because the coenzymes needed for one-carbon transfer reactions are not produced from tetrahydrofolic acid because there is no tetrahydrofolic acid. Again, without DNA, no cell division will be there (Van Scott *et al.,* 1960).

2. *5-Fluorouracil*: 5-Fluorouracil (5-FU; Adrucil, Fluorouracil, Efudex, Fluoroplex) is an effective pyrimidine antimetabolite. Fluorouracil is synthesized into the nucleotide, 5-fluoro-2-deoxyuridine. This product acts as an antimetabolite by inhibiting the synthesis of 2-deoxythymidine because the carbon - fluorine bond is extremely stable and prevents the addition of a methyl group in the 5-position. The failure to synthesize the thymidine nucleotide results in little or no production of DNA. Two other similar drugs include: gemcitabine (Gemzar) and arabinosylcytosine (araC). They all work through similar mechanisms (Longley *et al.*, 2003).

3. *Hydroxyurea*: Hydroxyurea blocks an enzyme which converts the cytosine nucleotide into the deoxy derivative (Stearns *et al.*, 1963). In addition, DNA synthesis is further inhibited because hydroxyurea blocks the incorporation of the thymidine nucleotide into the DNA strand.

4. *Mercaptopurine*: Mercaptopurine, a chemical analogue of the purine adenine, inhibits the biosynthesis of adenine nucleotides by acting as an antimetabolite (Pershin *et al.*, 1962). In the body, 6-MP is converted to the corresponding ribonucleotide. 6-MP ribonucleotide is a potent inhibitor of the conversion of a compound called inosinic acid to adenine. Without adenine, DNA cannot be synthesized. 6-MP also works by being incorporated into nucleic acids as thioguanosine, rendering the resulting nucleic acids (DNA, RNA) unable to direct proper protein synthesis.

5. *Thioguanine*: Thioguanine works as an antimetabolite in the synthesis of guanine nucleotides (Chojnacki *et al.*, 1975).

6. *Nitrosureas*: Cyclosporamide is a classical example of the role of the host metabolism in the activation of an alkylating agent and is one or the most widely used agents of this class. It was hoped that the cancer cells might possesses enzymes capable of accomplishing the cleavage, thus resulting in the selective production of activated nitrogen mustard in the malignant cells. Compare the top and bottom structures in the graphic on the left.

7. *Antibiotics*: A number of antibiotics such as anthracyclines, dactinomycin, bleomycin, adriamycin, mithramycin, bind to DNA and inactivate it. Thus the synthesis of RNA is prevented. General properties of these drugs include: interaction with DNA in a variety of different ways including intercalation (squeezing between the base pairs), DNA strand breakage and inhibition with the enzyme topoisomerase II. Most of these compounds have been isolated from natural sources and antibiotics. However, they lack the specificity of the antimicrobial antibiotics and thus produce significant toxicity. The anthracyclines are among the most important antitumor drugs available. Doxorubicin is widely used for the treatment of several solid tumours while daunorubicin and idarubicin are used exclusively for the treatment of leukaemia. These agents have a number of important effects including: intercalating (squeezing between the base pairs) with DNA affecting many functions of the DNA including DNA and RNA synthesis. Breakage of the DNA strand can also occur by inhibition of the enzyme topoisomerase II. *Dactinomycin* (Actinomycin D): At low concentrations dactinomycin inhibits DNA directed RNA synthesis and at higher concentrations DNA synthesis is also inhibited. All types of RNA are affected, but ribosomal RNA is more sensitive. Dactinomycin binds to double stranded DNA, permitting RNA chain initiation but blocking chain elongation. Binding to the DNA depends on the presence of guanine.

8. *Mitotic Disrupters*: Plant alkaloids like vincristine prevent cell division, or mitosis. There are several phases of mitosis, one of which is the metaphase. During metaphase, the cell pulls duplicated DNA chromosomes to either side of the parent cell in structures called "spindles". These spindles ensure that each new cell gets a full set of DNA. Spindles are microtubular fibers formed with the help of the protein "tubulin". Vincristine binds to tubulin, thus preventing the formation of spindles and cell division.

9. *Carboplatin and Cisplatin*: These related drugs covalently bind to DNA with preferential binding to the N-7 position of guanine and adenine. They are able to bind to two different sites on DNA producing cross-links, either intrastrand (within the same DNA molecule which results in inhibition of DNA synthesis and transcription.

Bioactive Compounds

Cancer Prevention by Fruits and Vegetables

The fact that only 5–10 per cent of all cancer cases are due to genetic defects and that the remaining 90–95 per cent are due to environment and lifestyle provides major opportunities for preventing cancer. Because tobacco, diet, infection, obesity, and other factors contribute approximately 25–30 per cent, 30–35 per cent, 15–20 per cent, 10–20 per cent, and 10–15 per cent, respectively, to the incidence of all cancer deaths in the USA, it is clear how we can prevent cancer. Almost 90 per cent of patients diagnosed with lung cancer are cigarette smokers; and cigarette smoking combined with alcohol intake can synergistically contribute to tumorigenesis. Similarly, smokeless tobacco is responsible for 400,000 cases (4 per cent of all cancers) of oral cancer worldwide. Thus avoidance of tobacco products and minimization of alcohol consumption would likely have a major effect on cancer incidence. Infection by various bacteria and viruses is another very prominent cause of various cancers. Vaccines for cervical cancer and HCC should help prevent some of these cancers, and a cleaner environment and modified lifestyle behaviour would be even more helpful in preventing infection caused cancers.

The first FDA approved chemopreventive agent was tamoxifen, for reducing the risk of breast cancer. This agent was found to reduce the breast cancer incidence by 50 per cent in women at high risk. With tamoxifen, there is an increased risk of serious side effects such as uterine cancer, blood clots, ocular disturbances, hypercalcemia, and stroke. Recently it has been shown that an osteoporosis drug raloxifene is as effective as tamoxifen in preventing estrogen-receptor-positive, invasive breast cancer but had fewer side effects than tamoxifen. Though it is better than tamoxifen with respect to side effects, it can cause blood clots and stroke. Other potential side effects of raloxifene include hot flashes, leg cramps, swelling of the legs and feet, flu-like symptoms, joint pain, and sweating.

The second chemopreventive agent to reach to clinic was finasteride, for prostate cancer, which was found to reduce incidence by 25 per cent in men at high risk. The recognized side effects of this agent include erectile dysfunction, lowered sexual desire, impotence and gynecomastia. Celecoxib, a COX-2 inhibitor is another approved agent for prevention of familial adenomatous polyposis (FAP). However, the chemopreventive benefit of celecoxib is at the cost of its serious cardiovascular harm. The serious side effects of the FDA approved chemopreventive drugs is an issue of particular concern when considering long-term administration of a drug to healthy people who may or may not develop cancer. This clearly indicates the need for agents, which are safe and efficacious in preventing cancer. Diet derived natural products will be potential candidates for this purpose. Diet, obesity, and metabolic syndrome are very much linked to various cancers and may account for as much as 30–35 per cent of cancer deaths, indicating that a reasonably good fraction of cancer deaths can be prevented by modifying the diet. Extensive research has revealed that a diet consisting of fruits, vegetables, spices, and grains has the potential to prevent cancer. The specific substances in these dietary foods that are responsible for preventing cancer and the mechanisms by which they achieve this have also been examined extensively. Various phytochemicals have been identified in fruits, vegetables, spices, and grains that exhibit chemopreventive potential, and numerous studies have shown that a proper diet can help protect against cancer (Divisi *et al.*, 2006). Below is a description of selected dietary agents and diet-derived phytochemicals that have been studied extensively to determine their role in cancer prevention.

Fruits and Vegetables

The protective role of fruits and vegetables against cancers that occur in various anatomical sites is now well supported (Divisi *et al.*, 2006). In 1966, Wattenberg (Wattenberg *et al.*, 1966) proposed for the first time that the regular consumption of certain constituents in fruits and vegetables might provide protection from cancer. According to a 1997 estimate, approximately 30–40 per cent of cancer cases worldwide were preventable by feasible dietary means. Several studies have addressed the cancer chemopreventive effects of the active components derived from fruits and vegetables. More than 25,000 different phytochemicals have been identified that may have potential against various cancers. These phytochemicals have advantages because they are safe and usually target multiple cell-signalling pathways (Aggarwal and Shishodia 2006). Major chemopreventive compounds identified from fruits and vegetables (Figures 7.1–7.3) include carotenoids, vitamins, resveratrol, quercetin, silymarin, sulphoraphane and indole-3-carbinol.

Carotenoids

Various natural carotenoids present in fruits and vegetables were reported to have anti-inflammatory and anticarcinogenic activity. Lycopene is one of the main carotenoids in the regional Mediterranean diet and can account for 50 per cent of the carotenoids in human serum. Lycopene is present in fruits, including watermelon, apricots, pink guava, grapefruit, rosehip, and tomatoes. A wide variety of processed tomato based products account for more than 85 per cent of dietary lycopene. The anticancer activity of lycopene has been demonstrated in both *in vitro* and *in vivo* tumor models as well as in humans. The proposed mechanisms for the anticancer effect of lycopene involve ROS scavenging, upregulation of detoxification systems, interference with cell proliferation, induction of gap-junctional communication, inhibition of cell-cycle progression, and modulation of signal transduction pathways. Other carotenoids reported to have anticancer activity include beta-carotene, alpha-carotene, lutein, zeaxanthin, beta-cryptoxanthin, fucoxanthin, astaxanthin, capsanthin, crocetin, and phytoene (Nishino *et al.*, 2002).

Resveratrol

The stilbene resveratrol has been found in fruits such as grapes, peanuts, and berries. Resveratrol exhibits anticancer properties against a wide variety of tumors, including lymphoid and myeloid cancers, multiple myeloma, and cancers of the breast, prostate, stomach, colon, and pancreas. The growth-inhibitory effects of resveratrol are mediated through cell-cycle arrest; induction of apoptosis via Fas/CD95, p53, ceramide activation, tubulin polymerization, mitochondrial and adenylyl cyclase pathways; up-regulation of p21 p53 and Bax; down-regulation of survivin, cyclin D1, cyclin E, Bcl-2, Bcl-xL, and cellular inhibitor of apoptosis proteins; activation of caspases; suppression of nitric oxide synthase; suppression of transcription factors such as NF-κB, AP-1, and early growth response-1; inhibition of cyclooxygenase-2 (COX-2) and lipoxygenase; suppression of adhesion molecules; and inhibition of angiogenesis, invasion, and metastasis. Limited data in humans have revealed that

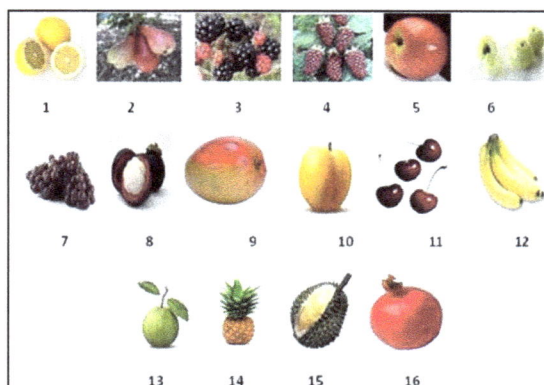

Figure 7.1

1: Citrus fruits; 2: Malay apple; 3: Blackberry; 4: Dessert date; 5: Apple; 6: Indian gooseberry; 7: Grapes; 8: Mangosteen; 9: Mango 10: Apricot; 11: Cherry; 12: Banana; 13: Guava; 14: Pineapple; 15: Durian; 16: Pomegranate:

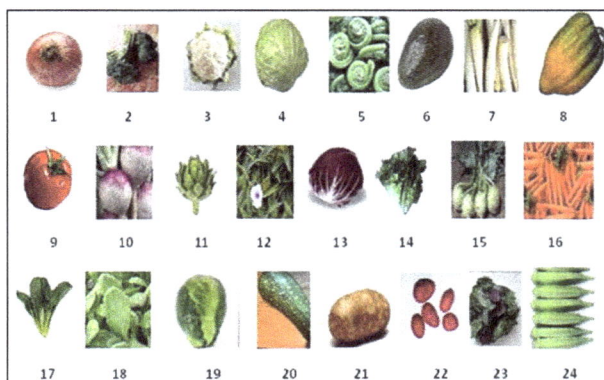

Figure 7.2

1: Onion; 2: Broccoli; 3: Cauliflower; 4: Cabbage; 5: Fiddle head; 6: Avocado; 7: Daikon; 8: Winter squash; 9: Tomato; 10: Turnip; 11: Artichoke; 12: Water cress; 13: Radicchio; 14: Lettuce; 15: Kohlrabi; 16: Carrot; 17: Komatsuna; 18: Salt bush; 19: Brussels sprout; 20: Zucchini; 21: Potato; 22: Ulluco; 23: Spinach; 24: Okra.

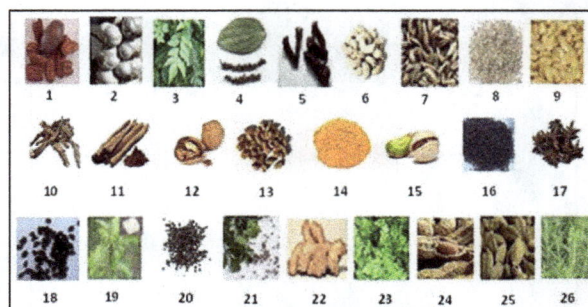

Figure 7.3

1: Pecan; 2: Garlic; 3: Curry leaves; 4: Black pepper; 5: Clove; 6: Cashew nut; 7: Fennel; 8: Sesame seed; 9: Flax seed; 10: Licorice; 11: Cinnamon; 12: Walnut; 13: Fenugreek; 14: Turmeric; 15: Pistachio; 16: Mustard; 17: Star anise; 18: Kalonji; 19: Camphor; 20: Black mustard; 21: Coriander; 22: Ginger; 23: Parsley; 24: Peanut; 25: Cardamom; 26: Rosemary.

resveratrol is pharmacologically safe. As a nutraceutical, resveratrol is commercially available in the USA and Europe in 50 μg to 60 mg doses. Currently, structural analogues of resveratrol with improved bioavailability are being pursued as potential chemopreventive and therapeutic agents for cancer (Harikumar *et al.*, 2008).

Quercetin

The flavone quercetin (3, 3, 4, 5, 7-pentahydroxyflavone), one of the major dietary flavonoids, is found in a broad range of fruits, vegetables, and beverages such as tea and wine, with a daily intake in Western countries of 25–30 mg. The antioxidant, anti-inflammatory, antiproliferative, and apoptotic effects of the molecule have been largely analyzed in cell culture models, and it is known to block NF-κB activation. In animal models, quercetin has been shown to inhibit inflammation and prevent colon and lung cancer. A phase 1 clinical trial indicated that the molecule can be safely administered and that its plasma levels are sufficient to inhibit lymphocyte tyrosine kinase activity. Consumption of quercetin in onions and apples was found to be inversely associated with lung cancer risk in Hawaii. The effect of onions was particularly strong against squamous cell carcinoma. In another study, an increased plasma level of quercetin after a meal of onions was accompanied by increased resistance to strand breakage in lymphocytic DNA and decreased levels of some oxidative metabolites in the urine (Russo 2007).

Silymarin

The flavonoid silymarin (silybin, isosilybin, silychristin, silydianin, and taxifolin) is commonly found in the dried fruit of the milk thistle plant *Silybum marianum*. Although silymarin role as an antioxidant and hepatoprotective agent is well known, its role as an anticancer agent is just emerging. The anti-inflammatory effects of silymarin are mediated through suppression of NF-κB-regulated gene products, including COX-2, lipoxygenase (LOX), inducible NO synthase, TNF, and IL-1. Numerous studies have indicated that silymarin is a chemopreventive agent *in vivo* against various carcinogens/

tumor promoters, including UV light, 7, 12-dimethylbenz anthracene (DMBA), phorbol 12-myristate 13- acetate, and others. Silymarin has also been shown to sensitize tumors to chemotherapeutic agents through downregulation of the MDR protein and other mechanisms. It binds to both estrogen and androgen receptors and downregulates prostate specific antigen. In addition to its chemopreventive effects, silymarin exhibits activity against tumors (*e.g.*, prostate and ovary) in rodents. Various clinical trials have indicated that silymarin is bioavailable and pharmacologically safe (Agarwal *et al.*, 2006).

Indole-3-carbinol

The flavonoid indole-3-carbinol (I3C) is present in vegetables such as cabbage, broccoli, brussels sprout, cauliflower, and daikon artichoke. The hydrolysis product of I3C metabolizes to a variety of products, including the dimer 3, 32-diindolylmethane. Both I3C and 3, 32-diindolylmethane exerts a variety of biological and biochemical effects, most of which appear to occur because I3C modulates several nuclear transcription factors. I3C induces phase 1 and phase 2 enzymes that metabolize carcinogens, including estrogens. I3C has also been found to be effective in treating some cases of recurrent respiratory papillomatosis and may have other clinical uses (Rogan 2006).

Sulforaphane

Sulforaphane (SFN) is an isothiothiocyanate found in cruciferous vegetables such as broccoli. Its chemopreventive effects have been established in both in vitro and in vivo studies. The mechanisms of action of SFN include inhibition of phase 1 enzymes, induction of phase 2 enzymes to detoxify carcinogens, cell-cycle arrest, induction of apoptosis, inhibition of histone deacetylase, modulation of the MAPK pathway, inhibition of NF-κB, and production of ROS. Preclinical and clinical studies of this compound have suggested its chemopreventive effects at several stages of carcinogenesis. In a clinical trial, SFN was given to eight healthy women an hour before they underwent elective reduction mammoplasty. Induction in NAD(P) H/quinine oxidoreductase and heme oxygenase-1 was observed in the breast tissue of all patients, indicating the anticancer effect of SFN (Juge *et al.*, 2007).

Prevention of Cancer by Teas and Spices

Spices are used all over the world to add flavour, taste, and nutritional value to food. A growing body of research has demonstrated that phytochemicals such as catechins (green tea), curcumin (turmeric), diallyldisulfide (garlic), thymoquinone (black cumin), capsaicin (red chilli), gingerol (ginger), anethole (licorice), diosgenin (fenugreek) and eugenol (clove, cinnamon) possess therapeutic and preventive potential against cancers of various anatomical origins (Figure 7.3). Other phytochemicals with this potential include ellagic acid (clove), ferulic acid (fennel, mustard, and sesame), apigenin (coriander, parsley), betulinic acid (rosemary), kaempferol (clove, fenugreek), sesamin (sesame), piperine (pepper), limonene (rosemary), and gambogic acid (kokum). Below is a description of some important phytochemicals associated with cancer.

Catechins

More than 3,000 studies have shown that catechins derived from green and black teas have potential against various cancers. Phase 1 trials of healthy volunteers have defined the basic biodistribution patterns, pharmacokinetic parameters, and preliminary safety profiles for short-term oral administration of various green tea preparations. The consumption of green tea appears to be relatively safe. Among patients with established premalignant conditions, green tea derivatives have shown potential efficacy against cervical, prostate, and hepatic malignancies without inducing major toxic effects. One novel study determined that even persons with solid tumors could safely consume up to 1 g of green tea solids, the equivalent of approximately 900 ml of green tea, three times daily. This observation supports the use of green tea for both cancer prevention and treatment (Chen *et al.*, 2007).

Curcumin

Curcumin is one of the most extensively studied compounds isolated from dietary sources for inhibition of inflammation and cancer chemoprevention, as indicated by almost 3000 published studies. Studies from our laboratory showed that curcumin inhibited NF-κB and NF-κB-regulated gene expression in various cancer cell lines. In vitro and in vivo studies showed that this phytochemical inhibited inflammation and carcinogenesis in animal models, including breast, esophageal, stomach, and colon cancer models. Other studies showed that curcumin inhibited ulcerative proctitis and Crohn's disease and one showed that curcumin inhibited ulcerative colitis in humans. Study conducted in patients with familial adenomatous polyposis showed that curcumin has a potential role in inhibiting this condition. In that study, all five patients were treated with curcumin and quercetin for a mean of 6 months and had a decreased polyp number (60.4 per cent) and size (50.9 per cent) from baseline with minimal adverse effects and no laboratory-determined abnormalities. The pharmacodynamic and pharmacokinetic effects of oral Curcuma extract in patients with colorectal cancer have also been studied. In a study of patients with advanced colorectal cancer refractory to standard chemotherapies, 15 patients received Curcuma extract daily for up to 4 months. Results showed that oral Curcuma extract was well tolerated, and dose-limiting toxic effects were not observed. Another study showed that in patients with advanced colorectal cancer, a daily dose of 3.6 g of curcumin engendered a 62 per cent decrease in inducible prostaglandin E2 production on day 1 and a 57 per cent decrease on day 29 in blood samples taken 1 h after dose administration. An early clinical trial with 62 cancer patients with external cancerous lesions at various sites (breast, 37; vulva,4; oral, 7; skin, 7; and others, 11) reported reductions in the sense of smell (90 per cent of patients), itching (almost all patients),lesion size and pain (10 per cent of patients), and exudates (70 per cent of patients) after topical application of an ointment containing curcumin. In a phase 1 clinical trial, a daily dose of 8,000 mg of curcumin taken by mouth for 3 months resulted in histologic improvement of precancerous lesions in patients with uterine cervical intraepithelial neoplasm (one of four patients), intestinal metaplasia (one of six patients), bladder cancer (one of two patients), and oral leukoplakia (two of seven patients). Results from another study showed that curcumin inhibited constitutive activation of NF-κB, COX-2, and STAT3 in peripheral blood mononuclear cells from the 29 multiple myeloma patients enrolled in this study. Curcumin was given in doses of 2, 4, 8, or 12 g/day orally. Treatment with curcumin was well tolerated with no adverse events. Of the 29 patients, 12 underwent treatment for 12 weeks and 5 completed 1 year of treatment with stable disease. Other studies from our group showed that curcumin inhibited pancreatic cancer. Curcumin down-regulated the expression of NF-κB, COX-2 and phosphorylated STAT3 in peripheral blood mononuclear cells from patients (most of whom had baseline levels considerably higher than those found in healthy volunteers). These studies showed that curcumin is a potent anti-inflammatory and chemopreventive agent (Anand *et al.*, 2008).

Diallyldisulfide

Diallyldisulfide, isolated from garlic, inhibits the growth and proliferation of a number of cancer cell lines including colon, breast, glioblastoma, melanoma, and neuroblastoma cell lines. Recent studies showed that this compound induces apoptosis in Colo 320 DM human colon cancer cells by inhibiting COX-2, NF-κB, and ERK-2. It has been shown to inhibit a number of cancers including dimethylhydrazine-induced colon cancer, benzo[a]pyrene-induced neoplasia, and glutathione S-transferase activity in mice; benzo[a]pyrene-induced skin carcinogenesis in mice; N-nitrosomethylbenzylamine-induced esophageal cancer in rats; N-nitrosodiethylamine-induced forestomach neoplasia in female A/J mice; aristolochic acid-induced forestomach carcinogenesis in rats; diethylnitrosamine-induced glutathione S-transferase positive foci in rat liver; 2-amino-3-methylimidazo[4,5-f]quinoline-induced hepatocarcinogenesis in rats; and diethylnitrosamine-induced liver foci and hepatocellular adenomas in C3H mice. Diallyldisulfide has also been shown to inhibit mutagenesis or tumorigenesis induced by vinyl carbamate and N-nitrosodimethylamine; aflatoxin B1-induced and N-nitrosodiethylamine-induced liver preneoplastic foci in rats; arylamine N-acetyltransferase activity and 2-aminofluorene-DNA adducts in human promyelocytic leukemia cells; DMBA-induced mouse skin tumors; N-nitrosomethylbenzylamine-induced mutation in rat oesophagus; and diethylstilbesterol-induced DNA adducts in the breasts of female ACI rats. Diallyldisulfide is believed to bring about an anticarcinogenic effect through a number of mechanisms, such as scavenging of radicals; increasing gluathione levels; increasing the activities of enzymes such as glutathione S-transferase and catalase; inhibiting cytochrome p4502E1 and DNA repair mechanisms; and preventing chromosomal damage (Khanum *et al.,* 2004).

Thymoquinone

The chemotherapeutic and chemoprotective agents from black cumin include thymoquinone (TQ), dithymoquinone (DTQ), and thymohydroquinone, which are present in the oil of this seed. TQ has antineoplastic activity against various tumor cells. DTQ also contributes to the chemotherapeutic effects of Nigella sativa. In vitro study results indicated that DTQ and TQ are equally cytotoxic to several parental cell lines and to their corresponding multidrug-resistant human tumor cell lines. TQ induces apoptosis by p53-dependent and p53-independent pathways in cancer cell lines. It also induces cell-cycle arrest and modulates the levels of inflammatory mediators. To date, the chemotherapeutic potential of TQ has not been tested, but numerous studies have shown its promising anticancer effects in animal models. TQ suppresses carcinogen-induced forestomach and skin tumor formation in mice and acts as a chemopreventive agent at the early stage of skin tumorigenesis. Moreover, the combination of TQ and clinically used anticancer drugs has been shown to improve the drug's therapeutic index, prevents nontumor tissues from sustaining chemotherapy-induced damage, and enhances the antitumor activity of drugs such as cisplatin and ifosfamide (Sethi *et al.,* 2008).

Capsaicin

The phenolic compound capsaicin (t8-methyl-N-vanillyl-6-nonenamide), a component of red chilli, has been extensively studied. Although capsaicin has been suspected to be a carcinogen, a considerable amount of evidence suggests that it has chemopreventive effects. The antioxidant, anti-inflammatory, and antitumor properties of capsaicin have been established in both in vitro and in vivo systems. Capsaicin can suppress the TPA-stimulated activation of NF-κB and AP-1 in cultured HL-60 cells. In addition, capsaicin inhibited the constitutive activation of NF-κB in malignant melanoma cells. Furthermore, capsaicin strongly suppressed the TPA-stimulated activation of NF-κB and the epidermal activation of AP-1 in mice. Another proposed mechanism of action of capsaicin is its interaction with xenobiotic metabolizing enzymes, involved in the activation and detoxification of various chemical carcinogens and mutagens. Metabolism of capsaicin by hepatic enzymes produces reactive phenoxy radical intermediates capable of binding to the active sites of enzymes and tissue macromolecules. Capsaicin can inhibit platelet aggregation and suppress calcium-ionophore–stimulated proinflammatory responses, such as the generation of superoxide anion, phospholipase A2 activity, and membrane lipid peroxidation in macrophages. It acts as an antioxidant in various organs of laboratory animals. Anti-inflammatory properties of capsaicin against carcinogen-induced inflammation have also been reported in rats and mice. Capsaicin has exerted protective effects against ethanol-induced gastric mucosal injury, hemorrhagic erosion, lipid peroxidation, and myeloperoxidase activity in rats that was associated with suppression of COX-2. While lacking intrinsic tumor-promoting activity, capsaicin inhibited TPA-promoted mouse skin papillomagenesis (Surh, 2002).

Gingerol

Gingerol, a phenolic substance mainly present in the spice ginger (Zingiber officinale Roscoe), has diverse pharmacologic effects including antioxidant, antiapoptotic, and anti-inflammatory effects. Gingerol has been shown to have anticancer and chemopreventive properties, and the proposed mechanisms of action include the inhibition of COX-2 expression by blocking of the p38 MAPK-NF-κB signaling pathway (Shukla et al., 2007).

Anethole

Anethole, the principal active component of the spice fennel, has shown anticancer activity. In 1995, Al-Harbi et al., studied the antitumor activity of anethole against Ehrlich ascites carcinoma induced in a tumor model in mice (Al-Harbi et al., 1995). The study revealed that anethole increased survival time, reduced tumor weight, and reduced the volume and body weight of the EAT-bearing mice. It also produced a significant cytotoxic effect in the EAT cells in the paw, reduced the levels of nucleic acids and MDA, and increased NP-SH concentrations. The histopathological changes observed after treatment with anethole were comparable to those after treatment with the standard cytotoxic drug cyclophosphamide. The frequency of micronuclei occurrence and the ratio of polychromatic erythrocytes to normochromatic erythrocytes showed anethole to be mitodepressive and nonclastogenic in the femoral cells of mice. Various studies showed the NF-κB inhibitory activity of a derivative of anethole and anetholdithiolthione (Sen et al., 1996). Their study results showed that anethole inhibited H_2O_2, phorbol myristate acetate or TNF alpha induced NF-κB activation in human jurkat T-cells studied the anticarcinogenic activity of anethole trithione against DMBA induced in a rat mammary cancer model. The study results showed that this phytochemical inhibited mammary tumor growth in a dose dependent manner. Nakagawa and Suzuki studied the metabolism and mechanism of action of trans-anethole (anethole) and the estrogen like activity of the compound and its metabolites in freshly isolated rat hepatocytes and cultured MCF-7 human breast cancer cells (Nakagawa et al., 2003). The results suggested that the biotransformation of anethole induces a cytotoxic effect at higher concentrations in rat hepatocytes and an estrogenic effect at lower concentrations in MCF-7 cells on the basis of the concentrations of the hydroxylated intermediate, 4OHPB. Results from preclinical studies have suggested that the organosulfur compound anethole dithiolethione may be an effective chemopreventive agent against lung cancer. Lam et al., conducted a phase 2b trial of anethole dithiolethione in smokers with bronchial dysplasia (Lam et al., 2002). The results of this clinical trial suggested that anethole dithiolethione is a potentially efficacious chemopreventive agent against lung cancer.

Diosgenin

Diosgenin, a steroidal saponin present in fenugreek, has been shown to suppress inflammation, inhibit proliferation, and induce apoptosis in various tumor cells. Research during the past decade has shown that diosgenin suppresses proliferation and induces apoptosis in a wide variety of cancer cells lines. Antiproliferative effects of diosgenin are mediated through cell-cycle arrest, disruption of Ca^{2+} homeostasis, activation of p53, release of apoptosis-inducing factor, and modulation of caspase-

3 activity. Diosgenin also inhibits azoxymethane-induced aberrant colon crypt foci, has been shown to inhibit intestinal inflammation, and modulates the activity of LOX and COX-2. Diosgenin has also been shown to bind to the chemokine receptor CXCR3, which mediates inflammatory responses (Shishodia *et al.*, 2006).

Eugenol

Eugenol is one of the active components of cloves. Studies showed that eugenol suppressed the proliferation of melanoma cells. In a B16 xenograft study, eugenol treatment produced a significant tumor growth delay, an almost 40 per cent decrease in tumor size, and a 19 per cent increase in the median time to end point. Of more importance, 50 per cent of the animals in the control group died of metastatic growth, whereas none in the eugenol treatment group showed any signs of cell invasion or metastasis (Ghosh *et al.*, 2005). Eugenol DMBA also induced skin tumors in mice (Sukumaran *et al.*, 1994). The same study showed that eugenol inhibited superoxide formation and lipid peroxidation and the radical scavenging activity that may be responsible for its chemopreventive action. Studies conducted by Imaida *et al.*, showed that eugenol enhanced the development of 1, 2-dimethylhydrazine-induced hyperplasia and papillomas in the forestomach but decreased the incidence of 1-methyl-1-nitrosourea-induced kidney nephroblastomas in F344 male rats (Imaida *et al.*, 1990). Another study demonstrated that, eugenol and related biphenyl (S)-6,62-dibromo- dehydrodieugenol elicit specific antiproliferative activity on neuroectodermal tumor cells, partially triggering apoptosis (Pisano *et al.*, 2007). Eugenol suppresses COX-2 mRNA expression (one of the main genes implicated in the processes of inflammation and carcinogenesis) in HT-29 cells and lipopolysaccharide-stimulated mouse macrophage RAW264.7 cells (Kim *et al.*, 2003). Another study showed that 12-hydroxyeugenol is a good inhibitor of 5-lipoxygenase and Cu (2+)-mediated low-density lipoprotein oxidation. *In vivo* treatment of rats with eugenol reduced the mutagenicity of benzopyrene in the Salmonella typhimurium mutagenicity assay, whereas in vitro treatment of cultured cells with eugenol increased the genotoxicity of benzopyrene (Rompelberg *et al.*, 1996).

Wholegrain Foods

The major wholegrain foods are wheat, rice, and maize; the minor ones are barley, sorghum, millet, rye, and oats. Grains form the dietary staple for most cultures, but most are eaten as refined-grain products in Westernized countries. Whole grains contain chemopreventive antioxidants such as vitamin E, tocotrienols, phenolic acids, lignans, and phytic acid. The antioxidant content of whole grains is less than that of some berries but is greater than that of common fruits or vegetables. The refining process concentrates the carbohydrate and reduces the amount of other macronutrients, vitamins, and minerals because the outer layers are removed. In fact, all nutrients with potential preventive actions against cancer are reduced. For example, vitamin E is reduced by as much as 92 per cent. Wholegrain intake was found to reduce the risk of several cancers including those of the oral cavity, pharynx, oesophagus, gallbladder, larynx, bowel, colorectum, upper digestive tract, breasts, liver, endometrium, ovaries, prostate gland, bladder, kidneys, and thyroid gland, as well as lymphomas, leukemias, and myeloma. Intake of wholegrain foods in these studies reduced the risk of cancers by 30–70 per cent. Whole grains reduce the risk of cancer by several potential mechanisms. For instance, insoluble fibers, a major constituent of whole grains, can reduce the risk of bowel cancer. Additionally, insoluble fiber undergoes fermentation, thus producing short-chain fatty acids such as butyrate, which is an important suppressor of tumor formation. Whole grains also mediate favourable glucose response, which is protective against breast and colon cancers. Also, several phytochemicals from grains and pulses were reported to have chemopreventive action against a wide variety of cancers. For example, isoflavones (including daidzein, genistein, and equol) are nonsteroidal diphenolic compounds that are found in leguminous plants and have antiproliferative activities. Findings from several, but not all, studies have shown significant correlations between an isoflavone-rich soy-based diet and reduced incidence of cancer or mortality from cancer in humans. Observational studies have suggested that a diet rich in soy isoflavones (such as the typical Asian diet) is one of the most significant contributing factors for the lower observed incidence and mortality of prostate cancers in Asia. On the basis of findings about diet and of urinary excretion levels associated with daidzein, genistein, and equol in Japanese subjects compared with findings in American or European subjects, the isoflavonoids in soy products were proposed to be the agents responsible for reduced cancer risk. In addition to its effect on breast cancer, genistein and related isoflavones also inhibit cell growth or the development of chemically induced cancers in the stomach, bladder, lung, prostate, and blood (Sarkar *et al.*, 2006).

Vitamins

Although controversial, the role of vitamins in cancer chemoprevention is being evaluated increasingly. Fruits and vegetables are the primary dietary sources of vitamins except for vitamin D. Vitamins, especially vitamins C, D, and E, are reported to have cancer chemopreventive activity without apparent toxicity. Epidemiologic study findings suggest that the anticancer/chemopreventive effects of vitamin C against various types of cancers correlate with its antioxidant activities and with the inhibition of inflammation and gap junction intercellular communication. Findings from a recent epidemiologic study showed that a high vitamin C concentration in plasma had an inverse relationship with cancer-related mortality. In 1997, expert panels at the World Cancer Research Fund and the American Institute for Cancer Research estimated that vitamin C can reduce the risk of cancers of the stomach, mouth, pharynx, oesophagus, lung, pancreas, and cervix. The protective effects of vitamin D result from its role as a nuclear transcription factor that regulates cell growth, differentiation, apoptosis, and a wide range of cellular mechanisms central to the development of cancer (Ingraham *et al.*, 2008).

Role of Medicinal Plants Derivatives in Therapy of Cancer

Over the past decade, herbal medicine has become a topic of global importance, making an impact on both world health and international trade. Medicinal plants continue to play a central role in the healthcare system of large proportions of the world's population. This is particularly true in developing countries, where herbal medicine has a long and uninterrupted history of use. Recognition and development of the medicinal and economic benefits of these plants are on the increase in both developing and industrialized nations. Continuous usage of herbal medicine by a large proportion of the population in the developing countries is largely due to the high cost of Western pharmaceuticals and healthcare. In addition, herbal medicines are more acceptable in these countries from their cultural and spiritual points of view. Use of plants for medicinal remedies is an integral part of the Indian cultural life, and this is unlikely to change in the years to come.

Among the human diseases treated with medicinal plants is cancer, which is probably the most important genetic disease. Every year, millions of people are diagnosed with cancer, leading to death in a majority of the cases. According to the American Cancer Society, deaths arising from cancer constitute 2–3 per cent of the annual deaths recorded worldwide. Cancer rates are increasing every year; breast cancer being the most common form of cancer in women worldwide and the second most common cancer amongst women. Despite the long history of cancer treatment using herbal remedies in the Province, the knowledge and experience of these herbalists have not been scientifically documented. There are wide varieties of medicinal plants like *Cinchona, Taxus, Calcalia delhiniifolia* etc. whose derived compounds are now proved anti cancer compounds (Figure 7.4).

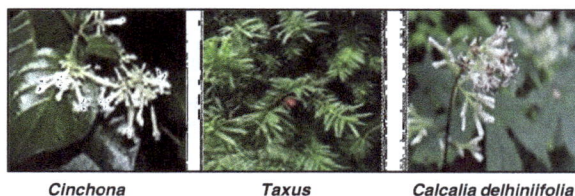

| Cinchona | Taxus | Calcalia delhiniifolia |

Figure 7.4: Photographs Showing Medicinal Plants.

Quinacrine and Chloroquine (*Cinchona*)

Quinacrine and chloroquine are bioactive compounds derived from bark of cinchona tree. Since 1920's these drugs were used as anti malarial agents and various other indications but recently these compounds were rediscovered as anti-cancer compounds in chemical library screening of small molecules that are able to activate p53 in tumour cells. QC intercalates in DNA and activates p53 in tumor cells without causing genotoxicity (DNA damage) and down regulates NF-κB, thereby decreasing the cell survival in renal cell carcinoma (RCC) cells. Various other QC related compounds also shows anti-cancer potentiality like amsacrine in anti-pancreatic cancer, cisplatin in head and neck squamous cell carcinoma, chloroquine in glioblastoma multiforme therapy. It was also found that novel substituted 9-AAs such as could inhibit cell proliferation of cell lines by inducing apoptosis (Gurova, 2009).

Taxol (*Taxus*)

Taxol is one of the most effective anti-cancer drugs ever developed. The natural source of taxol is the inner bark of several *Taxus* species, but it accumulates at a very low concentration and with a prohibitively high cost of extraction. Another problem is that the use of inner bark for taxol production implies the destruction of yew trees. Taxol can also be semisynthetically produced via the conversion of baccatin III or 10-deacethylbaccatinIII found in Taxus needles but the cost and difficulty of the extraction process of the semisynthetic precursors are also very high. The most promising approach for the sustainable production of taxol and related taxoids is provided by plant cell cultures at an industrial level. Taxol is currently being clinically used against different tumour processes but due to the difficulty of its extraction and formulation, as well as the growing demand for the compound, new taxol analogues with improved properties are being studied (Exposito *et al.,* 2009). For example, Paclitaxel (taxol) was first isolated from the bark of the Pacific Yew (Taxus brevifolia). Docetaxel is a more potent analogue that is produced semisynthetically. In contrast to other microtubule antagonists, taxol disrupts the equilibrium between free tubulin and mircrotubules by shifting it in the direction of assembly, rather than disassembly. As a result, taxol treatment causes both the stabilization of microtubules and the formation of abnormal bundles of microtubules. The net effect is still the disruption of mitosis.

Cacalol (*Calcalia delhiniifolia*)

Cacalol was isolated as a free radical-scavenging compound from *Cacalia delphiniifolia* which is a traditional Asian herbal plant and is believed to have medicinal effects on cancer. Cacalol has strong anti-proliferation effect on breast cancer cells and induces apoptosis by activating a pro-apoptotic pathway. Combination of cacalol and other chemotherapeutic drugs (Taxol and cyclophosphamide) also synergistically induced apoptosis and partially overcame chemo-resistance. A mechanistic insight of cacacol in breast cancer cells showed significantly modulated expression of the FAS gene, which resulted in apoptosis through activation of DAPK2 and caspase 3. In a xenograft model of nude mouse, when cacalol was administered intraperitoneally, tumor growth was significantly suppressed. Importantly, oral administration of cacalol before implanting tumors showed significant preventive effect on tumor growth in the same animal model. Furthermore, the treatment of mice with a combination of low dose of Taxol and cacalol significantly suppressed the tumor growth. Taken together cacalol induces apoptosis in breast cancer cells and impairs mammary tumor growth in vivo by blocking the expression of the FAS gene through modulation of Akt-SREBP pathway, suggesting that cacalol has potential utility as a chemopreventive and chemotherapeutic agent for breast cancer (Liu *et al.*, 2010).

Apart from these efficient medicinal plants derivatives, various other plants are also known for anti-cancer potentiality such as *Saraca Asoca* (Ashoka), *Terminalia arjuna* (Arjuna Herb), *Nigella Sativa, Gloriosa Superba, Embelia ribes etc.* Herbal medicines are of great importance with lots of benefits and least side effects. Usage of herbal medicines will be cost effective and good for health.

Natural Anticancer Agents *vs.* Synthetic Drugs

Currently to approve a new synthetic drug, the drug needs to go through clinical trials with a certain number of selected subjects for several years. However, the side effects of many of such drugs are undetected until they have entered the market and have been used by a larger population for a longer period of time. Many drugs have been withdrawn from the market after such broader usages because of their high toxicity. But spices and herbs have been tested by generations and generations of people for thousands of years, and their effects from various aspects have been very well documented, such as those in Chinese medicine. So clinically speaking, we actually have more knowledge about herbs than most of the newly approved synthetic drugs. In some herbal practices, such as in Chinese herbal medicine, several herbs are usually used together in a formula to treat one illness. The combination of herbs takes advantage of the interactions among different ingredients from multiple herbs for more balanced, less toxic, and more powerful effects. Spices and herbs act on multiple targets, unlike some synthetic drugs that target on only one molecule while their effects on other molecules in the pathways or systems are unknown. Such unknown effects can often lead to severe side effects of the synthetic drugs. Compared with synthetic drugs, herbs are quite safe if used correctly. For example, in Chinese medicine, different herbs are prescribed with different dosages for different patients, even if the patients have the same disease.

Because of the above reasons, spices and usually have fewer side effects than synthetic drugs.

Prevention is Better than Cure - Lifestyle Modification

Healthiness of a person is the complete reflection of his lifestyle. Apart from the consumption of fruits and vegetables, one should maintain a good lifestyle too. It's always advisable to prevent something before it strikes. A good food habit and little exercise to keep you away from the diseases like cancer that are better to be avoided than to be treated. Cancer prone lifestyle includes smoking, consumption of alcohol and no physical activity. Smoking is closely associated with lungs cancer and so is the alcohol consumption with that of liver.

There is extensive evidence suggesting that regular physical exercise may reduce the incidence of various cancers. A sedentary lifestyle has been associated with most chronic illnesses. Physical exercises and mental exercise like meditation play a very vital role to maintain a healthy lifestyle and hence to prevent cancer. Physical inactivity has been linked with increased risk of cancer of the breast, colon, prostate, and pancreas and of melanoma (Booth *et al.*, 2002). Physical activity like walk, exercises and meditation are much necessary along with the green and fresh fruits and vegetables to maintain a healthy life.

Exercise and diet are very closely related and show their effects if properly followed. Caloric restriction is much necessary for a healthy life as body gets all sorts of energy from the ingredients of diet. The link between diet and cancer is revealed by the large variation in rates of specific cancers in various countries and by the observed changes in the incidence of cancer in migrating. Fasting is a type of caloric restriction that is prescribed in most cultures. Perhaps one of the first reports that caloric restriction can influence cancer incidence was published in 1940 on the formation of skin tumors and hepatoma in mice (Tannenbaum *et al.*, 1940; Hursting *et al.*, 2003). Since then, several reports on this subject have been published (Ross *et al.*, 1971; Albanes 1987). The diet should be designed in such a manner that body should get the necessary amount of energy and no such extra material get deposited as fat, as that may interfere in maintaining a healthy life.

A healthy lifestyle will lead to good consequences like good health and long lifespan. A combination of routine life, controlled lifestyle and regular checkups will work like wonder to kick-out cancer.

A body of research supports the protective role of fresh fruits and vegetables, dietary fiber, and intake of a low-fat diet in reducing the risk for cancer. However there is a very restricted knowledge, about the cancer-preventing properties of some specific micronutrients, apart from β-carotene. The information about the optimal levels of intake of various micronutrients and reports regarding the patterns of food intake associated with reduced risk for cancer. The relationship between breast cancer recurrence and survival and dietary intakes in women diagnosed with breast cancer is revealed from many sources (Blackburn *et al.*, 2003; Rock *et al.*, 2002). Several studies have indicated the association between diagnosis of breast cancer and decreased physical activity (Irwin *et al.*, 2004), and relations among higher BMI, lower physical activity, and high estrogen levels have also been described (McTiernan *et al.*, 2006).

It's always preferable to prevent cancer through dietary modification than by the administration of other individual agents. Studies regarding the role of dietary modification in preventing cancer have yielded a success rate that is though vary a little but is generally quite promising. Researchers from the United Kingdom predicted that "realistic" lifestyle modifications involving diet and exercise would lead to a 26 per cent reduction in the number of cases of colorectal cancer in the British population. This would be expected to produce at least an equivalent decrease in the number of deaths, they add. The predictions were carried out by the Cancer Research UK Center at the Wolfson Institute of Preventive Medicine in London. A team headed by senior epidemiologist Max Parkin, MD, used results from epidemiologic studies showing the effect of diet on colorectal cancer, and then predicted the effect of lifestyle modifications on the incidence rates using a statistical method known as the Nordpred package (Moller *et al.*, 2003).

The lifestyle modifications involved:

☆ Reducing consumption of red and processed meat to less than 90 g/day.

☆ Increasing consumption of fresh fruits and vegetables to at least 5 portions per day.

☆ Exercising for at least 30 minutes per day on 5 or more days a week, at least at "moderate intensity" (similar to brisk walking).

The current study reveals that increase in the rate of cancer risk is due to a large population who are in excess of the consumption with respect of alcohol and red-meat and they do not meet the guidelines with respect to exercise and fruits and vegetables consumption.

Conclusion

On the basis of above described studies, we can say that there is a strong link between all lifestyle factors that cause cancer (carcinogenic agents) and all agents that prevent cancer (chemopreventive agents). Numerous agents in fruits and vegetables can interfere with various cell-signalling pathways, when used in their pure form for the therapy. These agents can also be used in their natural form for the prevention of cancer. Derivatives of medicinal plants are also very effective in both preventing and curing cancer. Most of the modern medicines currently available for treating cancers are very toxic, less effective and very expensive in treating the disease. Thus, further investigations and more clinical trials are still required for the traditional agents derived from natural sources to validate the usefulness of these agents either alone or in combination therapy. In summary, this review outlines the preventability of cancer based on the major risk factors for cancer.

References

Agarwal R, Agarwal C, Ichikawa H *et al.* (2006). Anticancer potential of silymarin: from bench to bed side. Anticancer Res 26: 4457–4498.

Aggarwal BB, Shishodia S (2006). Molecular targets of dietary agents for prevention and therapy of cancer. Biochem Pharmacol 71: 1397–1421.

Albanes D (1987). Total calories, body weight, and tumor incidence in mice. Cancer Res 47: 1987–1992.

Al-Harbi MM, Qureshi S, Raza M *et al.* (1995). Influence of anethole treatment on the tumour induced by Ehrlich ascites carcinoma cells in paw of Swiss albino mice. *Eur J Cancer Prev* 4: 307–318.

Anand P, Sundaram C, Jhurani S *et al.* (2008). Curcumin and cancer: An "old-age" disease with an "age-old" solution. Cancer Letters (in press).

Blackburn GL, Copland T, Khaodhiar L *et al.* (2003). Diet and breast cancer. Journal of Women's Health (Larchmt). 12: 183–192.

Booth FW, Chakravarthy MV, Gordon SE *et al.* (2002). Waging war on physical inactivity: using modern molecular ammunition against an ancient enemy. J Appl Physiol 93: 3–30.

Chen L, Zhang HY (2007). Cancer preventive mechanisms of the green tea polyphenol (")-epigallocatechin-3-gallate. Molecules 12: 946–957.

Chojnacki H, Sokalski WA (1975). Interactions of 6-thioguanine in B-DNA: possible mechanism of its mutagenic action. J Theor Biol 54: 167-174.

Divisi D, Di Tommaso S, Salvemini S *et al.* (2006). Diet and cancer. Acta Biomedica 77: 118–123.

Exposito O, Bonfill M, Moyano E *et al.* (2009). Biotechnological production of taxol and related taxoids: current state and prospects. *Anti-Cancer Agents* Med Chem 9: 109-121.

Ghosh R, Nadiminty N, Fitzpatrick JE *et al.* (2005). Eugenol causes melanoma growth suppression through inhibition of E2F1 transcriptional activity. J Biol Chem 280: 5812–5819.

Gurova K (2009). New hopes from old drugs: revisiting DNA-binding small molecules as anticancer agents. Future Oncol 5: 1685-1704.

Harikumar KB, Aggarwal BB (2008). Resveratrol: A multitargeted agent for age-associated chronic diseases. Cell Cycle 7: 1020–1037.

Imaida K, Hirose M, Yamaguchi S *et al.* (1990). Effects of naturally occurring antioxidants on combined 1, 2- dimethylhydrazine- and 1-methyl-1-nitrosourea-initiated carcinogenesis in F344 male rats. Cancer Letters 55: 53–59.

Ingraham BA, Bragdon B, Nohe A (2008). Molecular basis of the potential of vitamin D to prevent cancer. *Curr* Med Res *Opin* 24: 139–149.

Irwin M, McTiernan A, Bernstein L *et al.* (2004). Physical activity levels among breast cancer survivors. Med Sci Sports Exerc 36: 1484–1491.

Juge N, Mithen RF, Traka M (2007). Molecular basis for chemoprevention by sulforaphane: a comprehensive review. *Cell Mol Life Sci* 64: 1105–1127.

Khanum F, Anilakumar KR, Viswanathan KR (2004). Anticarcinogenic properties of garlic: a review. *Crit* Rev *Food Sci Nutr* 44: 479–488.

Kim SS, Oh OJ, Min HY *et al.* (2003). Eugenol suppresses cyclooxygenase-2 expression in lipopolysaccharide-stimulated mouse macrophage RAW264.7 cells. Life Science 73: 337–348.

Lam S, MacAulay C, Le Riche JC *et al.* (2002). A randomized phase IIb trial of anethole dithiolethione in smokers with bronchial dysplasia. *J* Natl Cancer Inst 94: 1001–1009.

Liu W, Furuta E, Shindo K *et al.* (2010). Cacalol, a natural sesquiterpene, induces apoptosis in breast cancer cells by modulating Akt-SREBP-FAS signaling pathway. Breast Cancer Res Treat [Epub ahead of print].

Longley DB, Latif T, Boyer J *et al.,* (2003). The interaction of thymidylate synthase expression with p53-regulated signaling pathways in tumor cells. Seminars in Oncology 30: 3-9.

McTiernan A, Wu L, Chen C *et al.* (2006). Relation of BMI and physical acitivy to sex hormones in postmenopausal women. Obesity (Silver Spring). 14: 1662–1677.

Moller B, Fekaer H, Hakulinen T *et al.* (2003). Prediction of cancer incidence in the Nordic countries: empirical comparison of different approaches. *Statistics in Medicine* 22: 2751-2766.

Nakagawa Y, Suzuki T (2003). Cytotoxic and xenoestrogenic effects via biotransformation of trans-anethole on isolated rat hepatocytes and cultured MCF-7 human breast cancer cells. Biochem Pharmacol 66: 63–73.

Nishino H, Murakosh M, Ii T *et al.* (2002). Carotenoids in cancer chemoprevention. Cancer Met Rev 21: 257–264.

Pagano JS, Blaser M, Buendia MA *et al.* (2004). Infectious agents and cancer: criteria for a causal relation. Seminars in Cancer Biology 14: 453–471.

Pershin GN, Shcherbakova LI (1962). On the mechanism of action of 6-mercaptopurine. Farmakologi i a i Toksikologi i a 25: 19-24.

Pisano M, Pagnan G, Loi M *et al.* (2007). Antiproliferative and pro-apoptotic activity of eugenol-related biphenyls on malignant melanoma cells. Molecula Cancer 6: 8.

Rock CL, Demark-Wahnefried W (2002). Nutrition and survival after the diagnosis of breast cancer: a review of the evidence. J Clin Oncol 20: 3302–3316.

Rogan EG (2006). The natural chemopreventive compound indole-3-carbinol: state of the science. In Vivo 20: 221–228.

Ross MH, Bras G (1971). Lasting influence of early caloric restriction on prevalence of neoplasms in the rat. J Natl Cancer Inst 47: 1095–1113.

Russo GL (2007). Ins and outs of dietary phytochemicals in cancer chemoprevention. Biochem Pharmacol 74: 533–544.

Sarkar FH, Adsule S, Padhye S *et al.* (2006). The role of genistein and synthetic derivatives of isoflavone in cancer prevention and therapy. *Mini-*Reviews *Med Chem* 6: 401–407.

Sen CK, Traber KE, Packer L (1996). Inhibition of NF-kappa B activation in human T-cell lines by anetholdithiolthione. *Biochemical and Biophysical Research Communications* 218: 148–153.

Sethi G, Ahn KS, Aggarwal BB (2008). Targeting NF-kB activation pathway by thymoquinone: Role in suppression of antiapoptotic gene products and enhancement of apoptosis. Mol Cancer Res (in press).

Shishodia S, Aggarwal BB (2006). Diosgenin inhibits osteoclastogenesis, invasion, and proliferation through the downregulation of Akt, I kappa B kinase activation and NF-kappa B-regulated gene expression. Oncogene 25: 1463–1473.

Shukla Y, Singh M (2007). Cancer preventive properties of ginger: a brief review. *Food Chem Toxicol* 45: 683–690.

Stearns B, Losee KA, Bernstein J (1963). Hydroxyurea: A New Type of Potential Antitumor Agent. J Med Chem 6: 201.

Sukumaran K, Unnikrishnan MC, Kuttan R (1994). Inhibition of tumour promotion in mice by eugenol. Ind J Physiol Pharmacol 38: 306–308.

Surh YJ (2002). Anti-tumor promoting potential of selected spice ingredients with antioxidative and anti-inflammatory activities: a short review. Food Chem Toxicol 40: 1091–1097.

Tannenbaum A, Silverstone H (1940). The initiation and growth of tumors. Introduction. I. Effects of underfeeding. A J Cancer 38: 335–350.

Van Scott EJ, Shaw RK, Crounse RG *et al.* (1960). Effects of methotrexate on basal-cell carcinomas. Arch Dermatol 82: 762-771.

Wattenberg LW (1966). Chemoprophylaxis of carcinogenesis: a review. Cancer Research 26: 1520-1526.

2014, Advances in Biochemistry and Biotechnology Volume 2

Edited by: Dr. Biplab Sarkar and Dr. Chiranjib Chakraborty

Published by: DAYA PUBLISHING HOUSE

Pages 121-142

8

HIV: As We Know

Anchal Singh[1†], Shishir Agrahari[1], Shruti Rastogi[1],
Amulya Mohan[2] and Ashish Swarup Verma[1]*

[1]*Amity Institute of Biotechnology, Amity University,*
Sector-125, Noida – 201 303, Uttar Pradesh, India
[2]*Department of Biology and Health Promotions, St. Francis College,*
180 Remsen Street, Brooklyn, New Your City, NY 11201, USA

ABSTRACT

Microbial infections have always created havoc and adversely affected humanity with their fatal and adverse consequences. Antibiotics have helped to improve our ability to fight against microbial infections. New disease and microorganism have emerged and they have their own impact. HIV/AIDS has been discovered almost 30 years. HIV is considered as one of the most studied virus and its significance can be realized that UN has to create a separate organization as UNAIDS to look after the HIV epidemic. In this article, an effort has been made to provide brief information about the history of HIV infection and its discovery along with molecular biology of HIV and an overview of HIV replication mechanism and strategies to develop drugs for treatment of HIV infection. The article will also provide a brief about epidemiology both at

† *Present address*: Department of Microbiology and Immunology, Kirksville College of Osteopathy, A. T. Still University of Health Sciences, 800 W Jefferson Street, Kirksville MO 63501, USA

* *Corresponding author.* E-mail: asverma@amity.edu; ashish-gyanpur@hotmail.com

global and Indian level. Limitation and utility of animal model for HIV research along with some of the common myths prevailing in different societies have also been discussed here. This manuscript also gives an update on new targets for development of new anti-HIV drugs. All the efforts to treat HIV infections available to us, even then *"HIV infection can be prevented but cannot be cured"* as we are still unable to develop a vaccine against HIV.

Introduction

The significance of infectious disease and its impact on human society cannot be denied. Impact of microbes was far beyond imagination, even before the discovery of antibiotics. Antibiotics have significantly reduced human sufferings caused by infections. Antibiotics discovery brought so optimism that, we started thinking that we had already won the war against microbial infections because of antibiotics. Undoubtedly, we have seen enormous development and improvements in antibiotics, still the question is "Have we won the war against microbes?" Answer is NO!!! Since the discovery of antibiotics, we have seen emergence of new infections to name a few *viz.*, bird flu, SARS, HIV, Ebola, etc. Many a times, these new infections are untreatable, but in the recent past human immunodeficiency virus (HIV) and acquired immunodeficiency syndrome (AIDS) have received unprecedented importance due to various socio-political reasons associated with this infections.

AIDS is a fatal disease and it is caused by infection of HIV. AIDS has received considerable attention because of two main reasons (1) firstly, it was reported in USA, and (2) secondly all the patients initially reported with this infection were homosexuals. Just 5 patients were reported with this disease, which was noticed by a pharmacy technician working at Center for Disease Control and Prevention, Atlanta, and that was the start of HIV saga.

Alertness of a drug technician, Ms. Sandra Ford at CDC, Atlanta, USA has to be credited to notice the outbreak of HIV in USA, although, HIV was not known at that time. Ms. Ford for the 1st time noticed a high number of requests to refill for a rare drug Pentamidine. Pentamidine is a rare drug which is commonly used to treat *Pneumocystis carinii* Pneumonia (PCP). She said to Newsweek,

"A doctor was treating a gay man in his 20s who had pneumonia. Two weeks later, he called to ask for a refill of a rare drug that I handled. This was unusual-nobody ever asked for a refill. Patients usually were cured in one 10-days treatment or they died."

On June 5, 1981 CDC has published 5 cases of PCP without any identifiable cause of PCP among 5 gay men from Los Angles, USA (Gottlieb *et al.,* 1981a; Gottlieb *et al.,* 1981b). This report is considered as "beginning" of AIDS. In reality, it should not be considered as the beginning of AIDS, as a matter of fact, it was the beginning of AIDS awareness. CDC was quick to recognize the importance of such a high numbers of PCP patients, therefore CDC formulated a Task Force on Kaposi's sarcoma and Opportunistic Infection (KSOI). Initially limited information was available for this new and emerging disease. At this point of time the disease did not had any official name, so it was called as Lymphadenopathy or KOSI, itself. All the initial cases showed a common association of this disease with gays, therefore various names were used *viz.* "GCS (Gay Compromise Syndrome)", GRID (Gay-Related Immune Deficiency), AIDS (Acquired Immunodeficiency Disease), "Gay Cancer" and "Community-Acquired Immune Dysfunction", *etc.* certainly these were different names for the same disease.

KOSI Task force started a close monitoring for these cases; soon numerous cases were reported from all over USA. Unfortunately, detection of AIDS in Haitian hemophiliac led to the speculation that this disease might have originated from Haiti. But the occurrence of this disease among non-homosexuals made names like GRID irrelevant. Finally, AIDS name was adopted in a meeting on July 24th in 1982 at Washington D.C. Since then AIDS word was frequently used in media and scientific literature. In the mean time, various voluntary organizations for AIDS had cropped up and they started advising gay men for safer sex practices. By the end of 1982, a 20 month old also died due to AIDS. Clinical history of this child suggested that this child had received multiple blood transfusions; therefore, a need for safe blood supply was realized. Ever increasing numbers of AIDS cases was helpful to clear the existing belief that only homosexuals are affected by AIDS. Shortly, it was recognized that AIDS also exists in other parts of the world which led to emphasis that there is a need for identification of the causative organism for AIDS. France and USA took a lead role to identify the infective agent for AIDS. In 1983, Luc Montagnier from Pasteur Institute, Paris, was the first one to identify the causative organism for AIDS and he named this virus as Lymphadenopathy Associated Virus (LAV). Montagnier published his work in May 20, 1983 issue of Science. Then, Robert Gallo from National Cancer Institute, Bethesda reported his work in May 4, 1984 issue of Science. But, Gallo named this virus as Human T-Lymphotrophic Virus (HTLV$_{III}$). Discovery of HIV is also surrounded with controversies. The major controversy about HIV is that who is the discoverer of HIV? Is it Luc Montagnier or Robert Gallo? This controversy was resolved by a meeting between Ronald Regan and Jacques Chirac and it was decided that Gallo and Montagnier both have equal contribution for the discovery of HIV (Gallo *et al.*, 2003). But, Montagnier contribution for HIV discovery was finally acknowledged by awarding him Nobel Prize for Physiology and Medicine in 2008. There were few names taking rounds in literature for this virus, therefore, International Committee on Taxonomy of Viruses decided to name of this virus as HIV (Human Immunodeficiency Virus). Since then, HIV word is in use while other names like LAV and HTLV became obsolete (Verma *et al.*, 2009).

AIDS as a disease has received enormous publicity because of ever increasing number of AIDS patients. This is the reason that AIDS became 1st disease to be debated in 1987 in UN General Assembly. AZT (Azidothymidine) was approved by Federal Drug Administration (FDA) to treat HIV infections and December 1st was declared as World AIDS Day in 1988. In 1991, Red Ribbon was adopted as a symbol for AIDS awareness (Figure 7.1). United Nation started a Joint United Nation Programme on HIV/AIDS (UNAIDS) in 1996. Efficacy of active antiretroviral therapy for the first time was presented at 11th International AIDS Conference in Vancouver, Canada. First efficacy trial for HIV vaccine was tried in 1999. AIDS was discussed UN Security Council in 2000 and Global Fund was launched by UN Secretary General to fight HIV/AIDS. 2005 summit of G8 decided to start a programme "Universal Access of Anti-retroviral Treatment by 2010" (Table 7.1).

HIV and AIDS: Epidemiology

First case of AIDS was reported in 1981, and its causative organism was identified in 1983, but a consistent increase in number of AIDS patients was noticed since 1983, which was a real concern. Therefore, UNAIDS was created under the umbrella of United Nation, since 1990, UNAIDS is monitoring AIDS epidemic globally and publish its report annually.

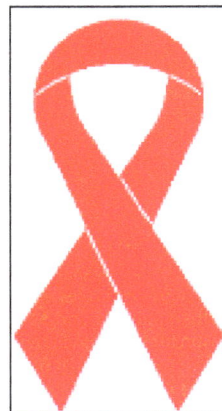

Figure 7.1: AIDS Awareness Campaign has Adopted "Red Ribbon" as a Symbol.

Advances in Biochemistry and Biotechnology, Vol. 2

Table 7.1: HIV: Important Facts.

Year	Events
1959	Oldest blood specimen with HIV positivity
1981	Failures of immune response in gay men
1982	AIDS was defined by CDC Center for Disease Control and Prevention, Atlanta, USA
1983	Luc Montagnier 1st identified HIV
1984	Robert Gallo reconfirmed HIV
1985	Zidovudine (Formerly known as AZT) was first anti-retroviral
1986	Luc Montagnier of France identified HIV-2
1988	World AIDS Day was declared
1990	NNRTI were discovered
1991	Red Ribbon becomes symbol for AIDS awareness
1995	Protease inhibitors, another group of drug approved to treat HIV
1996	AIDS incidences in USA start decreasing
2007	Integrase Inhibitors were discovered
2008	Nobel Prize was awarded to Luc Montagnier

So far >70 million people have been infected with HIV. As per UNAIDS Report (2009), ~33.3 million people are living with HIV. The expected range is in between 29.2-33.7 million, this estimate suggests that men and women are equally affected by HIV. ~2.1 million children under the age of 15 are living with HIV, which ranges between 1.2-2.9 millions (Table 7.2). As per UNAIDS (2009), report every year ~2.7 million get new infection, out of which ~0.43 million infections account for new infections among children. Every year, ~2.0 million die due to HIV/AIDS, while ~0.28 million children below the age of 15 also die every year due to HIV/AIDS. Regional analysis of epidemiological data suggests that sub-saharan Africa is the worst affected region. ~67 per cent of total HIV/AIDS infected individuals live in this area, while the highest number of new HIV infection are also reported from this region alongwith maximum numbers of death due to HIV/AIDS. Oceania region is the least affected region of the world, which only accounts for ~0.0001 per cent of world's total HIV/AIDS burden. Without any doubt there is still a dire need of special attention to educate and to provide better health care to the residents of those countries, which are badly affected with this epidemic.

HIV and Myths

As we know that AIDS was discovered in mysterious circumstances, and it was also associated with high incidences of death too. Such high incidences of deaths have led to spread of numerous myths about HIV and AIDS (Verma *et al.*, 2010). Fear against such an incurable disease was the main reason to spread myths about HIV/AIDS and the major reason for these myths was just to create fear among people, so that spread of HIV/AIDS can be minimized, if not to control it. Various educational campaigns and awareness programs were started, which have really helped to clear myths about HIV and AIDS up to some extent. Still some common myths do exist among both literate as well as in literature (www.thebody.com).

Myths about HIV can be divided into three categories: (A) Myths about transmission of HIV, (B) Myths about cure for HIV, and (C) Myths about HIV medication.

Table 7.2: HIV Statistics: A Global View†

		Total Infection (in millions)	New Infection (in millions)	Death (in millions)
A)	**Global**			
	Adults	**31.3** (29.2-33.7)	**2.3** (2.0-2.5)	**1.7** (1.4-2.1)
	Children	**2.1** (1.2-2.9)	**0.43** (0.24-0.61)	**0.28** (0.15-0.41)
	Total	**33.4** (31.1-35.8)	**2.7** (2.4-3.0)	**2.0** (1.7-2.4)
B)	**Worst Affected Area** Sub-Saharan Africa			
	Total	**22.4** (20.8-24.1)	**1.9** (1.6-2.2)	**1.4** (1.1-1.7)
C)	**Least Affected Area** Oceania			
	Total	**0.06** (0.05-0.07)	**0.004** (0.003-0.005)	**0.002** (0.001-0.003)

Values given in parenthesis is suggestive of range.

†; Adapted from UNAIDS, 2009.

(A) Myths about Transmission of HIV

(1) HIV can be transmitted by mosquito, by sharing a drinking glass, by hugging or kissing of an AIDS patients, *etc.* This is not true, because HIV is transmitted by exposure to infected body fluids like blood, semen, vaginal fluid or mother's milk. (2) HIV infected woman cannot give a birth to a child free of HIV. This was true earlier, now this is not true anymore. If, an infected pregnant woman is under proper anti-retroviral treatment, she can deliver a child free of HIV infection.

(B) Myths about Cure for HIV

(1) It is always difficult to predict the outcome of HIV infections. Some HIV infected patients get sicker in just few months, while some HIV infected patients can lead a healthy life up to 10 years or more. Anti-retroviral treatments have serious side effects, too. (2) The most unfortunate myth about HIV prevailing in some part of the world is that AIDS can be cured by having sex with a virgin girl. Many young girls became victims of this myth and they herself became AIDS patients. (3) Medications to treat HIV are poison, so do not use them. This myth made so many HIV patients to visit quacks, and it is not true, side effects of new anti-retroviral drugs have been significantly reduced. (4) Some myths labeled AIDS as a "death sentence." A high death rate among AIDS patients is the main reason behind this myth. But this myth is not true anymore, as HIV patients who are under proper anti-retroviral treatment can lead a healthy life style for 10 years or more after initial exposure to HIV. (5) There is another myth perpetuated among minorities that AIDS infection is a government conspiracy to eradicate minorities, this myth has no foundation, none whatsoever.

(C) Myths about Medications

One has to be very precise about taking medicine to treat HIV, missing a single dose can be disastrous to HIV patient, but improved medications have seen enormous improvements to overcome these limitations.

Routes of HIV Infections

HIV infections are transmitted by below mentioned routes:

(A) **Sexual Route:** It includes both heterosexual and homosexual intercourse. Unprotected sex and multiple sex partners is the main source for HIV infections.

(B) **Parenteral Routes:** Recipients of blood transfusions, blood products, accidental exposure with contaminated surgical implements. Sharing needles among drug addicts is the major mean for transmission of HIV.

(C) **Vertical Routes:** Vertical transmission is defined as transmission of HIV infection from mother-to-child. Usually this happens during pregnancy, presently, vertical transmission of HIV infection has been reduced significantly among those pregnant women who are under proper medication.

Clinical Stages of HIV Infection

HIV infections were found to be ever increasing; therefore, it was necessary to have a system for effective clinical management and development of correct epidemiological data base. To overcome these issues, CDC has developed a system for classification of different clinical stages of HIV infections; these are updated on regular basis (CDC 1992). CDC classified clinical stages of HIV infection into 4 stages (A) Stage I, (B) Stage II, (C) Stage III, and (D) Stage IV (Table 7.3). A typical correlation of CD4 counts with the viral load is depicted in Figure 7.2 and values of CD4 counts at different clinical stages are mentioned in Table 7.4.

Table 7.3: Clinical Stages of HIV Infection.

Stage	Symptoms
I	Primary infection stage
II	Asymptomatic phase stage
III	Persistent and generalized lymphoadenopathy stage
IV	Symptomatic infection stage

Table 7.4: CD4 Counts: Progression of HIV Infection

Stages	Lymphocyte Counts	
	Absolute ($/\mu L$)	Relative (per cent)
I	>500	>28
II	200-500	14-28
III	<200	<14

(A) Stage I: Primary HIV Infection

Primary HIV infection is known as seroconversion stage. At this stage, HIV patients show presence of antibodies against HIV. ~65 per cent patients at primary HIV infection are reported with mild symptoms of illness. Majority of clinical symptoms at this stage are fever, malaise, diarrhea, lymphadenopathy, sore throat, headaches, *etc.* Severe symptoms are rare at this stage. Detection of HIV antigens and antibodies in peripheral circulation is the main criteria for diagnosis.

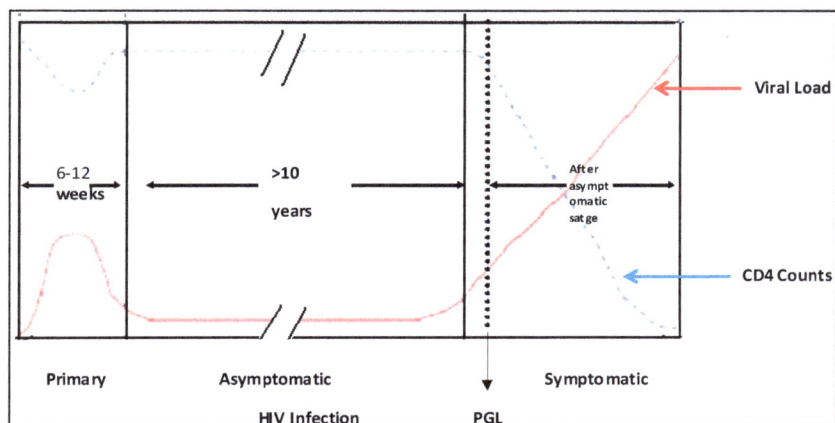

Figure 7.2: This Figure is a Generalized Representation of Progression of HIV Infection with Clinical Parameters like CD4 Counts and Viral Load. (Blue colour is representing viral load and red colour is representing for CD4 counts).

(B) Stage II: Asymptomatic Phase

Primary HIV infection stage lasts about 2-3 months, after these antibodies against HIV could be detected continuously and viral load falls to low levels. In these patients, viral replication does not stop, but slows down significantly. During asymptomatic stage CD4 counts are either close to normal or above normal *i.e.*, 350 x10^6 cells/L. Asymptomatic phase can persist up to 10 years or more. Asymptomatic phase can either be effectively maintained or prolonged with proper anti-retroviral medications. The choice of treatment should be based on CD4 counts and viral load. The main objective of treatment at this stage is to maintain normal immune functions by suppressing viral replication to minimal.

(C) Stage III: Persistent Generalized Lymphadenopathy

This stage persists for a short period and patients look healthy, otherwise. Non-specific adenopathy may persist but lymph node biopsies are not recommended as routine follow-ups. Lymphadenopathy does not show any differences between HIV and non-HIV patients for up to 3 month.

(D) Stage IV: Symptomatic HIV Infection

After clinical stage III, progression of HIV infection is fast resulting in rapid decline of immune competence due to enhanced HIV replication. This stage shows signs and symptoms of full-blown AIDS. At this stage, patients develop many constitutional symptoms *viz.* weight loss, fever, malaise, *etc.*, in general constitutional symptoms can be treated easily, but to control progression of disease is difficult. With time, these patients start showing neurological symptoms, opportunistic infections and AIDS defining cancer. These are signs and symptoms of terminal illness leaving patients and physician with limited choices of treatments (Rastogi *et al.,* 2011).

Diagnosis of HIV

It is now known that HIV starts its replication within 36 hours post infection but it cannot be detected in this period of time, and this delay is known as "Diagnostic Window". It takes a few weeks for the detection of antibodies against HIV. This delay in diagnosis of HIV is due to the time required for the production of antibodies post HIV infection. Mostly, 6 weeks are required to detect HIV in ~80 per cent of cases. By 12 weeks HIV can be detected in almost 100 per cent of cases. Various diagnostic tests are under development to curtail the period of diagnostic window as much as it is possible. These tests are based on simultaneous detection of p24 and anti-HIV antibodies. Diagnostic tests for HIV can be divided into 3 main categories: (A) HIV Antibody Test, (B) Confirmatory Test, and (C) Nucleic Acid Test.

(A) HIV Antibody Test

This test is performed to screen HIV positivity in patients. Patients with positive results are recommended for confirmatory test. Most of these screening tests are based on the principles of ELISA (enzyme linked immunosorbant assay), where antibodies present in serum/plasma samples can be detected. 'Rapid Tests' are also available for the diagnostic need in remote areas. Rapid tests are based on particle agglutinations and immunoblot method. Rapid Tests are convenient because they require a drop of blood, which can be drawn either from fingertip or from ear lobe, and results are available within 15-30 min. Patients turning out to be positive in preliminary test has to be confirmed with confirmatory test. Uni-Gold Recombingen HIV test is developed by Trinity Biotech PLC, Wicklow, Ireland (www.trinitybiotech.com), in which results can be achieved within 10-12 minutes after applying the test sample. Serum, plasma or whole blood can be used for diagnosis (Figure 7.3). Another kit has been developed by OraSure Technologies, Inc, USA, which gives the result in 20 min after application of test samples. With this test finger prick blood, venipuncture whole blood and even oral fluid can also be used for diagnosis of HIV (Figure 7.4). Nowadays some of the tests are available, which can even use urine sample for diagnosis of HIV.

(B) Confirmatory Tests

They are based on Western Blot methods to detect different HIV antigens on a nitrocellulose membrane. This method cannot be used as routine to screen patients, because it is expensive and time consuming.

(C) Nucleic Acid Test (NAT)

Nucleic Acid Test is very sensitive and technologically complex; therefore NAT is only used as confirmatory test. This test is based on principles of Polymerase Chain Reaction (PCR). Viral RNA is detected in cell free medium *e.g.,* serum/plasma and pro-viral cDNA after extracting DNA from in leukocytes (WBC). The cost of performing these tests is enormously high. NAT results are most useful as a prognostic marker to evaluate, (a) efficacy of anti-HIV drugs, and (b) disease progression.

Even though we have so many diagnostic tests, we still need to develop improved tests for HIV detection to reduce the time period of diagnostic window as much as it is possible.

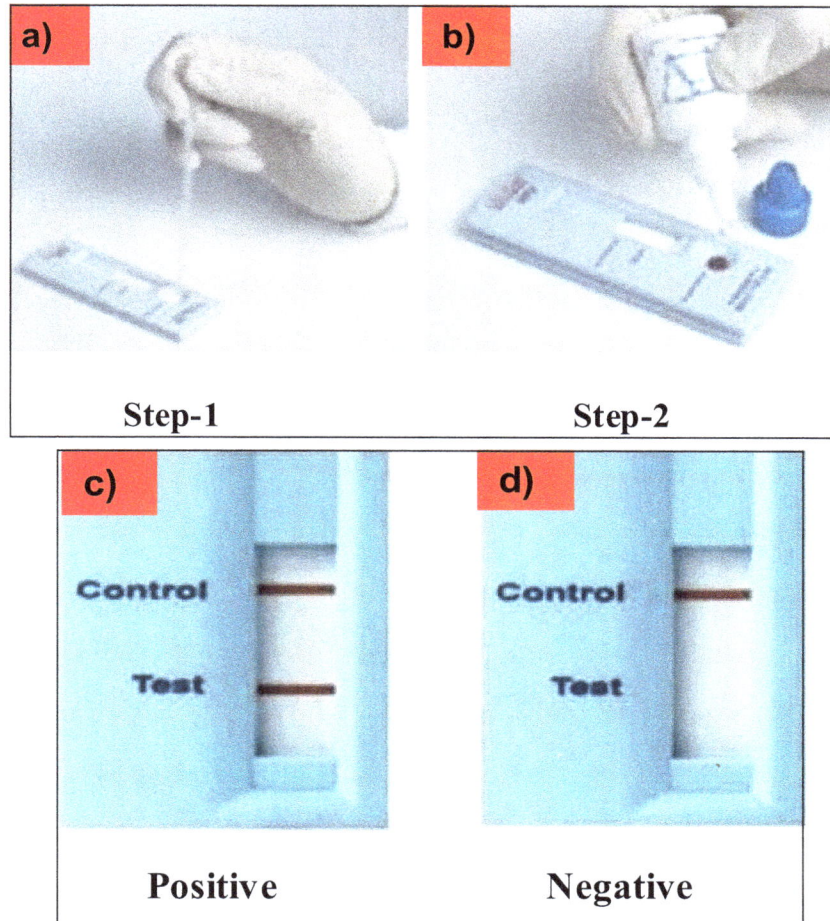

Figure 7.3: HIV Diagnostic Kit Developed by Trinity Biotech, Ireland.

a) 1st step one loading of test sample on the cassette, b) 2nd and final step loading washing solution and incubating for 10-12 min, c) Cassettes showing test sample as positive, two lines in the cassette, and d) Showing in case of negative sample there is only one line.

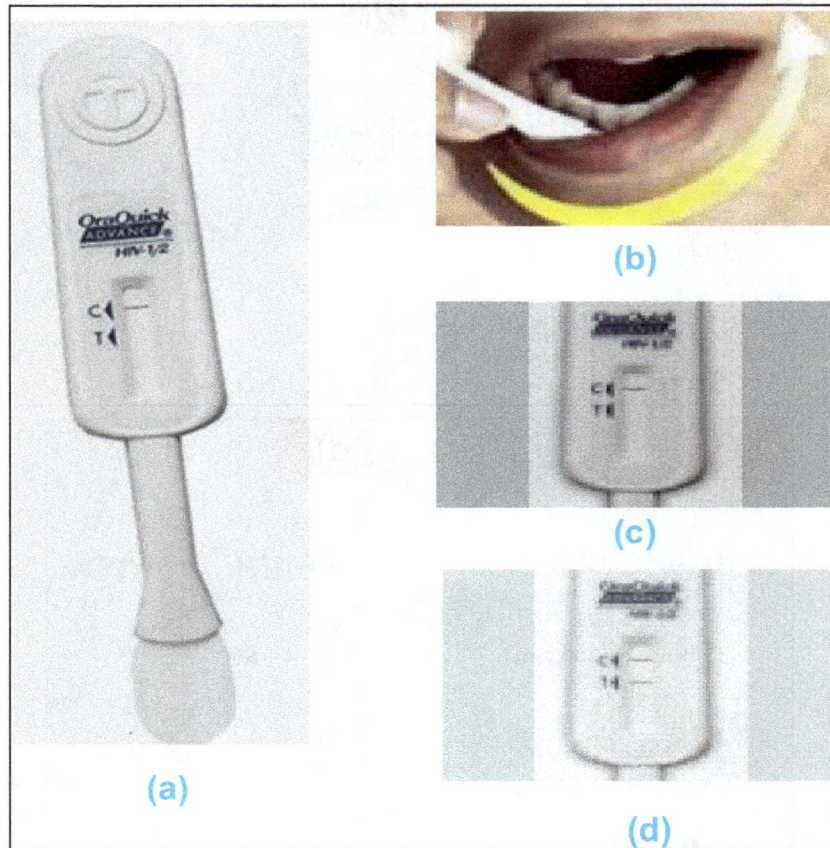

Figure 7.4: HIV Diagnostic Kit Developed and Commercialized by OraSure Technology, USA, where Oral Fluid, Finger Prick as well as Venipuncture Sample can be Used for Diagnosis for HIV.

a) Cassette provided with the kit for diagnosis, b) Procedure to show how to collect the oral fluid for testing, c) Cassettes is showing test sample as negative, because only one line developed, and d) Cassettes shows two lines in the window, which suggests that test sample is positive.

HIV: Classification, Structure and Molecular Biology

HIV is roughly spherical in shape and measures about 120 nm in diameter. HIV is a member of *Lentivirus* genus and belongs to *Retroviridae* family. HIV contains two copies of single-stranded, positive sense RNA with envelope and reverse transcriptase (RT) enzyme. The genetic information of HIV is transmitted *via,* RNA. Conversion of RNA into DNA takes place by RT enzyme (Costin, 2007) (Figure 7.5).

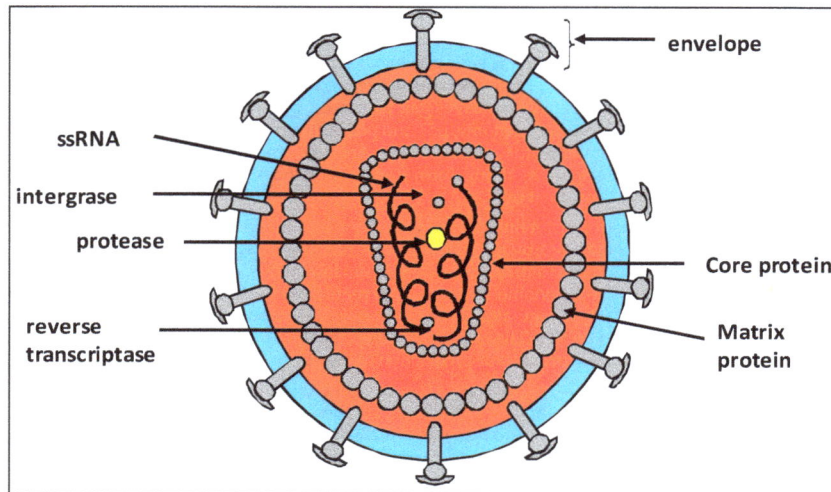

Figure 7.5: Structure of HIV-1 Virion.

Genome size of HIV is ~9.8 Kb, consists of 9 genes, which produces 15 different proteins during its life cycles. These proteins or genes can be divided into 3 sub-categories. Gag, Env, RT, and Pol, are structural proteins. Tat and Rev are regulatory proteins, while Nef, Vpr, Vif and Vpu are accessory proteins. The map of HIV genome is shown in Figure 7.6.

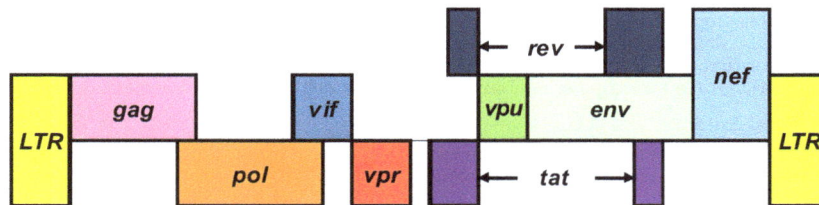

Figure 7.6: Genetic Organization of HIV-1.

Gag word is derived from "group-specific-antigen" and production of gag is regulated by *gag* gene. Primarily *gag* is responsible for production of structural components. A 53-kDa precursor protein is synthesized by *gag,* which produces 4 smaller proteins p7, p9, p17 and, p24, after enzymatic cleavage of precursor protein. Out of these proteins p17 is outer core protein, p24 is inner core protein, p9 is a components of nucleoid core, while p7 binds to genomic RNA. P24 protein has been used for detection of HIV in serum/plasma. Env word is derived from "envelope" and encoded by *env* gene and proteins encoded by *env* function as structural components of virion. A 160-kDa precursor protein is produced by *env,* which cleaves into two small proteins, *i.e.,* gp41 and gp120. These two proteins work for viral attachment and entry into CD4 cells. Pol word is derived from "polymerase" and encoded by *pol,* the major function of this gene product is structural in nature. A precursor protein which is encoded by *pol* gives rise to 4 different smaller cleaved products *viz.,* p10, p32, p51 and p64. Out of these p10 acts as protease which cleaves gag precursor, p32 acts as intergrase and it helps integration of proviral DNA into host genome, p51 and p64 both have reverse transcriptase activity, while p64 has an additional function to work as RNAse. Another gene in this category is Long Term Repeats (LTR) and it is also known as "Long Term Repeat Sequences". Main role of LTR is to help integration of proviral DNA into host cell DNA.

Tat and Rev are regulatory proteins in HIV. Functions of Tat and Rev are regulation of viral production. Tat protein is encoded by *tat* gene and this name is derived from "transactivator of transcription". Tat is 110 amino acid proteins present in nucleus and nucleolus of infected cells. Tat is essential for elongation of viral genome. Rev is another regulatory protein encoded by *rev* gene and this name has been derived from "regulator of viral expression." Unspliced transcripts from nucleus to cytoplasm are transported by Rev. The unspliced transcripts are spliced in predefined manner in cytoplasm, which is an essential process for production of infective new virions.

The third groups of genes are specified as "accessory gene", function of these genes is accessory in nature. These genes are not essential for replication, but they assist in efficient production of new virions. These 4 genes are *nef, vif, vpr* and *vpu.* Nef is a 27-kDa protein encoded by *nef,* its name has been derived from "negative factor." Nef gets detected at early stages of HIV infections. Nef induces ~10 fold increase in HIV infectivity. Vpr protein is also accessory protein and encoded by *vpr.* This name is derived from "Viral Protein R." Vpr is a 14-kDa protein and promote HIV infectivity in non-dividing cells. Vpu is also a gene of this category, which is derived from "Viral protein U" which down regulates CD4. The last gene in this category is *vif* and it is named as "Viral infectivity" its major role is to help in maintaining viral infectivity by completing viral assembly.

HIV Replication

HIV lacks its own synthetic machinery; therefore it has to exploit host cellular machinery for its replication, propagation and survival (Freed, 2001). HIV being a retrovirus, the genetic material in HIV is RNA. RNA being genetic material in HIV makes replication of HIV unique. The process of HIV replication can be divided into 5 stages. (A) Viral Entry, (B) Reverse Transcription, (C) Integration of pro-viral DNA, (D) Transcription and Translation, and (E) Completion and Release (Figure 7.7).

(A) Viral Entry

CD4 are the primary receptors for HIV infection that is the reason HIV infects T-cells which have CD4 receptor. CD4 is a 58-kDa glycoprotein present on cell surface of >60 per cent of T-lymphocytes in peripheral circulation. CD4 receptors are also present on other immune-cells *viz.,* monocytes, macrophages, dendritic cells, microglial, *etc.* CD4 is primary receptor for HIV-1. Viral entry begins

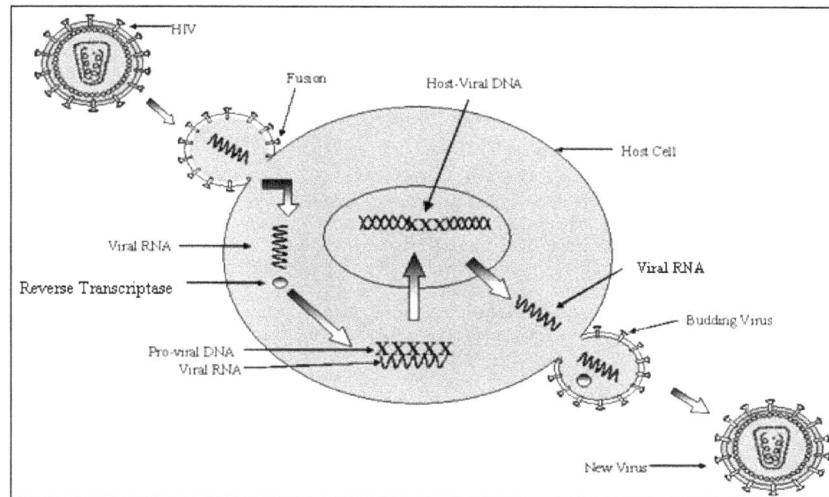

Figure 7.7: Life Cycle of HIV-1. The figure shows different steps of HIV replication.

with the attachment of virus to cell surface followed by its entry into the cell. The attachment of virus to cell surface takes place due to interaction with gp120 and gp41. gp120 and gp41 are envelop proteins of virus, which bind with CD4 and chemokine receptors, either CCR5 or CXCR4 depending upon virus type. The gp120 portion of HIV binds with high affinity to CD4 receptor on T-cell. After completion of HIV binding with CD4 and chemokine receptor, the viral envelop fuses with cell membrane of host cell, leading to the delivery of viral genome and other proteins into newly infected cells. This is the reason that viral attachment and fusion is an attractive target for drug development. Drugs are designed to interfere with any of these steps to stop viral entry.

(B) Reverse Transcription

After fusion, viral genome and enzymes of virus are released into cytoplasm of host cells. The genetic information of HIV is transmitted through RNA, therefore, HIV possesses Reverse Transcriptase (RT) enzyme, which copies single-stranded viral RNA into complementary DNA (cDNA). This newly synthesized DNA is now called as "Pro-viral DNA." RT lacks ability to proof-read; therefore, this step is highly error prone. High rate of mutations in HIV genome are commonly observed, which increases chances for survival of HIV, so that it can evade immune-system. High mutation rate is responsible for resistance against anti-HIV drugs. Reverse transcription has been mainly exploited as a drug target to treat HIV infections. NRTI, NtRTI and NNRTI drugs interfere with RT activity of virus and block viral replication.

(C) Integration of Pro-viral DNA

The newly synthesized pro-viral DNA integrates with cellular DNA with the help of Integrase enzyme. HIV carries 9 genes which are flanked by Long Term Repeat sequences (LTR). Long Term Repeat sequences along with integrase enzymes are essential for integration of provirus into host cell genome. Integration step is an attractive target for drug development.

(D) Transcription and Translation

The integrated pro-viral DNA may remain dormant in some cases, which is called as "latent HIV infection". Infective virus production requires presence of certain cellular transcription factors, which are up regulated by activation of T-cells; the most important transcription factor is NF-kB. The activation of NF-kB starts with the binding of LTR to promoter regions of cellular DNA. Binding of NF-kB at LTR initiates transcription of viral DNA into mRNA with the help of cellular RNA polymerases. The newly synthesized mRNA is now exported from nucleus to cytoplasm, where it gets translated into regulatory proteins Tat and Rev. At a later stage, structural proteins Env and Gag proteins are produced. The full-length RNA binds with Gag protein and gets finally packaged into a new virus particle.

(E) Assembly and Release

This is the final step of HIV replication. The Env polyprotein (gp160) passes through cytoplasmic endoplasmic reticulum and is transported to golgi complex, where it is cleaved by proteases and processed into two glycoproteins gp120 and gp41. These glyoproteins are transported to plasma membrane of host cell, where gp41 anchors gp120 to cell membranes of infected cells. Gag (p55) and Gag-pol (p160) polyproteins get associated to the inner surface of plasma membrane, along with genomic RNA and they help in budding of new virus. HIV protease cleaves polyproteins into various functional HIV proteins and enzymes, which completes maturation and release of HIV. This step is targeted by protease inhibitors which are used to block maturation of infective viruses.

Antiretroviral Drugs

Anti-retroviral drugs are primarily known to treat HIV infection. The development of these drugs has been possible because of better understanding of HIV replication. Scientists have been able to design new drugs, which interrupt different stages of HIV replication. These drugs have been classified into 5 categories: (A) NRTI, (B) NtRTI, (C) NNRTI, (D) PI, and (E) Integrase inhibitors (Table 7.5). Different anti-retroviral drugs target different stages of HIV replication as depicted in Figure 7.8.

(A) Nucleoside Reverse Transcriptase Inhibitors (NRTI)

Nucleoside analog acts as inhibitors of reverse transcriptase and these are the first available anti-retroviral drugs to treat HIV patients. NRTI targets activity of reverse transcriptase enzyme. NRTI interferes with cDNA synthesis by acting as 'False Building Bricks', because NRTI compete with physiological nucleosides for the synthesis of pro-viral DNA. NRTI lacks 3'-OH group on deoxyribose moiety, therefore, incorporation of these analogs during DNA synthesis results in chain termination. Chain termination halts further synthesis of DNA, therefore it stops viral replication. AZT, ddI, ddC, d4t, 3TC, ABC, FTC, INN and ATC belong to this group. Nucleoside variation exists among numerous NRTIs. Azidothymidine (AZT) was the first antiretroviral drug approved by FDA for HIV treatment. Promising results shown by AZT had led to the development of other drugs of this class. AZT and d4T are thymidine analogs, FTC and 3TC are cytidine analogs, ddI is an adenosine analog, ddC is a pyrimidine analog, while ABC is a guanosine analog. NRTIs are known to have side-effects, but alterations of different NRTI analogs during treatment have proven to be effective and with reduction in side-effects.

Table 7.5: Anti-HIV Drugs*.

Class	Generic Name	Chemical Name	Trade Name
NRTI	Zidovudine	ZDV	Retrovir/Retrovis
	Azidothymidine	AZT	Azitidin
	Didanosine	ddI	Videx/Videx EC
	Zalcitabine	ddC	Hivid
	Stavudine	d4T	Zerit
	Lamivudine	3TC	Epivir/Zettix/Heptovir/Epivir-HBV
	Abacavir	ABC	Ziagen
NtRTI	Tenfovir	TDF/PMPA	Viread
NNRTI	Nevirapine	NVR	Viramune
	Delavirdine	DLV	Rescriptor
	Efavirenz	EFV	Stocrin/Sustiva
PI	Saquniavir	SQV-hgc	Invirase
	Ritonavir	RTV	Norvir
	Indinavir	IDV	Crixivan
	Nelfinavir	NFV	Viracept
	Amphrenavir	APV	Agenerase
	Lponavir	LPV	Kaletra
Int.I	Raltegravir	RGV	Isentress

* It is not an exhaustive list of Anti-HIV drugs.

NRTI: Nucleoside Reverse Transcriptase Inhibitors; NtRTI: Nucleotide Reverse Transcriptase Inhibitors; NNRTI: Non-nucleoside Reverse Transcriptase Inhibitors; PI: Protease Inhibitors; Int.I: Integrase Inhibitors.

(B) Nucleotide Reverse Transcriptase Inhibitors (NtRTI)

Nucleotide reverse transcriptase inhibitors act similar to NRTI. Physiologically nucleoside inhibitors have to be converted into nucleotide analogs with the help of certain enzymes to perform their inhibitory activity. NtRTI skip the conversion step, therefore NtRTI are less toxic compared to NRTI. TDF and bis-POM PMPA belongs to NtRTI category. TDF is a monophosphorylated analog. NtRTIs also have some side-effects. A combination of TDF and ddI should be avoided.

(C) Non-Nucleoside Reverse Transcriptase Inhibitors (NNRTI)

NNRTI were first described in 1990. Their mode of action is different than both NRTI and NtRTI. NNRTI inhibits RT enzyme by directly binding to enzyme at a position closer to the binding site for nucleoside. Therefore, NNRTI blocks catalytic activation of binding site and reduce nucleoside binding. NNRTIs do not require activation for the inhibition of viral replication. Binding of NNRTI is non-competitive. Nevirapine, Delavirdine and Efavirenz are examples of NNRTI.

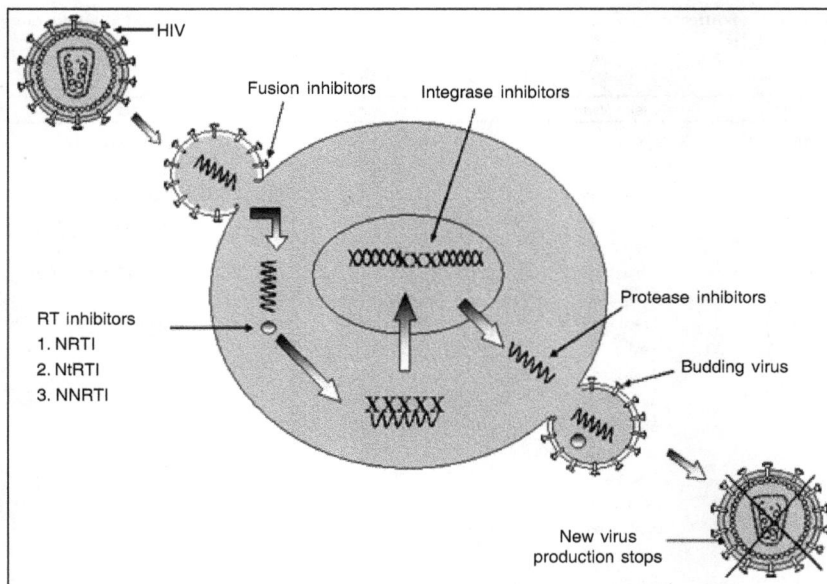

Figure 7.8: This Picture Shows Different Drugs Targets during HIV Replication.

(D) Protease Inhibitors (PI)

Protease inhibitors prevent viral replication by blocking the last steps of viral replication. PI inhibits activity of protease enzymes thus preventing production of new viruses. PIs prevent splicing of nascent proteins, which are required for final assembly of new virions. At molecular level, these drugs are designed in such a manner that they exactly fit to the active site of enzymes. PIs were initially criticized for their need to administer frequently, but this problem has been improved now. Caution has been advised for these drugs. In case of viral resistance PIs are better choice for treatment compared to NRTI and NtRTI. Saquinavir was the first approved PI. Ritonavir, Indinavir and Nelfinavir are other examples for protease inhibitors.

(E) Integrase Inhibitors (InI)

Integrase inhibitors target the activity of integrase enzyme. InI block the activity of integrase, therefore prevent pro-viral DNA integration to host cell genome. InI were primarily developed as anti-HIV drugs, but InI could also be used for other retroviral infections. The first integrase inhibitor Raltegravir was approved by FDA in 2007 for HIV treatment.

HAART

A highly active antiretroviral therapy is abbreviated as HAART. As a matter of fact, combination therapy to treat HIV infection has been given a new name as HAART. HAART uses an aggressive approach to treat HIV infections by targeting various steps of HIV replication simultaneously. HAART uses combination of 3-4 drugs from different classes of anti-retroviral drugs to control HIV infections. These drugs can be selected from NRTI, NtRTI, NNRTI, PI and InI. HAART has been designed to treat HIV by a panel of NIH experts and other international organizations. HAART regimen is helpful to reduce complexity of dose scheduling. A physician decides combination of different anti-retroviral drugs by evaluating potential risks and benefits to the patient. HAART regimen has an added advantage that it can overcome drug resistance. When HAART regimen fails in that case Mega-HAART or Salvage Therapy is the option for HIV patient. Salvage therapy is very expensive and associated with severe side effects.

New-target for Anti-HIV Drugs

The need for new class of antiretroviral drugs has become evident due to obvious reason for long-term treatment of HIV patients. Anti-retroviral drugs have limitations like (1) toxic effects of existing drugs, (2) development of resistance against drugs, (3) frequency of change in treatment *etc.* Combination therapy with reverse transcriptase and protease inhibitors is the most effective treatment protocol. Still there are various steps in HIV replication cycle, which can be targeted for treatment. The application of various molecular biology tools and improved understanding about HIV entry and fusion is helpful for the development of a new class of drugs which are known as Entry Inhibitors or Fusion Inhibitors. These new drugs can block HIV entry in to target cell or these drugs can block fusion of HIV with target cells. These entry inhibitors or fusion inhibitors cannot be used alone, as they may not be effective anti-retroviral drug, when administered alone. But in combination with other anti-retroviral fusion inhibitor can increase efficacy of anti-retroviral treatments (Table 7.6). These drugs interfere with the binding, fusion as well as entry of virus by targeting on viral envelope glycoproteins and their receptors. Each of the main steps in the process of HIV can be exploited as a potential target to develop entry inhibitors. The drugs which are currently under development can be categorized into three categories: (A) gp120-CD4 binding inhibitors, (B) gp120-co-receptors binding inhibitors, and (C) membrane fusion inhibitors, which interfere with the formation of six-helical bundle formed by activated gp41 (Ryser *et al.*, 2005).

(A) CD4 is the primary receptor used by HIV for its entry. The logical choice is to develop drugs which can block this stage are BMS806 (BMS378806) and BMS-488043 which have been shown to bind with gp120 and block entry of HIV. Effective concentration of BMS806 is in nanoMolar (nM) concentrations. Both these drugs are under clinical trial and have shown promising results. Another drug in this category is TNX355, a monoclonal antibody, that binds CD4 therefore, inhibits binding of gp120 to CD4. Some other compounds with similar activities are Pro542, CD4M33 and b12 and also CADA. Before mentioned compounds reduces HIV infection by down regulating CD4 receptors at post-translational level.

(B) Evidences from recent studies suggest that chemokine receptors CCR5 and CXCR4 are also valuable targets to block viral entry. The natural ligands for these co-receptors are RANTES, MIP-1α, MIP-1β and SDF-1α, which inhibit viral entry to host cells. Some compounds in this category like SCH-D, UK427, 85, AMD070/AMD1107 are under clinical trials. A few of these compounds like SCH-C, AMD3100, *etc.* have been withdrawn for further studies.

(C) An active state of gp41 is distinguished by formation of a six-helical-bundle which acts as fusogenic structure and fuses with cell membrane of host cell. T-20 a drug has been developed to inhibit HIV entry by attaching to a transient intermediate of gp41.

Table 7.6: Inhibitors of HIV Entry.

Compound	Mechanism	Manufacturer
gp-120-D4 Binding		
BMS-78806	gp120-binding	Bristol-Myers Squibb
BMS-488043	–do–	Bristol-Myers Squibb
Pro 542	–do–	Progenics
TNX-355	CD4-binding	Tanox/Bogen
gp-120-coreceptor binding		
SCH-C	**CCR5 binding**	Schering-Plough
SCH-D	–do–	Schering-Plough
Pro-140	–do–	Progenics
Tak-779	–do–	Takeda
Tak-220	–do–	Tekeda
GW873140	–do–	GSK
UK-427,857	–do–	Pfizer
AMD3100	**CXCR4 binding**	AnorMed
KRH-2731	–do–	Kureha
Fusion Inhibitors		
Fuzeaon	CHR mimic	Trimeris

Apart from HIV, target for viral entry have also been discovered on cell surface of host cells. Protein Disulphide Isomerase (PDI) is present on cell surface. PDI plays a crucial role for viral entry. During viral attachment on cell surface, it forms a PDI-CD4-gp120 complex. PDI causes conformational changes in gp120 leading to activation of fusogenic potential of gp 41. During this process gp120 bound to CD4 undergoing disulfide reduction, this can be prevented by PDI inhibitors. PDI inhibitors also prevent HIV envelope-mediated cell-cell fusion. Studies on PDI have suggested there are 3 steps which could be used as a target to stop viral entry: (1) PDI activity on cell surface, (2) Binding of PDI with CD4, and (3) Access of CD4-bound PDI to gp120 disulphide. Knocking out PDI gene in mammalian cells usually turned out to be lethal. Some PDI inhibitors like DTNB, PCMBS and APAO are under clinical investigation. BMS 806 is under trial because, it acts as antagonist to PDI and it competes with the binding site of gp120.

Genetic Diversity in HIV

General perception is that HIV is a one virus, but reality is far from this belief. Any infected person will not have all identical viruses. HIV genome shows enormous variability which is called as Genetic Diversity (genetic variation). The major reason for genetic diversity in HIV is a high rate of error during reverse transcription. Various selection pressures like host, environment and/or therapeutic selection pressure also contribute towards generation of diversity (Spira *et al.*, 2003).

HIV-1 is divided into 3 major classes, based on their genetic diversity and geographical distribution. The classes are named as M (major), O (outlying) and N (new). The M group accounts for >90 per cent of HIV/AIDS cases. M group is further divided into sub-types, known as "clade." There are 9 major clades of HIV, *viz.* A-D, F-H, J and K, other recombinant forms have been named as Mosaics. Mosaics are evolved due to recombination of 2 or more HIV subtypes (Table 7.7).

Almost all genes of HIV are vulnerable for mutation, but phylogenetic classification of HIV is primarily based on *env* gene. Envelop (*env*) nucleotide sequences differ ~20-50 per cent. M and O nucleotide sequences vary 30-50 per cent. Inter-clade variations of *env* gene are ~20-30 per cent and intra-clade variations are 10-15 per cent. *pol* region of HIV is about 2-3 times, less divergent compared to *env* gene. Less diversity in *pol* is crucial because excessive mutation of RT can make virus inoperative. *gag* is least mutable gene. Evolution of these clades supports the long term survival of HIV in host. Clade diversity is a major hurdle in designing efficient vaccines against HIV.

HIV and Animal Model

Majority of the data about HIV research has come either from *in vitro* studies or from *in vivo* results obtained from infected patients. Various animal models have been extensively used for HIV research. Medical Research Modernization Committee (MRMC) has identified fundamental problems with AIDS-related animal experimentation. Scientists failed to find any suitable non-human animal model for AIDS (Kaufman *et al.*, 2006), which can faithfully replicate natural history of AIDS. Nonhuman animals do not get AIDS in nature. In some animal models attempts were made to induce conditions which mimic AIDS partially. Chimpanzee is only non-human animal to have a healthy immune system, which can be infected with HIV. Over a period of more than 10 years more than 100 chimpanzees were infected with HIV, only two chimpanzees became sick. These numbers are so low that they cannot demonstrate any statistical significance for disease progression. This observation suggests that chimpanzee is not a suitable model for AIDS, because they rarely develop disease, even if they do, it is very slow. Some HIV vaccines studies have used chimpanzee as animal model. But this model has following limitations: (1) Chimpanzee show very little HMI and CMI, (2) Ratio of T4 and T8 lymphocytes in chimpanzee is different than human, (3) These animals were treated with laboratory HIV strain, which is different than naturally occurring HIV, (4) Due to limited replication of HIV in chimpanzee vaccination in laboratory conditions proves successful, which may not be true in human, (5) Chimpanzee being intelligent and highly social animal are kept in isolation for experimental purposes, and (6) They are an endangered species.

Monkeys are also commonly used for HIV research. Simian Immunodeficiency Virus (SIV) infects monkeys, but it does not cause any illness in monkey. Rhesus monkey can be artificially infected with sooty mangabey SIV strain (Lackner *et al.*, 2007). SIV markedly differs with HIV however anti-retroviral drugs works similarly for both HIV and SIV. Initially, SIV was considered a suitable model to study HIV vaccine, but it was observed that SIV infected monkeys do not produce antibodies against V3 loop

Table 7.7: HIV Clades and its Geographical Distribution.

Strain	Clade	Geographical Distribution
M (Major)	A*	West and Central Asia
	B$	Europe and USA
	C	South East Africa ad Asia
	D	East and Cental Africa
	E#	Never found alone
	F	Central Africa, South America and Eastern Europe
	G&	West and Eastern Africa and Central Europe
	H	Central Africa
	J	Central America
	K	Congo and Cameroon
N (New)		
O (Outlying)		

*: A and G recombinant variant, $: >40 per cent infection is non-B, because of increased migration, #: E always present as A/E recombinant, &: A/G variant also exist.

of HIV, which is in contrast to HIV and is essential for immune response. Later, Monkeys were infected with chimeric viruses called as SHIV (Simian Human Immunodeficiency Viruses). The SHIV has been developed by recombining with outer covering of HIV and rest is from SIV. This has shown a lot of similarity with HIV and has been used extensively to study the pathogenesis of SHIV in monkey model. Variability of results from one strain of SIV to another is so high that it is quite a task to extrapolate these results for HIV-1 infections.

In last decade scientists have developed different transgenic animal models using mice and rat to study the importance of individual HIV genes (Mindel *et al.,* 2001).

HIV/AIDS Vaccine

After identification of causative organism for AIDS, United States Health and Human Services Secretary Margaret Heckler declared that a vaccine against HIV infection would be available in two years. Since then it is more than 25 years, but we do not have a successful vaccine against HIV. Ms. Hecklers assumptions were based on some other successful examples of vaccination, with time, it was realized that the same principles are not applicable for the development of vaccine against HIV. Certainly, importance of vaccine against HIV can neither be denied nor be ignored. Various sincere efforts were tried to develop a vaccine against HIV (Sekaly, 2008). Unfortunately, all these efforts have to face an unprecedented problem, which was never imagined with any other vaccine program, so far. Even some of the clinical trials for vaccines have to be stopped in the middle, due to adverse results. Scientists are still optimistic that one day they may be able to crack complexity to develop HIV vaccine, which may eventually lead to development of a successful vaccine. To develop a successful vaccine against HIV, we may have to address some of the important issues at hand, like (1) To understand natural history of HIV, (2) To develop a suitable animal model, (3) To understand the significance and mechanism of long latency, (4) To control rapid mutation, and (5) Ethical issues related to placebo.

Acknowledgements

Authors are thankful to Mr. Dinesh Kumar for his secretarial and to Mr. Udai Pratap Singh for graphical designing.

References

Abbas KA, Lichtman AH, Pillai S (2008). Cellular and Molecular Immunology. Elsevier, New Delhi.

AIDS Myths Misunderstandings. AIDS InfoNet. http: //www.thebody.com/images/logo/ logo_notopics.gif Accessed 23 January 2012.

(1992). 1993 revised classification system for HIV infection and expanded surveillance definition for AIDS among adolescents and adults. MMWR Recomm Rep 41: 1-19.

Costin JM (2007). Cytopathic mechanisms of HIV-1. Virology J 4: 100.

Dandona L, Lakshmi V, Anil Kumar G *et al.* (2006). Is the HIV burden in India being overestimated? BMC Public Health 6: 308.

Freed EO (2001). HIV-1 Replication. Somat Cell Mol Genet 26: 13-33.

Gallo RC, Montagnier L (2003). The discovery of HIV as the causes of AIDS. N Engl *J Med* 349: 2283-2285.

Gottlieb MS, Schanker HM, Fan PT *et al.* (1981). Epidemiological notes and reports. MMWR 30: 1-3.

Gottlieb MS, Schroff R, Schanker HM (1981). Pneumocystis carinii pneumonia and mucosal candidiasis in previously healthy homosexual men: evidence of a new acquired cellular immunodeficiency. N Engl J Med 305: 1425-1431.

Kaufman SR, Murrey MJ, Simmons S (2006). Short comings of AIDS-related animal experimentation. Medical Research Modernization Committee, New York.

Khan FH (2009). The elements of immunology. Pearson, New Delhi.

Lackner AA, Veazey RS (2007). Current concepts in AIDS pathogenesis: Insights from SIV/Macaque Model. Ann Rev Med 58: 461-476.

Mindel A, Tenant-Flowers M (2001). ABC of AIDS natural history and management of early HIV infection. Brit Med J 322: 1290-1293.

Murphy K, Travers P, Walport M (2008). Immunobiology. Garland Sciences, New York.

Male D, Brostoff J, Roth DB *et al.* (2006). Immunology. Mosby Elsevier, Phildelphia.

Rastogi S, Agrahari S, Singh A *et al.* (2011). Clinical Stages of HIV. Biolixir (Accepted).

Rossi JJ, June CH, Kohn DB (2007). Genetic therapies against HIV. Nature Biotech 25: 1444-1453.

Ryser HJP, Fluckiger R (2005). Progress in targeting HIV-1 entry. Drug Discovery Today 10: 1085-1094.

Sekaly R (2008). The failed HIV Merck vaccine study: a step back or a launching point for vaccine development? J Exp Med 205: 7-12.

Shacklett BL (2008). Can the new humanized mouse models give HIV research a boost? PloS Med 5: e13.

Singh A, Singh UP, Varma A *et al.* (2011). Cure for HIV: New Possibility on Horizon J Pharm Bioall Sci 3: 461-464.

Spira S, Wainberg MA, Loemba H *et al.* (2003). Impact of clade on HIV-1 virulence, antiretroviral drug sensitivity and drug resistance. J Antimicrob Chemother 51: 229-240.

UNAIDS Annual Report, 2009.

Verma AS, Bhatt SM, Singh A *et al.* (2009). HIV: An Introduction. In: Chauhan AK and Varma A (ed). Text Book on Molecular Biotechnology, I.K. International Publishing House, New Delhi, pp. 853-877.

Verma AS, Singh A, Singh UP *et al.* (2010). NeuroAIDS in Indian Scenario. In: Gaur RK, Sharma P, Pratap R, Sharma KP, Sharma M, Dwivedi R (ed). Recent Trends in Biotechnology and Microbiology, Nova Scientific Publishers, USA, pp. 155-167.

Verma AS, Singh UP, Mallick P *et al.* (2010). HIV and NeuroAIDS. In: DBT Sponsored Training Program on Diagnosis and Management of Plant Viruses at AIMT, AUUP, NOIDA, June 15-25.

Verma AS, Singh UP, Dwivedi PD *et al.* (2010). NeuroAIDS: Role of cells of Central Nervous System (CNS). J Pharm Bioall Sci 2: 300-306.

Verma AS, Singh UP, Singh A (2010). NeuroAIDS: A Real Concern. IIOAB J 1: 28-31.

Verma AS, Singh A (2010). NeuroAIDS: A Worrisome Issue. Chron Young Sci 1: 33-35.

Verma AS, Singh A. (2011). Bone Marrow Transplantation: A New Avenue to Cure HIV. http://bloodjournal.hematologylibrary.org/content/117/10/2791/reply#content-block. Accessed 8 March 2011.

Verma AS, Singh UP, Mallick P *et al.* (2011). NeuroAIDS and Omics of HIV vpr. In: Barh D, Blum K, Madigan MA (ed). OMICS: Biomedical Perspectives and Applications (Accepted). CRC Press, Taylor and Francis LLC, USA.

Verma AS, Mallick P, Singh UP *et al.* (2010). HIV and Prevailing Myths. Science India 7-13.

Verma AS, Singh A (2011). Racial Discrimination done by HIV itself. Science India (Accepted).

2014, Advances in Biochemistry and Biotechnology Volume 2
Pages 143-162

Edited by: **Dr. Biplab Sarkar and Dr. Chiranjib Chakraborty**

Published by: **DAYA PUBLISHING HOUSE**

9

Recent Advances in Pathogenesis, Control and Prevention of Tuberculosis

Avinash Sonawane* and Soumitra Mohanty

School of Biotechnology, Campus-11, KIIT University, Bhubaneswar – 751 024, Orissa, India

ABSTRACT

Despite the discovery of tuberculosis bacillus for over 100 years ago and the availability of efficient drugs for over 50 years, tuberculosis still remains a major health problem around the world. There are 1.5 million deaths and 9 million new cases every year, and this number may increase if proper preventive and control measures are not taken. The emergence of multidrug-resistant (MDR) and extensively drug-resistant (XDR) *Mycobacterium tuberculosis* strains that are posing a threat for global tuberculosis (TB) control, the association of AIDS and tuberculosis, failure of health systems, greater mobility of people, and poverty further worsened the problem. For researchers the appearance of MDR and XDR strains has driven an increased interest in understanding the mechanisms of drug action and drug resistance, which could provide a

* *Corresponding author.* E-mail: asonawane@kiitbiotech.ac.in

significant contribution in the development of new antimicrobials. One of the major factors responsible for TB epidemiology is the lack of faster, more specific and sensible diagnostic methods. The current methodologies use molecular and immunological techniques, radioisotopes, and some others are based on fluorescence modifications of dyes. To win the fight against tuberculosis the major challenges lies ahead are understanding the pathology of drug-resistant TB strains, development of sensitive and specific detection methods, finding more potent drugs with adequate pharmacokinetics for shorter treatments for multidrug and latent forms of bacilli, new routes of administration and ways for increasing compliance.

Introduction

Tuberculosis (TB), a disease caused by the bacterium *Mycobacterium tuberculosis*, now asymptomatically infects one-third of the world's population and kills more than 1.5 million people every year (Small, 1996; WHO, 2011). TB has been a serious threat to humans for over 5000 years. Hippocrates, writing in the 5th century BCE, described *phthisis*-the Greek term for tuberculosis-as the most common disease of his time. Known as "white plaque" or "the consumption", TB took lives of so many people during Industrial Revolution, such that 1 out of 4 individuals in England were killed because of this disease. The causative agent of TB has been discovered almost 125 years back by Robert Koch still we are unable to win a fight against this disease. Consequently, today TB is the second-largest cause of death from an infectious agent worldwide (WHO, 20011). Despite steady drops in the number of cases in some parts of the world, the number of new cases appears to be growing, with an estimated 9 million new cases per year. Sub-Saharan Africa has the highest incidence rate, while one-half of the world's cases are in Bangladesh, China, India, Indonesia, and Pakistan (Kumar *et al.*, 2007; WHO, 20010). Today more than 90 per cent deaths occur in developing countries, among them individuals aged 15-60 accounts for three quarters of TB morbidity and mortality. Although, one out of three people is infected with bacilli that cause TB, but in most of the individuals bacilli lie dormant referred to as "latent TB" unless the infected individual's immune system becomes compromised or in malnourished or old age people.

TB usually attacks the lungs called pulmonary TB, the most common form of TB, but can also affect other parts of the body causing other kinds of TB collectively called as extrapulmonary tuberculosis (EPTB) (Golden and Vikram, 2005). EPTB infection sites include the pleura (pleurisy TB), central nervous system (meningitis TB), genitourinary system (urogenital TB), lymph nodes, and an especially serious form of disseminated TB called miliary tuberculosis (Regnier *et al.*, 2009). Extrapulmonary TB may co-exist with pulmonary TB as well (Golden and Vikram, 2005).

M. tuberculosis is an aerobic, non-motile, acid-fast bacillus with lipid rich cell wall, which is a unique clinical characteristic of this pathogen. The generation time of this bacterium is 16 to 20 hours, an extremely slow growth rate compared with other bacteria, which usually divide in less than an hour (Cox, 2004). The *M. tuberculosis* complex includes four other TB-causing mycobacteria: *M. bovis*, *M. africanum*, *M. canetti* and *M. microti* (van Soolingen *et al.*, 1997). *M. bovis* was once a common cause of tuberculosis, but the introduction of pasteurized milk has largely eliminated this as a public health problem in developed countries (Thoen *et al.*, 2006). *M. africanum* is not widespread, but in parts of Africa it is a significant cause of tuberculosis (Niemann *et al.*, 2002; Niobe-Eyangoh *et al.*, 2003). *M. canetti* is rare and seems to be limited to Africa, although a few cases have been seen in African emigrants (Pfyffer *et al.*, 1998), whereas *M. microti* is mostly seen in immunodeficient people (Niemann *et al.*, 2000). Other known pathogenic mycobacteria include *M. leprae, M. marinum, M. avium* and *M. kansasii.* The last two are part of the non-tuberculous mycobacteria (NTM) group. Non-tuberculous mycobacteria cause neither TB nor leprosy, but they do cause pulmonary diseases resembling TB.

Mode of Transmission and Pathogenesis of TB

The tubercle bacilli are carried in airborne particles, or droplet nuclei, that can be generated when persons who have pulmonary TB sneeze, cough, speak or sing. The particles are an estimated 1-5 mm in size. The risk of becoming infected after a small number of contacts with TB bacilli is low, but it increases in people who are exposed over long periods or whose immune system is weakened by ill health or immunosuppressive diseases such as HIV/AIDS. Infection occurs when a susceptible person inhales droplet nuclei containing *M. tuberculosis,* and these droplet nuclei traverse the mouth or nasal passages, upper respiratory tract, and bronchi to reach the alveoli of the lungs (Behr *et al.*, 1999; Nicas *et al.*, 2005). Once in the alveoli, the organisms are taken up by alveolar macrophages and spread from the site of initial infection in the lung through lymphatics or blood to other parts of the body. Usually within 2-10 weeks after initial infection with *M. tuberculosis,* the immune response limits further multiplication and spread of the tubercle bacilli; however, some of the bacilli remain dormant (called latent TB) and viable for many years. People with latent TB infection cannot transmit the microbes onto others except in environments where HIV/AIDS is widespread, less than one out of 10 individuals with TB infection will develop active TB disease in their life times. This risk is greatest during the first 2 years after infection. When TB disease does develop symptoms include coughing blood, fatigue, fever, persistent cough, weight loss, and night sweats (WHO, 2009).

Emerging Threats in Tuberculosis

HIV-TB Co-infection

Tuberculosis and HIV have been closely linked since the emergence of AIDS. HIV infection has contributed to a significant increase in the worldwide incidence of tuberculosis (Raviglione *et al.*, 1992). By producing a progressive decline in cell-mediated immunity, HIV alters the pathogenesis of tuberculosis, greatly increasing the risk of developing disease in co-infected individuals and leading to more frequent TB infection. Although HIV-related tuberculosis is both treatable and preventable, incidence rates continue to climb in developing nations where HIV infection and tuberculosis are endemic and resources are limited. By weakening the immune system, AIDS sharply increases susceptibility in people with latent TB disease. Those infected with HIV are up to 50 times more likely to develop TB disease each year. WHO estimates that 200,000 of those infected with HIV die from TB each year than HIV-uninfected individuals with the majority of these deaths occurring in Sub-Saharan Africa (Wells *et al.*, 2007).

Emergence of MDR and XDR-TB Strains

Another relatively new threat is the emergence of drug-resistant TB strains (Seung *et al.*, 2009). In all countries, strains of TB have been found that are resistant to one or another of the first-line TB drug treatment. Problems with treatment such as stopping a treatment course early have allowed the TB bacillus to mutate and develop resistance. Consequently multidrug-resistant (MDR) and extremely drug-resistant (XDR) TB has emerged (Gandhi *et al.*, 2006; Gandhi *et al.*, 2010). MDR-TB is due to bacteria that are resistant to at least isoniazid (INH) and rifampicin (RIF), the two most powerful first-line anti-TB drugs (WHO, 2006; Pillay, M; Sturm, 2007). MDR-TB is treatable using second-line drugs, although the treatment takes longer (up to two years as opposed to six months for non-resistant TB) and has more serious side effects than first-line drugs. There are now more than 500,000 new cases of MDR-TB each year, accounting for 4 per cent of all TB cases worldwide.

If these drugs are also misused or mismanaged, extensively drug-resistant TB (XDR-TB) can develop. In the year 2006, XDR-TB has been reported for the first time (Gandhi *et al.*, 2006). XDR-TB is resistant to first line drugs or the most commonly used second-line drugs, therefore, treatment options are seriously limited and so are the chances of cure. MDR- and XDR-TB is most common in Africa, China, Eastern Europe and Central Asia. Although overall XDR incidences are currently low, it has been detected in all world regions and it may become more prevalent as MDR-TB. Combination therapy, using at least two drugs in the initial stages of treatment, is used to counter such resistance.

Host Immune Responses against Mycobacteria

Innate Immune Responses

Receptor Mediated-Endocytosis

Phagocytosis of *M. tuberculosis* by alveolar macrophages is the first event following entry of the bacilli in the body (Schorey *et al.*, 1997). This host-pathogen interaction decides the outcome of the infection. Macrophage-*Mycobacterium* interactions involve surface receptor mediated binding of the bacilli to the phagocytes (Figure 9.1). These receptors involve complement receptors (CR1, CR2, CR3 and CR4), mannose receptors (MR) and Toll-like receptors (TLRs) (Heldwein and Fenton, 2002). The interaction between MR on the macrophages and mycobacteria is mediated through the pathogen surface glycoprotein lipoarabinomannan (LAM) (Chan *et al.*, 1991). Prostaglandin E2 and interleukin-4 are known to induce the expression of CR and MR receptors and function. Interaction between *M. tuberculosis* and TLRs is complex and it appears that distinct mycobacterial components interact with different members of the TLR family mainly TLR2 and TLR4. Following phagocytosis, microorganisms are enclosed into vesicle like structures called as "phagosomes". The engulfed bacteria are then subjected to degradation by lysosomal milieu (such as hydrolases and acidic environment) upon phagolysosome fusion (Figure 9.1). It is well known that pathogenic mycobacteria prevent the phagolysosome fusion by which *M. tuberculosis* survives inside macrophages. Several mycobacteria associated molecules such as multiacylated trehalose 2-sulphate, sulphatides, LAM plays a crucial role in inhibition of phagolysosomal fusion. In addition, *M. tuberculosis* is equipped with numerous immune evasion strategies, including modulation of antigen presentation to avoid elimination by T cells. *M. tuberculosis*-infected macrophages appear to be diminished in their ability to present antigen to CD4+ T cells, which leads to persistent infection (Selvaraj *et al.*, 1988). Another mechanism by which macrophages contribute to impaired T cell proliferation and function is by the production of cytokines such as TGF-b, IL-10 (Rojas *et al.*, 1999) and IL-6 (van Heyningen *et al.*, 1997).

Antibacterial Molecules Involved in Handling Mycobacteria inside Macrophages

In addition to the phago-lysosome fusion mechanism many other anti-mycobacterial effector molecules of macrophages are involved in resisting mycobacterial growth. These include generation of reactive oxygen intermediates (ROI), reactive nitrogen intermediates (RNI), mechanisms involving activation of macrophages by cytokines. Hydrogen peroxide (H_2O_2), one of the ROI intermediate generated via oxidative burst by macrophages, mediate mycobactericidal activity of phagocytes (Walker and Lowrie, 1981). Phagocytes, upon activation by interferon-g (IFN-g) and tumor necrosis factor-a (TNF-a), generate nitric oxide (NO) and RNI via inducible nitric oxide synthease (iNOS2). These toxic nitrogen oxides have been shown critical in host defense under *in vitro* and *in vivo* conditions against

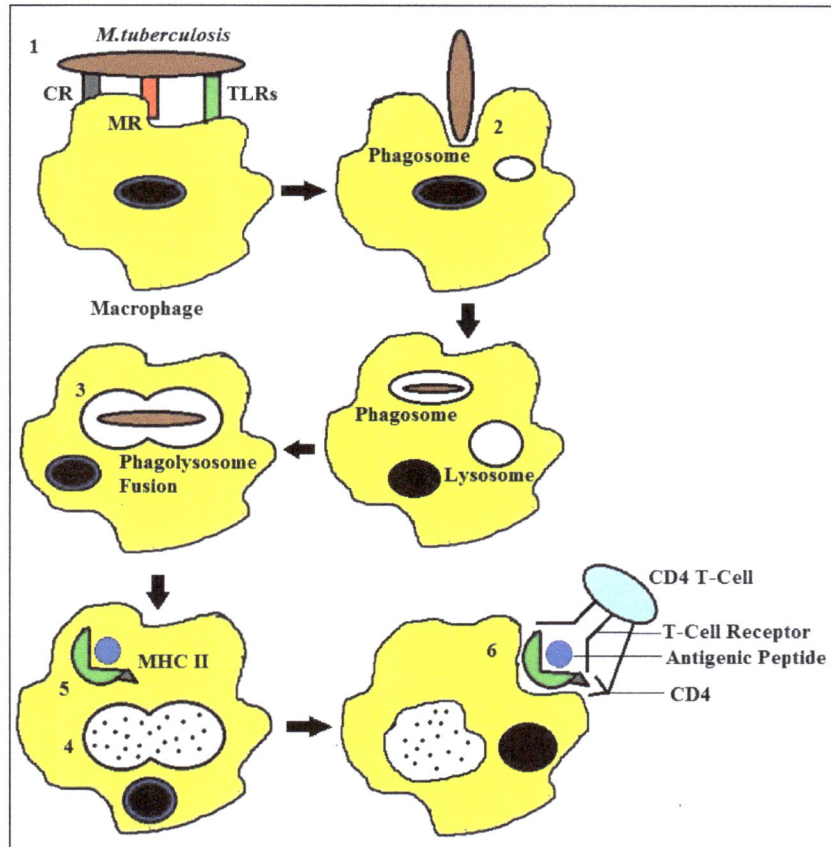

Figure 9.1

(1) Antigen interacts with macrophage receptors (2) Engulfment of antigen by phagosome (3) Fusion of phagosome and lysosome *i.e.* phagolysosome (4) Antigen processed to peptides in phagolysosome (5) Peptides bind to MHC II (6) Phagolysosome fuse with plasma membrane. Peptide MHC II complex is presented to CD4 helper T cell.

mycobacteria, particularly in murine system (Chan and Flynn, 1999). The role of RNI in human infection is controversial and differs from that of mice.

Macrophage Apoptosis

Another potential mechanism involved in macrophage defense against mycobacteria is induction of programmed cell death or apoptosis. Molloy *et al.* (1994) have shown that macrophage apoptosis results in reduced intracellular viability of mycobacteria. Klingler *et al.* (1997) have demonstrated that TB infection down regulate bcl-2, an inhibitor of apoptosis, expression resulting in stimulation of apoptosis process.

The other components of innate immunity are neutrophils, natural killer cells (NK), and antimicrobial peptides (AMPs) such as cathelicidins and defensins.

Neutrophils

M. tuberculosis replicates in, and in turn is controlled by macrophages. Neutrophils, the first cells to migrate to the site of infection followed by NK cells, are endowed with an array of antimicrobial substances. Recently it has been shown that macrophages phagocytose apoptotic neutrophils and thereby deploy neutrophil peptides with antimycobacterial activity (Tan *et al.*, 2006). Increased accumulation of neutrophils in the TB granuloma and increased chemotaxis has been suggested a role for neutrophils in TB infection. Several studies have demonstrated that neutrophils provide agents such as AMPs, which is lacking for macrophage-mediated killing (Ogata *et al.*, 1992) Two such classes of AMPs have been identified to date in human: the a defensins human neutrophil peptides (HNPs) 1-3 (Fu *et al.*, 2003), human cathelicidin LL-37 (Liu *et al.*, 2006, Martineau *et al.*, 2007), lipocalin 2, which binds to soluble mycobacterial siderophores. These molecules have found to exert potent mycobactericidal activities under *in vitro* and *in vivo* conditions.

Natural Killer (NK) Cells

NK cells are also the effector cells of innate immunity. During early infection, NK cells are capable of activating phagocytic cells. NK cells lyse the pathogen or infected macrophages through the action of toxins such as perforin and granulysin and by production of IFN-γ. However, lowered NK activity was demonstrated during TB infection (Nirmala *et al.*, 2001).

Cell Mediated Immunity (CMI)

Cell mediated immunity plays an important role in eliciting protective immune response against *M. tuberculosis* infection. Since *M. tuberculosis* is an intracellular pathogen, the bacteria are shielded from antibodies. Although many researchers have dismissed a role for B cells or antibody in protection against TB (Johnson *et al.*, 1997), several studies suggest that these may contribute to the response to TB (Bosio *et al.*, 2000). Within 2 to 8 weeks of infection, various *M. tuberculosis* specific antigens stimulate CMI response resulting in infiltration of lymphocytes, neutrophils and activated macrophages into the lesion resulting in the formation of a solid mass like structure called as "granuloma". The metabolic activities and growth of the bacilli is lowered and dead macrophages form caseous structures surrounding the bacilli. The bacilli may remain dormant forever within the granuloma, get re-activated if the immune system of the person is compromised or may get discharged into the airways.

Various mycobacterial antigens are known to induce CMI in humans. Among different immune cells, CD4+ and CD8+ T cells are crucial components of CMI against mycobacteria infection.

CD4 T Cells

Antigen presentation is mediated by two classical pathways namely endogeneous and exogeneous antigen presentation pathways. *M. tuberculosis* resides primarily in a vacuole within macrophage, and thus, major histocompatibility complex (MHC) class II presentation of mycobacterial antigens to CD4[+] T cells is obvious mode of antigen presentation (Figure 9.1).These cells are most important in the protective response against *M. tuberculosis* infection. In humans, the pathogenesis of HIV infection has demonstrated that the loss of CD4[+] T cells greatly increases susceptibility to both acute and re-activation TB (Selwyn *et al.,* 1989). The primary function of CD4[+] T cells is the production of IFN-g and other cytokines, which activate macrophages. Apoptosis or lysis of infected cells by CD4[+] T cells may also play a role in controlling infection (Keane *et al.,* 1997).

CD8 T Cells

CD8 T cells are also capable of secreting cytokines such as IFN-γ and thus may play a role in regulating the balance between Th1 and Th2 cells in the lungs of patients with pulmonary TB. The mechanism by which mycobacterial proteins gain access to the MHC class I molecules is still ill defined. Recently it has been shown that bacilli in macrophages are found outside phagosomes 2-3 days after infection (van der Wel *et al.,* 2007). It has been hypothesized that mycobacteria induce pore or break in the vesicular membrane surrounding the bacilli that might allow mycobacterial antigen to enter the cytoplasm of the infected cell (Teitelbaum *et al.,* 1999). Separate studies (Yu *et al.,* 1995; Taha *et al.,* 1997) showed increase in CD8 T cells in the bronchoalveolar lavage (BAL) of active TB patients, along with increase in the number of BAL expressing IFN-γ, and lysis of infected dendritic cells and macrophages. The killing of intracellular bacteria was dependent on preforin/granulysin, toxins secreted by cytotoxic T lymphocytes. Many studies support the notion that CD8[+] as well as CD4[+] T cell responses must be stimulated to provide protective immunity. However, a variety of pathogens can weaken CMI by inducing T cell apoptosis. Several evidences indicate that apoptosis of T cells does occur in murine (Kremer *et al.,* 2000) and human TB (Hirsch *et al.,* 2001). The observed apoptosis is associated with reduced *M. tuberculosis*-stimulated IFN-g and IL-2 production.

Cytokines

Production of several interleukins is induced following phagocytosis of *M. tuberculosis* by macrophages and dendritic cells (Ladel *et al.,* 1997), which leads to development of a T cell response with production of IFN-γ. Humans with reduced IFN-γ production from T cells are found more susceptible to *M. bovis*-BCG and *M. avium* infections (Ottenhof *et al.,* 1998). McDyer *et al.* (McDyer *et al.,* 1997) found that stimulated peripheral blood monocyte cells from MDR-TB patients had less secretion of IFN-γ and IL-2. IFN-γ, a key cytokine in control of *M. tuberculosis* infection is produced by both CD4[+] and CD8[+] T cells. IFN-γ might augment antigen presentation, leading to recruitment of CD4[+] T-lymphocytes and cytotoxic T-lymphocytes, which participate in mycobacterial killing. Although IFN-γ production alone is insufficient to control *M. tuberculosis* infection, it is required for the protective response to this pathogen. IL-4, IL-6 could also bring about *in vitro* killing of mycobacteria by macrophages either alone or in synergy with IFN-γ. TNF-α is also believed to play multiple roles in immune responses against *M. tuberculosis* infection. *M. tuberculosis* induces TNF-α secretion by macrophages, dendritic cells and T cells. In mice deficient in TNF-α, *M. tuberculosis* resulted in rapid death of the mice, with substantially higher bacterial burdens (Flynn *et al.,* 1995). TNF-a in synergy with IFN-γ induces nitric oxide synthase 2 (NOS2), an inducible enzyme responsible for production of anti-mycobacterial reactive free radical nitrogen oxide, expression (Flynn *et al.,* 1995). TNF-α is important in preventing dissemination of TB, granuloma formation (Flynn *et al.,* 1995; Garcia *et al.,*

1997), cell migration and localization within tissues in *M. tuberculosis* infection. TNF-α along with IL-1 plays an important role in the acute phase response in TB. Another cytokine IL-2 has a pivotal role in generating an immune response by inducing an expansion of the pool of lymphocytes specific for an *M. tuberculosis* antigen. IL-2 secretion by the protective CD4 Th1 cells can influence the course of mycobacterial infections, either alone or in combination with other cytokines (Blanchard *et al.*, 1989). IL-6 has also been implicated in the host response to *M. tuberculosis*. This cytokine has multiple roles in the immune response, including inflammation, hematopoiesis and differentiation of T cells. Early increase in lung burden in IL-6 $^{-/-}$ mice suggests that IL-6 is important in the initial innate response to the pathogen (Saunders *et al.*, 2000).

IL-10 is considered as an anti-inflammatory cytokine. This cytokine, produced by macrophages and T cells during *M. tuberculosis* infection, possesses macrophage deactivating properties, including downregulation of IL-12 production, which in turn decreases IFN-γ production by T cells. IL-10 also directly involved in inhibition of CD4[+]T cell responses, as well as by inhibiting antigen presenting function of cells infected with mycobacteria (Rojas *et al.*, 1999).

Diagnosis

In ancient days primitive methods like medical history, physical examination were used, but these tests could not be used to confirm the TB. Definitive diagnosis of TB involves demonstration of the organism by microbiological, cytopathological or histopathological methods. Commonly used diagnostic tests involve chest X-ray, microbiological examination of sputum and other biological samples depending up on the type of TB, tuberculin skin test (Mantoux test), surgical biopsy and assays based on the release of specific cytokines after stimulation with *M. tuberculosis* antigens.

Radiography

TB is marked with scarring (fibrosis) or hardening (calcification) in the lungs Lesions may appear anywhere in the lungs. In disseminated TB a pattern of many tiny nodules throughout the lung fields is seen - the so called miliary TB. Abnormalities on chest radiographs may be suggestive of, but are never diagnostic of, TB. However, chest radiographs may be used for the diagnosis of pulmonary TB in conjunction with other methods such as sputum smear analysis and staining. The pattern of chest radiography depends upon the type of TB. For example in patients with pleural TB, the chest radiograph usually reveals a unilateral pleural effusion encysted in the costoparietal regions. In acute disseminated TB nodules of 2-3 mm size are seen. Some patients with TB, however, may have normal chest radiographs and some may have patterns that are indistinguishable from interstitial pneumonia (Sharma *et al.*, 1995).

A variant of the chest X-Ray, abreugraphy (also called miniature mass radiography (MMR) or miniature chest radiograph), invented by Dr. Manuel Dias de Abreu in 1935, is used for the accurate diagnosis of TB. MMR is much less expensive than traditional X-ray. It is a photofluorography technique for mass screening of tuberculosis using a miniature (50 to 100 mm) photograph of the screen of X-ray fluoroscopy of the thorax.

Microbiological Examinations

TB diagnosis can be done by culturing *M. tuberculosis* from specimens taken from patients. Most often sputum, cerebrospinal fluid, and biopsied tissues are taken for examinations.

Sputum

M. tuberculosis is an acid-fast bacterium, therefore, a special bacteriological method Acid-fast staining is used to identify this organism since its lipid rich cell wall makes it resistant to Gram stain

(Darrow *et al.*, 1948). This method was first described by two German doctors: Franz Ziehl (1859 to 1926) and Friedrich Neelsen (1854 to 1894). Sputum smears are prepared for acid-fast bacilli and are stained with Ziel-Neelsen staining. Acid-fast bacilli will appear bright red after staining Samples of the sputum also are usually taken and cultured on different types of media such as Middlebrook (7H9, 7H10) or Löwenstein-Jensen (LJ) medium. More recently new automated and faster systems have been developed, which includes the MB/BacT, BACTEC 9000, and the Mycobacterial Growth Indicator Tube (MGIT). However, the major limitation of this method is the sensitivity. It cannot detect the bacteria below 10^4 per ml and is unable to distinguish between live and dead bacteria.

In patients incapable of producing a sputum sample, alternative sample sources for the diagnosis of TB includes laryngeal swab, bronchoscopy (with bronchoalveolar lavage or bronchial washings), and fine needle aspiration of transtracheal or transbronchial fluids. In some cases, more invasive techniques are necessary, including tissue biopsies during thoracoscopy.

PCR

M. tuberculosis is a slow growing organism with a generation time of approximately 16-20 h. The organism can take up to four to six weeks to grow in culture. A special test to diagnose TB called the polymerase chain reaction (PCR) detects the genetic material of the bacteria. This test is fast, specific and sensitive (it detects minute amounts of the bacteria). Using this test the results can be obtained within a few days.

Tuberculin Skin Test (Mantoux Test)

Several types of skin tests are used to screen for TB infection. The Mantoux test (also known as the Tuberculin test, Pirquet test, or PPD test for Purified Protein Derivative) is one of the widely used tests for the diagnosis of TB. In this test, a small amount of purified extract (ca. 5 tuberculin units) from dead tuberculosis bacteria is injected intradermally and observed 48 to 72 hours later (WHO, 1963). Person who has been exposed to the bacteria is expected to mount an immune response in the skin containing the bacterial proteins. If a person is infected with tuberculosis, a raised and induration occurs around the site of the injection (A TH *et al.*, 1996). In contrast, no reaction will occur at the site of the injection if a person is not infected with TB. When only the skin test is positive, or evidence of prior TB is present on chest X-rays, the disease is referred to as "latent tuberculosis."

However, Montoux test has certain limitations. A false positive result may be seen if the person is exposed to non-tuberculous mycobacteria or previously has been administered with a BCG vaccine. Those that are immunologically compromised, especially those with HIV and low CD4 T cell counts, frequently show negative results from the PPD test. This is because the immune system needs to be functional to mount a response to the protein derivative injected under the skin. Similarly, if the infection with tuberculosis has occurred recently, the skin test can be falsely negative because it usually takes 2 to 10 weeks after the time of infection with tuberculosis before the skin test becomes positive. TB skin test cannot determine whether the disease is active or not. This determination requires the chest X-rays and/or sputum analysis (smear and culture) in the laboratory.

Interferon-γ Release Assays

Interferon-gamma (IFN-γ) release assays (IGRAs) have been recently developed for the diagnosis of latent TB (LTB) infection (Pai *et al.*, 2004). Due to the lack of a gold standard for the diagnosis of LTB, the IGRA is compared to the Mantoux Tuberculin Skin Test (TST), which yields discordant results in varying numbers. Three IGRAs QuantiFERON®-TB Gold test (QFT-G), QuantiFERON®-TB Gold In-Tube test (QFT-GIT), T-SPOT® are used for TB diagnosis. IGRAs are based on the ability of the

M. tuberculosis antigens early secretory antigen target-6 (ESAT-6) and culture filtrate protein 10 (CFP-10) to stimulate host production of interferon-γ. Because these antigens are not present in non-tuberculous mycobacteria or in any BCG vaccine variant, these tests can distinguish latent tuberculosis infection (LTBI).

The blood tests QuantiFERON-TB Gold In Tube and T-SPOT-TB use these antigens to detect people with tuberculosis. Lymphocytes from the patient's blood are incubated with the *M. tuberculosis* antigens. If the patient has been exposed to tuberculosis before, T lymphocytes produce interferon in response. The QuantiFERON-TB Gold In Tube uses an ELISA format to detect the whole blood production of interferon γ with great sensitivity (89 per cent). The distinction between the tests is that QuantiFERON-TB Gold quantifies the total amount of interferon when whole blood is exposed to the antigens (ESAT-6, CFP-10). The enzyme-linked immunospot assay (ELISPOT) is another blood test is also available that may replace the skin test for diagnosis. T-SPOT-TB, a type of ELISPOT assay counts the number of activated T lymphocytes that secrete interferon γ.

Tuberculosis Treatment

Treatment of mycobacterial infections differs from that of other bacterial diseases due to several properties possessed by the mycobacteria. A hallmark of the mycobacteria is the complex lipid-rich cell wall envelop that protects the organism from the host response and antimycobacterial therapy (Figure 9.2). In addition, mycobacteria are slow growing, facultative intracellular parasites which generally cause a chronic infection. These properties add greater constraints to efficient therapy. To be effective, drugs must be able to penetrate the host macrophage and have reduced toxicity and be effective at low doses.

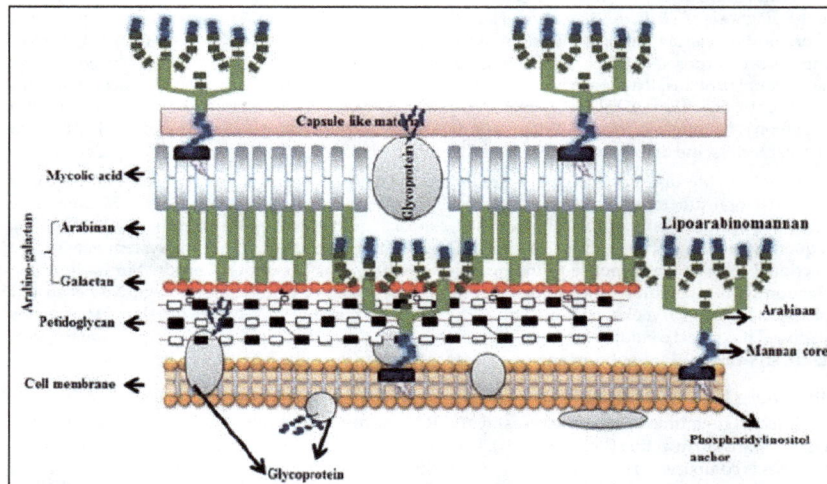

Figure 9.2: Schematic Diagram of Cell Wall of *Mycobacterium tuberculosis*.

Historically, those who contracted TB disease had a high risk of death. Pulmonary TB, the most common form of TB diseases, is fatal in over 50 per cent of cases when untreated. However, in the second half of the 19th century the " sanatorium cure" was discovered, which involved moving patients outside and exposing them to fresh air and sunlight, but the mechanism behind this was unknown. However, recently it was shown that interaction of a 19-kDa lipopeptide of *M.tuberculosis* with Toll-like receptor-2 on macrophage surface up-regulates the expression of vitamin D receptor that leads to induction of a antimicrobial peptide cathelicidin and resulting in killing of intracellular *M. tuberculosis* (Liu *et al.,* 2006). This is an important finding since it begins to explain the long-observed finding that vitamin D improves anti-tuberculosis therapy in humans.

Nonadherence of anti-TB therapy is the main reason for treatment failure and the development of drug-resistant strains of *M. tuberculosis*. Therefore, WHO recommends Directly Observed Therapy (DOT), whereby a treatment partner administers therapy to ensure adherence to the treatment regimen. Patients who are on DOTS are put on a course of four medicines (isoniazid, rifampicin, pyrazinamide and ethambutol) for two months called killing phase, followed by four months taking just the first of these drugs called sterilizing phase. This practice increases treatment effectiveness and reduces the risk that an individual patient develops drug-resistant TB. For latent TB the recommended regimens are 9 months of isoniazid or 2 months of rifampin plus pyrazinamide. For children, isoniazid for 9 months is the only recommended regimen.

Treatment of Mycobacterial Infections

For over 50 years combination of antibiotics is the most commonly used mode for the treatment of tuberculosis. TB patients are put on combination antibiotic therapy for nine to 12 months depending upon the type and progression of TB. Treatment of TB is classified into two classes of antibiotics: First line antibiotics and second line antibiotics. First line antibiotics include ethambutol (EMB), isoniazid (INH), pyrazinamide (PZA), rifampicin (RIF) and streptomycin (STM). There are six classes of second-ling drugs used for the treatment of TB. A drug is classified as second-line on the basis of its effectiveness as compared to first-line drugs, toxic side-effects, and availability in developing countries. These include aminoglycosides *e.g.* amikacin (AMK), kanamycin (KM) and fluoroquinolones *e.g.* ciprofloxacin (CIP), levofloxacin, moxifloxacin (MXF).

In the treatment of disease caused by *M. tuberculosis* susceptible to all agents, a 6-month course of treatment is effective. INH and RIF are used throughout the entire course of therapy, with pyrazinamide added during the first 2 months. Only patients with military, meningeal, or bone and joint disease require longer therapy. There are several reasons for supporting combination therapy. The different drugs in the regimen have different modes of action. INH is bactericidal against replicating bacteria (Inderlied and Nash, 1996). EMB is bacteriostatic at low doses, but is used in TB treatment at higher, bactericidal doses (Kilburn and Takayama, 1981). RMP is bactericidal and has a sterilizing effect (Olliaro *et al.,* 1995). PZA is only weakly bactericidal, but is very effective against bacteria located in acidic environments, inside macrophages, or in areas of acute inflammation

Isoniazid

INH is an analogue of nicotinamide, and is most effective against *M. tuberculosis,* with relatively low toxicity (Inderlied and Nash, 1996). INH is able to inhibit mycolic acid synthesis and is believed to be primarily responsible for mycobacterial cell death.

Ethambutol

EMB is a synthetic drug that was developed from N, N'-diisopropylethyl-enediamine. EMB prevents the polymerization of cell wall arabinan by inhibiting the incorporation of D-arabinose into arabinogalactan and lipoarabinomannan (Kahoo *et al.*, 1996; Kilburn *et al.*, 1981; Mikusova *et al.*, 1995).

Pyrazinamide

PZA is the amide of pyrazinoic acid that is metabolized to 5-hydroxypyrazinamide after absorption from the gastrointestinal tract (Inderlied and Nash, 1996). PZA is converted to pyrazinoic acid by nicotinamidase. PZA functions as prodrug of pyrazinoic acid. Susceptibity of *M. tuberculosis* to PZA is due to a deficient pyrazinoic acid efflux mechanism.

Rifamycins

Rifamycins are a group of bactericidal antimicrobials that were originally isolated from a species of *Streptomyces*. The target for rifamycins is the beta subunit of the DNA-dependent RNA polymerase (Olliaro *et al.*, 1995). Rifampin has the ability to kill both the actively growing extracellular mycobacteria and the slower growing semi-dormant extracellular mycobacteria found in caseous material (Friedman and Selwyn, 1995). Rifampin has the fastest onset of action (15-20 min), as compared to the other antituberculous drugs.

Aminoglycosides

Aminoglycosides are characterized by combinations of six-membered aminocyclitol rings with varying attached side chains. The mode of action of aminoglycosides is inhibition of protein synthesis. Inhibition is accomplished by irreversible binding of the drug to the bacterial 30S ribosomal subunit, thus freezing the initiation complex and preventing further elongation of polypeptide chains.

Fluoroquinolones

The fluoroquinolones are heterocyclic carbonic acid derivatives, which are structurally related to nalidixic acid. The primary target for the quinolones is the bacterial DNA gyrase (Inderlied and Nash, 1996). Binding of the drug to the enzyme prevents subsequent processes that depend upon the proper maintenance of DNA superhelical twists, such as replication and transcription (Chopra and Brennan, 1998).

New Strategies for Antimycobacterial Drug Development

A number of effective and reliable antimycobacterial drugs are currently available for treatment of several mycobacterial infections. The primary reason for the loss of efficacy of some of these drugs is the emergence of drug resistant strains. Development of resistance is an important variable to be considered in the eradication of mycobacterial disease. However, the recent advances in genomics, proteomics and emergence of antimicrobial peptides as potential therapeutic agents suggest a promising future with regard to development of effective drugs for control and/or eradication of mycobacterial diseases.

Genomics

The genome *M. tuberculosis* genome has been sequenced in 1998, therefore, development of new and better drugs should be possible. This is extremely important for *M. tuberculosis* because of the increasing numbers of drug resistant strains that are developing. Given the expanding genetic knowledge base, it should be possible to utilize sophisticated technologies to identify new drug targets and design new and improved therapeutic regimens for mycobacterial infections.

Proteomics

The next level of technological platforms being developed for drug discovery and development involves techniques that can analyze protein arrays. Unlike DNA and RNA arrays, proteomics addresses the final gene products. The benefit of this technology is that the major shortcomings of DNA microarray *i.e.* failure to consider pre-translational events and post-translational modifications of proteins is overcome.

Antimicrobial Peptides as Potential Drug Targets

At present, the antimycobacterial activities of the antimicrobial peptides have highlighted their potential as alternative therapeutic agents against mycobacteria. Therapeutic potential of human neutrophil peptide 1 against tuberculosis has already been reported (Sharma *et al.*, 2001). Recently, it has been reported that LL-37, human antimicrobial peptide cathelicidin, is capable of inhibiting mycobacterial growth in human cells and this will aid in the development of novel therapeutic agents for treatment of mycobacterial infections, and to develop an alternative/adjunct therapeutic strategy against tuberculosis (Méndez-Samperio *et al.*, 2008). In support of this, it has been shown that exogenous administration or transfer of the hCAP18 gene into mouse airways protected mice from microbial infection (Bals *et al.*, 1999; Bals, 2000; Bals and Wilson, 2003). To date, there are several patents, which have been related to the method of identifying peptides that have antimicrobial activity, including the use of cathelicidin LL-37 and its derivatives and/or synthetic analogs for wound healing (Zaiou *et al.*, 2007).

A different approach utilizes natural antimicrobial peptides as templates for the development of synthetic analogs with optimized biological functions, such as pexiganan acetate a synthetic analog of the cathelicidin LL-37 (Lamb and Wiseman, 1998). This approach represents an important alternative for bacterial resistance to conventional antibiotics, such as the multidrug resistant mycobacterial pathogens. It is important to consider that further studies are needed to investigate the costs of peptide production, the possible toxicities that might accompany systemic administration of peptides. However, the combination of the therapeutic use of antimicrobial peptides or their synthetic analogs and conventional antimycobacterial drugs (*e.g.* isoniazid and rifampicin) might be a result of reduced the prolonged (6–9 mo) treatment courses in antituberculosis drug therapy.

Nanoparticles as an Antimycobacterial Agent

Recently nanoparticles have gained a lot of attention as a strong antibacterial agent. These particles include many metallic nanoparticles like silver, zinc, gold, iron and titanium and also biopolymer like chitosan. Researchers have shown unprecedented interest as a therapeutic agent as bacteria are not able to develop resistance against these particles. For example silver nanoparticles bind to bacterial membrane and make pore in the bacterial membrane which in turn kills the bacteria. Although the mechanism by which silver exerts a toxic effect is not well understood till today but recent report says starch and chitosan coated silver nanoparticles effectively kills *Mycobacterium smegmatis* (Mohanty *et al.*, 2012, Jena *et al.*, 2012) with no toxicity to host cell. Similarly Plant biomass coated and fungal biomass coated silver nanoparticles in synergies with cationic antimicrobial peptides also efficiently kill *Mycobacterium smegmatis* and *Mycobacterium marinum* without damaging mouse macrophages. (Mohanty *et al.*, 2013). Poly rifampicin nanoparticles also efficiently clears *Mycobacterium bovis* BCG infection from macrophages. (Kalluru R *et al.*, 2013). In future these nanoparticles will help in combating M.tuberculosis and will also help in preventing the emergence of drug resistance problem.

Recent Advances in Anti-TB Drug Development

Fluoroquinolones

The fluoroquinolones are a promising second-line drugs for the treatment of TB (Gillespie and Kennedy, 1998). Moxifloxacin and gatifloxacin are candidates for shortening TB treatment, since they have the lowest MICs (Gillespie and Billington, 1999; Gillespie et al., 2001; Fung-Tome et al., 2000) and greatest bactericidal activity. Moxifloxacin and gatifloxacin inhibits bacterial DNA gyrase, an enzyme that is essential for the maintenance of DNA supercoils, which are necessary for chromosomal replication. Recently, a new generation of quinolone TBK 613 is being developed in preclinical research.

TMC207

TMC207 has shown equal activity in susceptible and MDR strains. It inhibits the mycobacterial ATP synthase enzyme (Andries et al., 2005; de Jonge et al., 2007).

Nitroimidazopyrans

The nitroimidazopyrans are derived from the bicyclic nitroimidazofurans that were originally developed for cancer chemotherapy but also exhibited activity against actively growing and dormant M. tuberculosis (Papadopoulou et al., 2007; Stover et al., 2000). The compounds are structurally related to metronidazole (Barry and O'Connor, 2007; Stover et al., 2000). PA-824 (a nitroimidazo-oxazine) and OPC-67683 (a dihydroimidazo-oxazole) are currently being investigated in clinical trials (Spigelman, 2007). Activated PA-824 inhibits the synthesis of proteins and cell wall lipids. OPC-67683 is a mycolic acid biosynthesis inhibitor (Sasaki et al., 2006). While isoniazid inhibits the synthesis of all mycolic acid subclasses, OPC-67683 inhibits methoxy and ketomycolic acid synthesis only (Matsumoto et al., 2006).

Pyrroles

Several pyrrole derivatives have shown potent mycobactericidal activities. LL3858 is being investigated in phase I clinical trials (Arrora et al., 2004). LL3858 is active against M. tuberculosis strains that are resistant to available anti-TB drugs A fixed-dose combination called LL3848, containing LL3858 and the standard, first-line anti-TB drugs, is also being developed (Protopopova et al., 2007). The mycobacterial target of LL3858 is not yet known.

Future Perspectives

Despite the progresses in the management of TB, important obstacles, uncertainties, and unmet priorities remain. An extraordinary and special effort is required in sub-Saharan Africa and Asia, where TB-related morbidity and mortality is increasing at an alarming rate. In April 2008, WHO convened a meeting of experts who concluded that the "Three I's for TB—isoniazid preventive therapy, intensified case finding for TB, and infection control for TB—should be an essential aspect of providing TB services. Priorities for TB include the further expansion of DOTS and addressing MDR and XDR disease as a matter of urgency. This highlights the huge problem of infrastructure, for without laboratory capacity, drug resistance cannot be tackled because it cannot be diagnosed.

Several new drugs for TB treatment are being evaluated in clinical trials. Moxifloxacin and gatifloxacin might shorten TB treatment. Co-administration of moxifloxacin and PA-824 could be active against latent TB. To overcome drug-resistance problem an important approach should be to use combination therapy of conventional drugs and antimicrobial peptides.

Unfortunately, shorter treatment regimens based on the new agents are likely to take at least another decade to be fully developed and implemented in clinical practice. Since not all new agents will succeed in clinically useful regimens, and since only a few drugs are currently in preclinical development, more new agents are needed. Therefore, urgent attention should be paid to the development of new drugs; this requires more involvement of large pharmaceutical industries. The development of new drugs should get a programmatic approach in which a series of consecutive studies are properly planned, while keeping the desired end product in mind. Moreover, the development of various agents must be coordinated, since a single new drug might not be very promising in a regimen with the standard anti-TB drugs, but could be highly active in combination with other new drugs. Ways to shorten clinical trials with new TB drugs should be explored. To facilitate clinical trials, research capacity should be strengthened in developing countries, where the TB burden is highest.

Finally, control of the TB epidemic implies more than developing new drugs. The diagnostic and therapeutic facilities of health care centers in developing countries should be improved, and the socio-economic status and general welfare of patients should be addressed to help eradicate TB.

Acknowledgements

We are grateful to Sonawane lab members for excellent discussions and technical support.

References

A TH, Reider HL, Trebucq A, Waaler HT (1996). Guidelines for conducting tuberculin skin test surveys in high prevalence countries. *Tubercle and Lung Disease* 77: 1-20.

Andries KP, Verhasselt J, Guillemont HW, Gohlmann JM, Neefs H, Winkler GJ *et al.* (2005). A diarylquinoline drug active on the ATP synthase of *Mycobacterium tuberculosis*. Science 307: 223–227.

Arrora SK, Sinha N, Sinha R, Bateja R, Sharma S, Upadhayaya RS (2004). Design, synthesis, modelling and activity of novel anti tubercular compounds, abstr. 63. Abstr. Am. Chem. Soc. Meet.

Bals R, Weiner DJ, Meegalla RL, Wilson JM (1999). Transfer of a cathelicidin peptide antibiotic gene restores bacterial killing in a cystic fibrosis xenograft model. J Clin Invest 103: 1113–7.

Bals R, Wilson JM (2003). Cathelicidins-a family of multifunctional antimicrobial peptides. Cell Mol Life Sci 60: 711–20.

Bals R (2000). Epithelial antimicrobial peptides in host defense against infection. Respir Res 1: 141–50.

Barry PJ, Connor TMO (2007). Novel agents in the management of *Mycobacterium tuberculosis* disease. Curr. Med. Chem. 14: 2000–2008.

Behr MA, Warren SA, Salamon H, *et al.* (1999). Transmission of *Mycobacterium tuberculosis* from patients smear-negative for acid-fast bacilli. Lancet 353: 444–9.

Blanchard DK, Michelini-Norris MB, Friedman H, Djeu JY (1989). Lysis of mycobacteria-infected monocytes by IL-2 activated killer cells: role of LFA-1. Cell Immunol 119 : 402-11.

Bosio CM, Gardner D, Elkins KL (2000). Infection of B cell deficient mice with CDC1551, a clinical isolate of *Mycobacterium tuberculosis*: delay in dissemination and development of lung pathology. J Immunol 164 : 6417-25.

Chan J and Flynn, J (1999). Nitric oxide in *Mycobacterium tuberculosis* infection. In: Fang FC, editor, Nitric oxide and infection, New York: Kluwer Academic Plenum: 281-310.

Chan J, Fan X, Hunter SW, Brennan PJ and Bloom BR (1991). Lipoarabinomannan, a possible virulence factor involved in persistence of *Mycobacterium tuberculosis* within macrophages. Infect Immun 59: 1755–1761.

Chopra I, Brennan P (1998). Molecular action of anti-mycobacterial agents. Tubercle and Lung Disease 78: 89-98.

Cox R (2004). Quantitative relationships for specific growth rates and macromolecular compositions of *Mycobacterium tuberculosis, Streptomyces coelicolor* A3(2) and *Escherichia coli* B/r: an integrative theoretical approach. Microbiology 150: 1413–26.

Darrow MA (1948). Staining the tubercle organism in sputum smears. Stain Technol 24: 93–94

De Jonge MR, Koymans LH, Guillemont JE, Koul A, Andries K (2007). A computational model of the inhibition of *Mycobacterium tuberculosis* ATPase by a new drug candidate R207910. Proteins 67: 971–980.

Edson M, Souza AS, Franquet T, Muller NL (2005). Diffuse High-Attenuation Pulmonary Abnormalities: A Pattern-Oriented Diagnostic Approach on High-Resolution CT. American Journal of Roentgenology 184: 273-282.

Flynn JL, Goldstein MM, Chan J, Triebold KJ, Pfeffer K, Lowenstein CJ, *et al.* (1995).Tumour necrosis factor-a is required in the protective immune response against *Mycobacterium tuberculosis* in mice. Immunity 2: 561-72.

Friedman LN, Selwyn (1994). PA Pulmonary tuberculosis: primary, reactivation, HIV related, and non-HIV related. In Friedman LN, ed.Tuberculosis: current concepts and treatment. CRC Press. Boca Raton, FL 93-112.

Fu LM (2003). The potential of human neutrophil peptides in tuberculosis therapy. *Int J Tuberc Lung Dis* 7: 1027–1032.

Fung-Tomc J, Minassian B, Kolek B, Washo T, Huczko E, BonnerD (2000). *In vitro* antibacterial spectrum of a new broad-spectrum 8-methoxy fluoroquinolone, gatifloxacin. J Antimicrob Chemother 45: 437–446.

Gandhi NR, Moll A, Sturm AW, Pawinski R, Govender T, Lalloo U, Zeller K, Andrews J, Friedland G (2006). Extensively drug-resistant tuberculosis as a cause of death in patients co-infected with tuberculosis and HIV in a rural area of South Africa. Lancet 368: 1575-80.

Gandhi NR, Shah NS, Andrews JR, Vella V, Moll AP, Scott M, Weissman D, Marra C, Lalloo UG, Friedland GH (2010). HIV coinfection in multidrug- and extensively drug-resistant tuberculosis results in high early mortality. Am J Respir Crit Care Med 181: 80-6.

Garcia I, Miyazaki Y, Marchal G, Lesslauer W, Vassalli P (1997). High sensitivity of transgenic mice expressing soluble TNFR1 fusion protein to mycobacterial infections: synergistic action of TNF and IFN-gamma in the differentiation of protective granulomas. Eur J Immunol 27 : 3182-90.

Gillespie SH, Kennedy N (1998). Fluoroquinolones: a new treatment for tuberculosis. Int. J. Tuberc. Lung Dis. 2: 265–271.

Gillespie SH, Billington O (1999). Activity of moxifloxacin against mycobacteria. J Antimicrob Chemother 44: 393–395.

Gillespie SH, Morrissey I, Everett D (2001). A comparison of the bactericidal activity of quinolone antibiotics in a Mycobacterium fortuitum model. J. Med. Microbiol 50: 565–570.

Golden MP, Vikram HR (2005). Extrapulmonary tuberculosis: An overview. Am Fam Physician 72: 1761-8.

Heldwein KA, Fenton MJ (2002). The role of Toll-like receptors in immunity against mycobacterial infection. Microbes Infect. 4: 937-44.

Hirsch CS, Toossi Z, Johnson JL, Luzze H, Ntambi L, Peters P, et al. (2001). Augmentation of apoptosis and interferong production at sites of active *Mycobacterium tuberculosis* infection in human tuberculosis. J Infect Dis 183 : 779-88.

Inderlied CB, Nash KA (1996). Antimycobacterial agents. *In vitro* susceptibility testing, spectra of activity, mechanisms of actions and reistance and assays for activity in biologic fluids. In antibiotics in laboratory medicine,4th ed (V.Lorian,ed).Wiliams and Wilkins. Baltimore 127-175.

Jena P, Mohanty S, Mallick R, Jacob B, Sonawane A. (2012). Toxicity and antibacterial assessment of chitosan-coated silver nanoparticles on human pathogens and macrophage cells. Int J Nanomedicine.7: 1805-18.

Johnson CM, Cooper AM, Frank AA, Bonorino CBC, Wysoki LJ, Orme IM (1997). *Mycobacterium tuberculosis* aerogenic rechallenge infections in B cell-deficient mice.Tuber Lung Dis 78 : 257-61.

Kalluru R, Fenaroli F, Westmoreland D, Ulanova L, Maleki A, Roos N, Paulsen Madsen M, Koster G, Egge-Jacobsen W, Wilson S, Roberg-Larsen H, Khuller GK, Singh A, Nyström B, Griffiths G. (2013). Poly(lactide-co-glycolide)-rifampicin nanoparticles efficiently clear *Mycobacterium bovis* BCG infection in macrophages and remain membrane-bound in phago-lysosomes. J Cell Sci. 2013 Jul 15; 126(Pt 14): 3043-54.

Keane J, Balcewicz-Sablinska MK, Remold HG, Chupp GL, Meek BB, Fenton MJ *et al.* (1997). Infection by *Mycobacterium tuberculosis* promotes human alveolar macrophage apoptosis. Infect Immun 65 : 298-304.

Khoo KH, Douglas E, Azadi P, Inamine JM, Besra GS, Mikusova K, Brennan PJ,Chatterjee D (1996). Truncated Structural Variants of Lipoarabinomannan in Ethambutol Drug-resistant Strains of *Mycobacterium smegmatis*: Inhibition of arabinan biosynthesis by ethambutol. *J. Biol. Che* 271: 28682-28690.

Kilburn JO, Takayama K (1981). Effects of ethambutol on accumulation and secretion of trehalose mycolates and free mycolic acid in *Mycobacterium smegmatis*. Antimicrob. Agents Chemother 20: 401-404.

Kingler K, Tchou-Wong KM, Brandi O, Aston C, Kim R, Chi C *et al.* (1997). Effects of mycobacteria on regulation of apoptosis in monouclear phagocytes. Infect Immun 65, 5272-8.

Kremer L, Estaquier J, Wolowczuk I, Biet F, Ameisen JC, Locht C (2000). Ineffective cellular immune response associated with T-cell apoptosis in susceptible *Mycobacterium bovis* BCG-infected mice. Infect Immun 68 : 4264-73.

Ladel CH, Szalay G, Riedel D, Kaufmann SH (1997). Interleukin-12 secretion by *Mycobacterium tuberculosis* infected macrophages. Infect Immun 65: 1936-8.

Lamb HM, Wiseman LR. Pexiganan acetate. Drugs 56: 1047–52.

Liu PT, Stenger S, Li H, Wenzel L, Tan BH, Krutzik S *et al.* (2006). Toll-like receptor triggering of a vitamin D-mediated human antimicrobial response. *Science* 311: 1770–1773.

Martineau AR, Wilkinson KA, Newton SM, Floto RA, Norman AW, Skolimowska K *et al*. (2007). IFN-gamma- and TNF-independent vitamin D-inducible human suppression of mycobacteria: the role of cathelicidin LL-37. *J Immunol* 178: 7190–7198.

Matsumoto M, Hashizume H, Tomishige T, Kawasaki M, Tsubouchi H, Sasaki H, Shimokawa Y, Komatsu M (2006). OPC-67683, a nitrodihydro- imidazooxazole derivative with promising action against tuberculosis *in vitro* and in mice. PLoS Med. 3: 466.

McDyer JF, Hackley MN, Walsh TE, Cook JL, Seder RA (1997). Patients with multidrug-resistant tuberculosis with low CD4+ T cell counts have impaired Th1 responses. J Immunol 158 : 492-500.

Méndez-Samperio P, Miranda E, Trejo A (2008). Expression and secretion of cathelicidin LL-37 in human epithelial cells after infection by *Mycobacterium bovis* Bacillus Calmette-Guérin. Clin Vaccine Immunol 15: 1450–5.

Mikusova K, Slayden RA, Besra GS, Brennan PJ (1995). Biogenesis of the mycobacterial cell wall and the site of action of ethambutol. Antimicrob. Agents Chemother 39: 2484-2489.

Mohanty S, Jena P, Mehta R, Pati R, Banerjee B, Patil S, Sonawane A. (2013). Cationic Antimicrobial Peptides and Biogenic Silver Nanoparticles Kill Mycobacteria without Eliciting DNA Damage and Cytotoxicity in Mouse Macrophages. Antimicrob Agents Chemother. Aug; 57(8): 3688-98.

Mohanty S, Mishra S, Jena P, Jacob B, Sarkar B, Sonawane A. (2012). An investigation on the antibacterial, cytotoxic, and antibiofilm efficacy of starch-stabilized silver nanoparticles. Nanomedicine.; 8(6): 916-24.

Molly A, Laochumroonverapog P, Kaplan G (1994). Apoptosis but not necrosis of infected monocytes is coupled with killing of intracellular bacillus Calmette Guerin. J. Exp. Med. 180: 1495-1509.

Nicas M, Nazaroff WW, Hubbard A (2005). Toward understanding the risk of secondary airborne infection: emission of respirable pathogens. J Occup Environ Hyg 2: 143–54.

Niemann S, Richter E, Dalügge-Tamm H, Schlesinger H, Graupner D, Königstein B, Gurath G, Greinert U, Rüsch-Gerdes S (2000). Two cases of *Mycobacterium microti* derived tuberculosis in HIV-negative immunocompetent patients. Emerg Infect Dis 6: 539–42.

Niemann S, Rüsch-Gerdes S, Joloba ML *et al*. (2002). *Mycobacterium africanum* subtype II is associated with two distinct genotypes and is a major cause of human tuberculosis in Kampala, Uganda. J Clin Microbiol 40: 3398–405.

Niobe-Eyangoh SN, Kuaban C, Sorlin P, *et al*. (2003). Genetic biodiversity of *Mycobacterium tuberculosis* complex strains from patients with pulmonary tuberculosis in Cameroon. J Clin Microbiol 41: 2547–53.

Nirmala R, Narayanan PR, Mathew R, Maran M, Deivanayagam CN (2001). Reduced NK activity in pulmonary tuberculosis patients with/without HIV infection: Identifying the defective stage and studying the effect of interleukins on NK activity. Tuberculosis. 81: 343-52.

Ogata K, Linzer BA, Zuberi RI, Ganz T, Lehrer RI,Catanzaro A (1992). Activity of Defensins from humanneutrophilic granulocytes against *Mycobacterium avium-Mycobacterium intracellulare*. Infect Immun 60: 4720-5.

Olliaro P, Dolfi L, Morelli P, Della-Bruna C, Sarolin-Benedelli M, Sassella D (1995). Rifabutin for prevention and treatment of mycobacterial diseases: a review of microbiology, clinical pharmacology, efficacy and tolerability data. Eur Respir Rev 5: 77-83.

Ottenhof TH, Kumararatne D, Casanova JL (1998). Novel human immunodeficiencies reveal the essential role of type-1 cytokines in immunity to intracellular bacteria. Immunol Today 19: 491-4.

Papadopoulou MV, Bloomer WD, McNeil MR (2007). NLCQ-1 and NLCQ-2, two new agents with activity against dormant *Mycobacterium tuberculosis*. Int. J. Antimicrob. Agents 29: 724–727.

Pfyffer GE, Auckenthaler R, van Embden JD, van Soolingen D (1998). *Mycobacterium canettii*, the smooth variant of *M. tuberculosis*, isolated from a Swiss patient exposed in Africa. Emerging Infect Dis 4: 631–4.

Pillay M, Sturm AW (2007). Evolution of the extensively drug-resistant F15/LAM4/KZN strain of *Mycobacterium tuberculosis* in KwaZulu-Natal, South Africa. Clinical infectious diseases: an official publication of the Infectious Diseases Society of America 45: 1409–14.

Protopopova M, Bogatcheva E, Nikonenko B, Hundert S, Einck L, Nacy CA (2007). In search of new cures for tuberculosis. Med. Chem 3: 301–316.

Raviglione MC, Narain JP, Kochi A (1992). HIV-associated tuberculosis in developing countries: clinical features, diagnosis, and treatment. Bull World Health Organ. 70: 515-26.

Regnier S, Ouagari Z, Perez ZL, Veziris N, Bricaire F, Caumes E (2009). Cutaneous miliary resistant tuberculosis in a patient infected with human immunodeficiency virus: case report and literature review. Clin Exp Dermatol 34: 690-2.

Rojas M, Olivier M, Gros P, Barrera LF, Garcia LF (1999). TNF-a and IL-10 modulate the induction of apoptosis by virulent *Mycobacterium tuberculosis* in murine macrophages. J Immunol 162: 6122-31.

Rojas RE, Balaji KN, Subramanian A, Boom WH (1999). Regulation of human CD4+ ab T cell receptor positive (TCR+). and gd (TCR +T-cell responses to *Mycobacterium tuberculosis* by interleukin-10 and transforming growth factor β. Infect Immun 67: 6461-72.

Sasaki H, Haraguchi Y, Itotani M, Kuroda H, Hashizume H, Tomishige T *et al.* (2006). Synthesis and antituberculosis activity of a novel series of optically active 6-nitro-2,3-dihydroimidazo[2,1-β] oxazoles. J. Med. Chem. 49: 7854–7860.

Saunders BM, Frank AA, Orme IM, Cooper AM (2000). Interleukin-6 induces early gamma interferon production in the infected lung but is not required for generation of specific immunity to *Mycobacterium tuberculosis* infection. Infect Immun 68: 3322-6.

Schorey JS, Carroll MC, Brown EJ (1997). A macrophage invasion mechanism of pathogenic mycobacteria. Science 277: 1091–1093.

Selvaraj P, Swamy R, Vijayan VK, Prabhakar R, Narayanan PR (1988). Hydrogen peroxide producing potential of alveolar macrophages and blood monocytes in pulmonary tuberculosis. Indian J Med Res 88: 124-9.

Selwyn PA, Hartel D, Lewis VA, Schoenbaum EE, Vermund SH, Klein RS, *et al.* (1989). A prospective study of the risk of tuberculosis among intravenous drug users with human immunodeficiency virus infection. N Engl J Med 320: 545-50.

Seung KJ, Omatayo DB, Keshavjee S, Furin JJ, Farmer PE, Satti H (2009). Early outcomes of MDR-TB treatment in a high HIV-prevalence setting in Southern Africa. PLoS One 25: 7186.

Sharma S, Verma I, Khuller GK (2001). Therapeutic potential of human neutrophil peptide 1 against experimental tuberculosis. Antimicrob Agents Chemother 45: 639–40.

Sharma SK, Mohan A, Prasad KL, Pande JN, Gupta AK, Khilnani GC (1995). Clinical profile, laboratory characteristics and outcome in miliary tuberculosis. *Q J M 88*: 29-37.

Small PM (1996). Tuberculosis research: Balancing the portfolio. JAMA. 276: 1512-3.

Spigelman MK (2007). New tuberculosis therapeutics: a growing pipeline. J. Infect. Dis 196: S28–S34.

Stover CK, Warrener P, VanDevanter DR, Sherman DR, Arain TM, Langhorne MH e tal (2000). A small-molecule nitroimidazopyran drug candidate for the treatment of tuberculosis. Nature 405: 962–966.

Taha RA, Kotsimbos TC, Song YL, Menzies D, Hamid Q (1997). IFN-gamma and IL-12 are increased in active compared with inactive tuberculosis. Am J Respir Crit Care Med 155: 1135-9.

Tan BH, Meinken C· Bastian M· Bruns H· Legaspi A· Ochoa M T *et al.* (2006). Macrophages acquires neutrophil granules for antimicrobial activity against intracellular pathogens. Immunol 177: 1864-1871.

Teitelbaum R, Cammer M, Maitland ML, Freitag NE, Condeelis J, Bloom BR (1999). Mycobacterial infection of macrophages results in membrane permeable phagosomes. Proc Natl Acad Sci USA 96: 15190-5.

Thoen C, Lobue P, de Kantor I (2006). The importance of *Mycobacterium bovis* as a zoonosis. Vet. Microbiol 112: 339–45.

VanderWel N, Hava D, Houben D, Fluitsma D, van Zon M, Pierson J, Brenner M, Peters PJ (2007). *M. tuberculosis* and *M. leprae* translocate from the phagolysosome to the cytosol in myeloid cells. *Cell* 129: 1287-1298.

Van Heyningen TK, Collins HL, Russell DG (1997). IL-6 produced by macrophages infected with *Mycobacterium* species suppresses T cell responses. J Immunol 158: 303-7.

van Soolingen D, Hoogenboezem T, de Haas PE, *et al.* (1997). A novel pathogenic taxon of the *Mycobacterium tuberculosis* complex, Canetti: characterization of an exceptional isolate from Africa. Int. J. Syst. Bacteriol 47: 1236–45.

Vinay K, Abbas AK, Nelson F, Mitchell RN (2007). Robbins Basic Pathology (8th ed.) Saunders Elsevier. pp. 516–522.

Walker L and Lowrie DB (1981). Killing of *Mycobacterium microti* by immunologically activated macrophages. Nature 293: 69-70.

Wells CD, Cegielski JP, Nelson LJ, Laserson KF, Holtz TH, Finlay A, Castro KG, Weyer K (2007). HIV infection and multidrug-resistant tuberculosis: the perfect storm. J Infect Dis 15: Suppl 1: S86-10.

World Health Organisation (2006). Press release: "WHO Global Task Force outlines measures to combat XDR-TB worldwide.

World Health Organization (2009). "Epidemiology". Global tuberculosis control: epidemiology, strategy, financing. pp. 6–33.

World Health Organization (1963). Standard tuberculin test. WHO/TB/Technical Guide Geneva, Switzerland.

Yu CT, Wang CH, Huang TJ, Lin HC, Kuo HP (1995). Relation of bronchoalveolar lavage T lymphocyte subpopulations to rate of regression of active pulmonary tuberculosis. Thorax 50: 869-74.

Zaiou M (2007). Multifunctional antimicrobial peptides: therapeutic targets in several human diseases. J Mol Med 85: 317–29.

2014, Advances in Biochemistry and Biotechnology Volume 2   *Pages 163-181*

Edited by: **Dr. Biplab Sarkar and Dr. Chiranjib Chakraborty**

Published by: **DAYA PUBLISHING HOUSE**

10

Circulating miRNAs as Biomarker for Early Diagnosis of Esophageal Cancer

Rinu Sharma

University School of Biotechnology, Guru Gobind Singh Indraprastha University,
Sector-16C, Dwarka, New Delhi – 110 075, India

ABSTRACT

In most cases, esophageal cancer is diagnosed and treated only in the advanced stage, when the cancer cells have already invaded and metastasized throughout the body. At this stage, therapeutic modalities are limited in their success. Detecting cancers in early stages even in the premalignant state, means that current or future treatment modalities might have a higher likelihood of a true cure. In spite of the use of modern surgical techniques combined with various adjuvant treatment modalities, such as radiotherapy and chemotherapy, the overall 5-year survival rate of esophageal cancer patients still remains less than 10 per cent. Hence, early detection of esophageal cancer lacks a specific symptom, a specific biomarker and accurate and reliable diagnostic, non-invasive modalities. MicroRNAs (miRNAs) are a class of small non-coding endogenous RNA molecules whose altered expression has been reported in various cancers. Recent innovations in miRNAs profiling technology have shed new light on their importance in the pathology of esophageal carcinoma. This chapter focuses on the potential role of miRNAs in detection of esophageal cancer and also the recent progresses in evaluating the levels of circulating cancer-associated miRNAs indicating their potential clinical use as novel minimally invasive biomarkers for esophageal cancer.

Keywords: *miRNA, Esophageal cancer, Biomarker, Oncogenes.*

Introduction

Esophageal cancer (EC) is one of the most lethal malignancies characterized with dramatic geographic difference in its incidence worldwide. Esophageal cancer is the eighth most common cancer worldwide and the sixth most common cause of death from cancer (Parkin *et al.*, 2008; Enzinger *et al.*, 2003). In India it ranks second most common cancer among males and the fourth most common cancer among females (Gajalakshmi *et al.*, 2001). It has extremely poor prognosis owing to insidious symptomatology, late clinical presentation and rapid progression (Landis *et al.*, 1999). Esophageal Squamous Cell Carcinoma (ESCC) and Esophageal Adenocarcinoma (EAC), the two main forms of EC, have different etiologic and pathologic characteristics. Although there is a rapid increase in incidence of Barrett's adenocarcinoma in Western countries, ESCC still remains the predominant subtype of EC in East Asia (Mathe *et al.*, 2009). Esophageal cancer has been known to be asymptomatic till it reaches the advanced stage and more than 10,900 (~ 4 per cent of all cancer cases) deaths have been expected in US for esophageal cancer in 2007 (American Cancer Society, 2008). In spite of the use of modern surgical techniques combined with various adjuvant treatment modalities, such as radiotherapy and chemotherapy, due to late stage of diagnosis and poor efficacy of treatment, the prognosis for patients with ESCC still remains poor with an average 5-year survival of less than 10 per cent globally (Montesano *et al.*, 1996; Parkin *et al.*, 2000) and less than 12 per cent in India (Gupta *et al.*, 2001; Yeole *et al.*, 2004).

It is observed that in most cases, cancer is diagnosed and treated only in the advanced stage, when the cancer cells have already invaded and metastasized throughout the body. At this stage, therapeutic modalities are limited in their success. Detecting cancers in early stages even in the premalignant state, means that current or future treatment modalities might have a higher likelihood of a true cure. Nevertheless, to date, efforts to identify molecular markers useful for diagnosis/prognosis of esophageal cancer have proven to be primarily unsuccessful for translation into clinics. Consequently, early detection of esophageal cancer lacks a specific symptom, a specific biomarker and accurate and reliable diagnostic, non-invasive modalities. The need for early detection of esophageal cancer has been established among clinicians and scientists for years. More than 90 per cent of early EC show enhanced 5-year survival rate (Enzinger *et al.*, 2003; Reed 1999; Headrick *et al.*, 2002), about 50 per cent of cancers extend beyond the primary local region at the time of diagnosis and almost 75 per cent of surgically treated patients have proximal lymph node metastasis (Guo *et al.*, 2008). Although considerable diagnostic and therapeutic advances have been made in treatment of ESCCs in recent years, till date, gastrointestinal endoscopy remains the primary screening tool, to histopathologically examine the biopsy specimens taken from the individuals suspected to be suffering from EC. This invasive test, even though it is proved to increase the detection of early tumor and therefore, can prolong the survival of the patient, is generally considered to be inconvenient and painful. Moreover, the invasive, unpleasant and inconvenient nature of the current diagnostic procedures limits the application of till date proven tumor markers. Hence, there is a pressing need for establishment of novel non-invasive biomarkers for early tumor diagnosis of EC and provide the clinician with useful information concerning patient prognosis and possible therapeutic options. Keeping in view the above, it is desirable to provide an effective, clinically useful biomarker measurable in a readily accessible body fluid and tissues. Development of better preventive and diagnostic approaches as well as more effective treatment modalities requires in-depth understanding of molecular mechanisms implicated in the complex process of esophageal carcinogenesis.

miRNAs are approximately 22 nt long evolutionarily conserved endogenous non-coding RNAs that regulate gene expression by posttranscriptional gene silencing. miRNAs are found in intergenic region, introns or exons of noncoding region as well as in introns of protein coding regions (Rodriguez *et al.,* 2004). Lin-4 was the first miRNA which was identified in *C. elegans* by Victor Ambros and colleagues (Ambros 1989; Lee *et al.,* 1993). The biogenesis of miRNAs is a multistep process involving a complex protein system (Kim *et al.,* 2006). The miRNA genes are generally transcribed by RNA pol-II to pri-mirna (Primary transcript of miRNA). Pri-miRNA is then cleaved by RNase III enzyme called Drosha to pre-miRNA which are ~60-70 nt long RNA molecules having hairpin structures. Pre-miRNAs are then transported to cytoplasm where Dicers cleave them to mature miRNAs. miRNA then binds to RISC complex and guides it to complementary mRNA. RISC either degrades target mRNA or blocks its translation depending upon miRNA-mRNA complementarity. If the complementarity is enough then target mRNA is degraded otherwise its translation is blocked. The specific region in miRNA, which is important for messenger RNA target recognition, is referred to as the "seed sequence", and located at the 52-end of the mature miRNA sequence, from bases 2 to 8 (Bartel 2004). With the seed sequence, we can search for the complementary sequences in the 32-untranslated regions (32-UTRs) of known genes that exhibit conservation across species (Bartel, 2004). In animals, most miRNAs are thought to form imperfect base pairs with their target mRNA(s) and these interaction sites are enriched in 32-UTRs (Bartel, 2004). To date, in the human genome, over 700 mature miRNAs have been identified, and the number is still increasing with the future studies. Up to 1000 miRNAs have been predicated by the bioinformatics studies of the human genome (Berezikov *et al.,* 2005).

MicroRNAs (miRNA) are involved in biological and pathologic processes including cell differentiation, proliferation, apoptosis and metabolism, and are emerging as highly tissue-specific biomarkers with potential clinical applicability for defining cancer types and origins (Rosenfeld *et al.,* 2008).

Role of miRNA in Cancer

miRNA are short non coding RNAs that control biological and pathological processes as cell growth, differentiation, apoptosis and metabolism. Therefore, altered miRNA expression results in uncontrolled cell division or proliferation leading to tumorigenesis. miRNAs are either upregulated or downregulated in different types of cancers. Those miRNAs whose expression is increased in tumors may be considered as oncogenes. These oncogene miRNAs, called "oncomirs", usually promote tumor development by negatively inhibiting tumor suppressor genes and/or genes that control cell differentiation or apoptosis (Zhang *et al.,* 2006). For example mir-17-92 cluster is located at chromosome 13q31, a genomic locus that is amplified in lung cancer and lymphomas, including diffuse large B-cell lymphoma (Hayashita *et al.,* 2005; He *et al.,* 2005). Co-expression of miR-17–19b, a truncated portion of miR-17-92, strongly accelerated lymphomagenesis (Hammond 2006) suggesting that miR-17-92, a polycistron acts as an oncogene. Further Donell *et al.,* demonstrated that the expression of miR-17–92

Table 10.1: Expression of miRNA in Esophageal Cancer Tissues Analyzed by different Techniques.

Sl.No.	Sample Size	Pathology	Population	miRNA Analysed	Upregulated miRNA	Downregulated miRNA	Targets	References
Array Profiling								
1.	31 Tumor v/s adjacent normal	ESCC	Chinese	435	hsa-miR-25, hsa-miR-424, hsa-miR-151	hsa-miR-100, hsa-miR-99a, hsa-miR-29c, hsa-miR-140	Not Determined	Guo et al., 2008
2.	35	ESCC	Japanese	Array had 328 miRNA probe	miR-342, miR21, miR-93	miR-205, miR-203	Not Determined	Feber et al., 2008
	35	EAC	Japanese		MiR-192, miR-194, miR-21, miR-93	miR-200c, miR-205, miR-203	Not Determined	
3.	32	EAC		470	hsa-miR-126, hsa-miR-143, hsa-miR-145, hsa-miR-146a, hsa-miR-181a, hsa-miR-181b, hsa-miR-195, hsa-miR-199a, hsa-miR-199a*, hsa-miR-199b, hsa-miR-28, hsa-miR-29c, hsa-miR-30a-5p, hsa-miR-424	hsa-miR-149, hsa-miR-203, hsa-miR-205, hsa-miR-210, hsa-miR-221, hsa-miR-27b, hsa-miR-494, hsa-miR-513, hsa-miR-617, hsa-miR-99a	Not Determined	Yang et al., 2009
4.	100	EAC	US, Canada, Japan	Chip had 329 human miRNA and 249 mouse miRNA probe	miR-21, miR-192, miR-194, miR-223	miR-203	Not Determined	Mathe et al., 2009
	70	ESCC	US, Canada, Japan		miR-21	MiR-375	Not Determined	
5.	10 pairs of tissue samples, and Human ESCC cell lines (TE2, TE3, TE12 and TE13)	ESCC	–	365 mature miRNAs		miR-375, -let-7c, miR -145, -143, -100, -133a, -99a, -133b, -1, -30a-3p, -504, -139-5p, -204, -203, -326	miR-145 and miR-133a/b target FSCN1	Kano et al., 2010

Contd...

Table 10.1–Contd...

Sl.No.	Sample Size	Pathology	Population	miRNA Analysed	Upregulated miRNA	Downregulated miRNA	Targets	References
6.	Cell lines and Biopsy	ESCC	–	–	miR-205	miR-10A	E-cadherin through ZEB2	Matsushima et al., 2011
7.	Cell lines	ESCC	–	–	miR-205, miR-21		–	Kimura et al., 2010
8.	16, 32 for RT-PCR	EC	–	377	miR-21, miR-143, miR-145, miR-194, miR-203, miR-205 and miR-215: upregulated in columnar	miR-143, miR-145, miR-215 lower in EAC	Not Determined	Wijnhoven et al., 2010
9.		ESCC	Chinese		miR-296		Cyclin D1 or p27	Hong et al., 2010
10.	22	BE	Caucasian	–	9 (miR-15b, -21, -192, -205, -486-5p, -584, 1246, -let7a, and -7d) identified by microarray and miR-15b, -21, -486-5p and let7a confirmed by qRT-PCR		Not Determined	Bansal et al., 2011
11.	ESCC Cell lines and 86 tissue specimens	ESCC	–	–	33 upregulated in microarray, miR-21	40 downregulated in microarray, miR-143, miR-145, miR-203, miR-99a, miR-100	Proteins involved in cell mobility, CD1, RARβ, and c-Met	Wu et al., 2011
qRT-PCR								
1.	11	EAC			miR-196a		KRT5, SPRR2C, S100A9	Luthra et al., 2008
2.	Cell lines	ESCC	Chinese		miR-let-7d, miR-330, miR-340, miR-373			Lee et al., 2009

Contd...

Table 10.1—Contd...

Sl.No.	Sample Size	Pathology	Population	miRNA Analysed	Upregulated miRNA	Downregulated miRNA	Targets	References
3	30	ESCC	Japanese	73	miR-9, miR-15b, miR-16, miR-17-5p, miR-20b, miR-20A, miR-21, miR-25, miR-34b, miR-34c, miR-103, miR-106a, miR-107, miR-127, miR-129, miR-130b, miR-130a, miR-132, miR-134, miR-137, miR-138, miR-151	miR-133a, miR-133b, miR-139, miR-145	–	Ogawa et al., 2009
4.	20 ESCC samples	20 ESCC and 7 ESCC cell lines	–	miR-21	miR-21	–	PDCD4	Hiyoshi et al., 2009
5.	38 ESCC paired tissues and 15 esophageal cancer cell lines (TE 1-15)	ESCC	Japanese	miR-21	miR-21		–	Mori et al., 2009
6.		BE, BM, EAC			miR-196a			Maru et al., 2009
7.		ESCC and Cell lines			miR-21, miR-10	miR-375		Tian et al., 2010
8.	98 Esophageal cancer pateints	EC	–	9	MiR-200c, miR-21	miR-145	PPP2R1B of miR-200C	Hamano et al., 2011
9.	40	EC	Chinese	1		MiR-375	PDK1	Li et al., 2011

Contd...

Table 10.1–Contd...

Sl.No.	Sample Size	Pathology	Population	miRNA Analysed	Upregulated miRNA	Downregulated miRNA	Targets	References
10.	Cell line Eca109 and paired fresh ESCC and normal adjacent tissue. And 150 paired tissues for IHC	ESCC	Chinese	1		let-7	HMGA2	Liu et al., 2011
11.	55 patients	ESCC	Japanese	5	Mature miR-21, mature-miR-145			Akagi et al., 2011
12.	ESCC cell lines, Eca109 and TE-1	ESCC	Cell line	miR-203	–	–	miR-203 down-regulates ΔNP63 at post-transcriptional level	Yuan et al., 2011
13.	107 ESCC patients, cell lines KYSE150, KYSE410, KYSE450, KYSE510 and EC9706	ESCC	Chinese	miR-92a	miR-92a		CDHI	Chen et al., 2011
14.	43	22 EAC		4- miR-21, miR-106a, miR-148a, miR-205		miR-148- when EAC was more proximal	Not Determined	Hummel et al., 2011
		21 ESCC			miR21	miR-148, miR106a	Not Determined	

Northern Blotting and in situ hybridization

1.	10 esophageal cancer cell lines and 158 tissue specimens	EAC	–	10	mir-16-2, miR-30e, miR-200a, miR-126, miR-195p		–	Hu et al., 2010

is related to the expression of c-Myc gene and both miR-17–92 and c-Myc regulate the expression of cell cycle transcription factor gene E2F1 (O'Donnell *et al.*, 2005), which controls transition from G1 to S phase of the cell cycle by regulating genes that are involved in cell division and apoptosis.

The first indication that miRNAs could function as tumor suppressors came from a study conducted by Calin *et al.* (2002). They showed that patients who were diagnosed with a common form of adult leukaemia, B-cell chronic lymphocytic leukemia (CLL), often have deletions or downregulation of two clustered miRNA genes, mir-15a and mir-16-1. Deletions occurred in 13q14 locus which is a 30-kb region. The down-regulation of miR-15a and miR-16-1 induces over-expression of the anti-apoptotic BCL2 protein in leukaemia cells (Cimmino *et al.*, 2005) suggesting their role in tumor-suppression. let-7 negatively regulates the expression of RAS and MYC which are key oncogenes of P53 pathway by targeting their mRNAs for translation repression (Johnson *et al.*, 2005). Felli *et al.* (2005) reported that miR-221 and miR-222 regulate erythropoiesis by downregulating KIT oncogene and inhibit growth of an erythroleukaemic TF-1 cell line in a KIT-dependent manner. Thus, miRNAs play a very crucial role in regulation of gene expression.

Clinical Potential of miRNAs

Previous studies demonstrating the altered expression of miRNAs in cancers and the fact that approximately half of the miRNA genes are localized in cancer-associated genomic regions/fragile sites (Calin *et al.*, 2004) indicates their potential clinical applicability as tissue specific biomarkers for defining cancer types and origins (Rosenfeld 2008). Various experimental techniques are available for analysis of miRNAs in tumor tissue samples. One of the most predominant methods is the oligonucleotide miRNA microarray analysis which has been used as a high throughput method for monitoring the cancer specific expression levels in a large number of samples (Kim *et al.*, 2006; Calin *et al.*, 2006; Liu *et al.*, 2004). Other techniques such as bead based flowcytometry, quantitative real time polymerase chain reaction and microarray platform with locked nucleic acid modified captured probes provide high specificity for closely related miRNAs and can discriminate with even single nucleotide differences (Lu *et al.*, 2005; Castoldi *et al.*, 2006). Advent of these techniques has facilitated the researchers to analyse the expression of miRNAs in tumors as compared with normal profile further providing insight into the, mechanism behind tumorigenesis and paving way for their application as novel biomarkers.

As discussed earlier, most of the methods available for diagnosis of cancer, especially esophageal cancer are invasive in nature. One of the major challenges in cancer research is identification of easily accessible, consistent, non-invasive, stable and reliable biomarker. miRNA profiles can be used to classify tumor type, discriminate human tumors based on the lineage and site of origin (Lu *et al.*, 2005; Volinia *et al.*, 2006). miRNAs, thus appear to be promising class of biomarkers. Moreover, stable expression of circulating miRNAs in human sera and plasma samples makes them attractive targets for minimally invasive diagnosis/prognosis of cancer.

miRNA Expression in Esophageal Cancer

Esophageal cancer is a complex multi-step disease wherein risk factor induced cumulative aberrations in the genetic material of a cell leads to preneoplastic condition of hyperplasia, dysplasia or barrett's esophagus. Further different sequential changes in the gene expression progresses these lesions into in-situ carcinoma followed by local nodal invasion and distant organ metastasis. As discussed earlier ESCC and EAC have distinct etiologic and pathologic characteristics and thus show different miRNA expression profiles (Zhou *et al.*, 2010).

Aberrant expression of several miRNAs has been reported in various cancers. In esophageal cancer miRNA expression has been analysed mainly in Chinese, Japanese and Caucasian populations. Table 10.1 summarizes expression of various miRNAs analyzed so far, both in ESCCs and EACs, using different techniques.

miRNA expression profile in esophageal cancer for the first time was reported by Guo et al. (2008). Microarray analysis of 31 pairs of ESCC tissues and adjacent normal tissues revealed a set of seven miRNA as classifier out of which three (hsa-miR-25, hsa-miR-424 and hsa-miR-151) were up-regulated and four (hsa-miR-100, hsa-miR-99a, hsa-miR29c and hsa-miR140*) were down-regulated. Also hsa-miR-103/107 showed a strong correlation between low expression and high overall survival period (Guo et al., 2008). They found that five miRNAs (miR-335, miR-181d, miR-25, miR-7 and hsa-miR-495) correlate with gross pathologic classification (fungating vs medullary) and two miRNAs (miR-25 and miR-130b) correlate with differentiation classification (high vs middle vs low) (Guo et al., 2008). In another study conducted by Feber et al. (2008) prediction analysis of microarray (PAM) were performed to classify 35 esophageal specimens according to their histological type. All 10 SCC and 10 AC samples were classified correctly. Also miR-203 and miR-205 were found to be expressed 2-10 fold lower in SCC and AC compared with NSE whereas miR-21 expression was 3-5 fold higher in tumor specimens compared to normal specimens (Feber et al., 2008).

In another study Microarray-based expression was measured in 100 ADC and 70 SCC patients. In ADC patients, miR-21, miR-192, miR-194 and miR-223 were elevated while miR-203 expression was reduced in cancer compared to non-cancer tissue. Similarly, In ESCC miR21 was elevated while miR-375 expression level was reduced in cancerous compared to non-cancerous tissue (Mathe et al., 2009). While comparing ADC vs SCC, miR-194 and miR-375 were elevated in ADC patients. Ogawa et al. (2009) quantified the expression of 73 miRNA in 30 primary ESCC specimens using qRT-PCR. The expression levels of 6 miRNA (miR-20b, miR-34b, miR-34c, miR-129, miR-130b and miR-138) were higher (4 fold) while expression of 4 miRNA (miR-133a, miR-133b, miR-139 and miR-145) were less than half in tumor tissues compared to normal esophageal tissues. Among these the expression levels of miR-34b were considerably higher in tumor tissue than normal. On the other hand miR-139 was seen less often in tumor tissue compared to normal tissue suggesting miR-34b and miR-139 as potential biomarker for EC.

Matsushima et al., analyzed miRNA extracted from ESCC and EAC cell lines as well as in other malignant cell lines (gastric adenocarcinoma, colorectaladenocarcinoma, lung adenocarcinoma etc) using microarray based technique followed by qReal-time PCR validation. miR-205 levels were found to be exclusively increased in each ESCC cell line than those in other malignant cell types whereas miR-10a expression was decreased substantially compared to non-malignant Het1A cells. Suggesting miR-205 and 10a are potential biomarkers for esophageal cancer (Matsushima et al., 2010; Matsushima et al., 2011).

Levels of miR-143 and miR-145 in 86 clinical samples of esophageal carcinoma and their matched normal tissue were evaluated using qRT-PCR. On average, miR143 was downregulated by 4.3 fold while miR-145 was downregulated by 3.2 fold. In same study, miR-21 was observed to be the most upregulated miRNA (with 24.4 fold change) whereas miR-203 was the most downregulated (with 4.3 fold change) miRNA (Wu et al., 2011). In a study conducted by Hiyoshi et al. (2009), out of 20 paired tissues 18 cancer tissues over expressed miR-21. Barrett's esophagus (BE) is a metaplastic condition in which the normal squamous epithelium of the lower esophagus is replaced by a small intestinal-like columnar linig. BE starts as a pre-malignant metaplastic lesion progresses to low-grade dysplasia (LGD), high-grade dysplasia (HGD), and finally to esophageal adenocarcinoma (EAC). Maru et al.

(2009) reported that miR196a was upregulated in EAC specimens and concluded that it targets annexin A1 which promotes pro-apoptotic mechanisms in cells. Kan *et al.*, discovered that miR-25, miR-93 and miR-106b were progressively activated at successive stages of neoplasia from normal epithelium to BE and finally to EAC (Kan and Meltzer, 2009). miR-143, miR-145 and miR-215 are downregulated in esophageal adenocarcinoma than in Barrett's oesophagus (Wijnhoven *et al.*, 2010). Yang *et al.* (2009) analysed the expression profile of miRNAs in tissues of Barrett's esophagus and Esophageal adenocarcinomas using miRNA microarray. Significant differences were observed in miRNA expression profiles of normal, dysplastic and adenocarcinoma tissues (Yang *et al.*, 2009). hsalet-7b, hsa-let-7a, hsalet-7c, hsa-let-7f, hsa-miR-345, hsamiR-494, and hsa-miR-193a were found to beassociated with progression of high grade dysplasia to EAC. In order to study miRNA expression pattern in patients with different stages of Barrett's esophagus and esophageal adenocarcinoma Yang *et al.* (2009) carried out microarray analysis followed by real-time PCR and identified 11 significant miRNA out of which five were upregulated and six were downregulated in progression from LGD to HGD. However, seven miRNA were downregulated in progression from HGD to EAC. Array profiling in 14 BE, 14 BM, 14 normal, 7 low grade neoplasia, 5 high grade neoplasia and 11 Adenocarcinoma conducted by Fassan *et al.* (2010) revealed that 6 miRNA were upregulated whereas 7 miRNA were downregulated. In a recent study miR-148a expression levels were found to be inversely correlated with cancer differentiation in EA patients (Hummel *et al.*, 2011).

Functional Significance of miRNAs in Esophageal Carcinomas

Guo *et al.* (2008) predicted putative targets of hsa-miR-103/107 by using Gene ontology, Biocarta, KEGG and Gene MAPP databases. Among these targets YWHAH is a tumor suppressor and regulates the cell cycle, TGFBR3 is involved in the transforming growth factor β signalling pathway, AXIN2 is involved in the Wnt signalling pathway, TAF5 is a transcription factor and CAPZA2 is involved in cell motility. Hiyoshi *et al.* (2009) reported an inverse correlation between levels of PDCD4 protein and miR-21 expression. Also down-regulation of endogenous miR-21 with anti micro-RNA-21 resulted in significant increase in levels of Programmed cell death protein 4 (PDCD4) mRNA suggesting that miR-21 targets PDCD4. Furthermore, in order to determine whether the 32 untranslated region of PDCD4 mRNA is a functional target of microRNA-21, a reporter plasmid driven by the SV40 promoter was cloned. Plasmid was constructed having full-length 32 untranslated region of PDCD4 mRNA at the 32 position of the luciferase reporter gene, and was transfected in TE10 cells along with anti–microRNA-21 inhibitor which led to a significant increase of reporter activity in comparison with the negative control. These findings suggest that the PDCD4 is negatively regulated by microRNA-21 at the posttranslational level via binding the 32 untranslated region of PDCD4 mRNA. Other targets of miRNA-21 are phosphatase and Tensin homolog PTEN (Meng *et al.*, 2006), tumor suppressor gene tropomyosin-1 TPM1 and Sprouty-2. Gandellini *et al.*, reported that down-regulation of miR-205 could represent an oncogenic event that results in an altered cell phenotype with reduced E-cadherin expression and enhanced invasive properties. EMT *i.e.* epithelial to mesenchymal transition represents the molecular and phenotypic changes that lead to conversion of immotile epithelial cells to motile mesenchymal cells. EMT leads to loss of cell-cell adhesion as well as altered cell-extracellular matrix interaction resulting in invasion and metastasis. Loss of E-cadherin has been reported as main cause of EMT. According to recent studies, Zinc Finger E-box binding Homeobox (ZEB1 and ZEB2) directly binds to E-cadherin promoter and represses its transcription. It was reported that miR-205 mediates regulation of EMT, via the repression of ZEB1 and ZEB2. Reporter assay using ZEB2-32UTR-luciferase plasmid confirmed ZEB2 as a target of miR-205 However ZEB1 32UTR was unable to reduce the luciferase reporter expression (Matsushima *et al.*, 2011). MiR-10A has been reported to be a suppressor of homeobox (HOX) genes in ESCC as well as in other cancers. In esophageal cancer cell lines FSCN1 has been proved to be a target of miR-145 (Kano *et al.,* 2010). Wu *et al.* (2011) reported that miR143 and miR145 inhibit cell-mobility. Wound healing assay showed that the cells transfected with miR-145 and miR-143 migrated very small distances and were unable to achieve wound closure. miR-143 suppresses colorectal cancer cell growth by targeting KRAS oncogene (Chen *et al.,* 2009). In breast cancer cell line miR-145 has been shown to regulate apoptosis by inhibiting TP53 and RTKN. Maru *et al.* (2009) conducted luciferase reporter assay and reported that miR-196a directly targets the 32untranslated region (UTR) of small proline-rich protein 2C (SPRR2C), S100A9 and KRT5 mRNA. S100A9 codes for calcium-binding protein and change in its expression has been implicated in epithelial cancers. Experimentally validated targets of miR-375 as listed in tarbase are Mxi1, Jak2 and Ahr (Papadopoulos *et al.,* 2009). Mxi1 was reported to be over-expressed in EAC (Boult *et al.,* 2008). Role of miR-34a was studied by Yuxin *et al.* (2011) in esophageal cancer cell lines (HCE-4, HCE-7, Seg-1 and Bic-1) by tranfecting expression vector containing 34-a into cell lines followed by western blotting. Western blotting revealed that miR-34a inhibited c-Met and cyclin D1 expression. Also, transfection of miR-16-2 inhibited RAR-β2 expression suggesting that Rar- β2 is a potential target of miR-162. Recently, Ding *et al.* (2011) have reported that miR-29c induces cell cycle arrest in ESCC by targeting cyclin E at its 32UTR. According to Kan and Meltzer (2009) the miR-106b-25 polycistron is a likely oncomiR involved in BE-EAC carcinogenic progression and may act via regulation of 2 specific target genes, p21 and Bim. By using bioinformatics target prediction programme two tumor suppressor genes PTEN (phosphatase and tensin homolog deleted on chromosome ten) and RB2 were predicted to be targeted by miR-17–92 cluster (Lewis *et al.,* 2003). PTEN promotes apoptosis through the P13K-Akt-PKB pathway (Hammond, 2006).

miRNA Signature Associated with Prognosis and Progression in EC

Guo *et al.* (2008) reported that 5 miRNA (hsa-miR-335, hsa-miR-181d, hsa-miR-25, hsa-miR-7 and hsa-miR-495) correlated with gross pathologic classification (fungating versus medullary) while two miRNA (hsa-miR-25 and hsa-miR-130b) correlated with differentiation classification (high versus middle versus low). Also in same study hsa-miR-103/107 showed a strong correlation between low expression and high overall survival period (Guoet al. 2008). miR-200C and mir-21 were over-expressed in esophageal cancer while miR-145 was found to be under-expressed in a study conducted by Hamano *et al.* (2011) and all these three miRNA correlated significantly with shortened overall duration of survival. Yuxin *et al.* (2010) studied expression of 10 miRNA in 10 esophageal cancer cell lines and 158 tissue spemiens using northern blotting and in-situ hybridization respectively. In this study miR-126 expression was found to be associated with tumor cell differentiation and lymph node metastasis while miR-16-2 expression was associated with lymph node metastasis and miR-195p was associated with higher pathologic disease stages. Moreover, in esophageal cancer miR-16-2 and miR-30e expressions were found to be significantly associated with poor overall and disease free survival (Yuxin *et al.,* 2010). The expression of 73 miRNA in 30 cancer patients was explored by Ogawa *et al.,* and they showed that higher expression of miR-129 detected in a significant fractions of ESCC specimens were associated with shorter postoperative survival suggesting that miR-129 may be a potential independent prognostic marker in surgically treated ESCC patients. Maru *et al.* (2009) identified miR-196 as a potential marker of BE progression to low-grade dysplasia, high grade dysplasia and EA. Progressive increase was noted in miR-196 levels with each stage of progression from normal mucosa to EA. In same year, a large study was conducted by Mathe *et al.* (2009) to measure miRNA expression in cancerous and adjacent non-cancerous tissue specimens collected from 70 SCC and 100 ADC patients. In this study, Kalpan-Meier analysis revealed significant association between elevated levels of miR-21 expression in non-cancerous tissue of SCC patients and worse prognosis. Also, reduced levels of miR-375 in cancerous tissue of ADC patients with BE were found to be strongly associated with worse prognosis. Mir-21 is known to be oncogenic while miR-148 is considerd as anti-oncogenic. Hummel *et al.* (2011) studied relationship of miR-148a, miR-21 and miR-106a with tumor stages and survival in 43 patients undergoing esophagectomy and reported that miR-148a expression levels were inversely associated with cancer differentiation. miR-21 expression levels were higher if distant lymph node metastasis were present while miR106a and miR-148a were linked to tumor recurrence and outcome. Their study was consistent with previous literature that miR-106a has antitumor activity and miR-148a is a tumor-suppressor.

miRNA and Response to Therapy in Esophageal Cancer

Hamano *et al.* (2011) reported a significant correlation between miR-200c expression and response to chemotherapy (P = 0.009 for clinical response and P = 0.007 for pathologic response). MTT assay was carried out and inhibition of miR-200c expression with anti-miR-200c resulted in reduced IC-50 value for cisplastin suggesting that miR-200c mediates chemo-resistance in esophageal cancer cells. Furthermore in same study, targets of miR-200c were explored and it was found that miR-200c regulates chemo-sensitivity of esophageal cancer cells by targeting PPP2R1B, a subunit of protein phosphatase 2A, which inhibits phosphorylation of Akt and thus results in upregulation of Akt signalling. Akt is a serine/threonine kinase which has been known to play an important role in oncogenesis. On the other hand miR-148 was found to sensitize chemotherapy-resistant esophageal cancer cells to cisplastin and 5-FU in vitro. Potential targets which have already been reported and through which miR-148 mediates its effect include mitogen and stress activated kinase-I (MSK1), de-novo DNA methylation and pregame X receptor (PXR) (Hummel *et al.*, 2011).

Circulating miRNA as Ideal Class of Blood Based Biomarkers

As mentioned before, one of the major challenges in EC is to detect the disease at an early stage so that the efficacy of treatment can be enhanced. At diagnosis nearly 50 per cent of patients have cancer that extends beyond the primary locoregional confines and approximately 75 per cent of patients requiring surgery have proximal lymphnode metastases. The present diagnostic methodologies, mainly invasive in nature, provide little therapeutic biological information such as metastatic potential or sensitivity or resistance of the tumor to radiotherapy and chemotherapy. Thus, there is an urgent need for discovery of accurate diagnostic and prognostic indicators to distinguish the high risk patients in order to design optimal therapeutic modalities. In addition to frequent tissue specific dysregulation in esophageal cancer, tumor derived miRNAs have unusually high stability in serum and plasma (Mitchell *et al.*, 2008).

While miRNA presence is relevant for the regulation of cancer-associated genes in tissues, the possibility to extract and reliably determine cell-free miRNA content in body fluids like serum was first shown in 2008 (Lawrie *et al.*, 2008). This finding was confirmed by a subsequent study revealing that miRNAs are enriched in the small RNA fraction isolated from serum samples (Chen *et al.*, 2008). Cell-free miRNAs in body fluids are stable under harsh conditions including boiling, low/high pH, extended storage and multiple freeze-thaw cycles (Chen *et al.*, 2008; Mitchell *et al.*, 2008; Taylor *et al.*, 2008; Gilad *et al.*, 2008; Ho *et al.*, 2010). In contrast, synthetic miRNAs were found to be quickly degraded by the high levels of RNAse activity in plasma (Mitchell *et al.*, 2008). Filtering and differential centrifugation experiments suggest that miRNAs are not derived from cells circulating in the blood (Mitchell *et al.*, 2008). At present, there are at least two possible explanations for the stability and origin of circulating miRNAs: One hypothesis is that passive release occurs during tissue injury. For example, miRNA-208 was shown to be exclusively expressed in the heart and was measured in the serum after heart tissue injury (Ji *et al.,* 2009). The same unspecific release could also exist in cancer, since the high rate of proliferation and cell lysis in tumors might contribute to the abundance of miRNAs in the blood stream. Alternatively, miRNAs are contained in small particles and are therefore protected against RNase activity. Recently, it has been shown that a transfer of mRNA and miRNA between cells can be accomplished through microvesicles (Valadi *et al.,* 2007). These are small (50 nm to 100 nm) particles, which are shed from the cell plasma membrane into the extracellular space and released into the blood stream (Caby *et al.,* 2005; Van *et al.,* 2006). Microvesicles are derived from different cell types, *e.g.* reticulocytes, dendritic cells, B/T cells and mast cells (Escola *et al.,* 1998; Andre *et al.,* 2002; Valenti *et al.,* 2006; Thery *et al.,* 1999; Raposo *et al.,* 1996). Additionally, it was shown that non-hematopoietic cells like intestinal epithelial cells and neuroglial cells are capable to release microvesicles (Fevrier *et al.,* 2004; Van *et al.,* 2001).

Tumor derived miRNAs can be readily accessed in patient sera or plasma samples. In healthy individuals also, the levels of cell free miRNAs present in sera are stable and more than 100 miRNAs can be detected in sera of healthy individuals (Mitchell *et al.,* 2008; Chen *et al.,* 2008; Gilad *et al.,* 2008).

Potential of circulating miRNA as non-invasive tumor specific biomarker was first reported by Lawrie *et al.* (2008) who compared miRNA profile in serum from diffuse large B-cell lymphoma (DLBCL) patients ($n = 60$) with healthy controls ($n = 43$). High *MIRN21* expression was found to be associated with relapse-free survival. Mitchell (2008) implanted a human prostate cancer cell line into mice to show that there were tumor-derived miRNAs circulating in blood. In various studies it has been reported that serum mi-RNA are stable and their expression profiles are reproducible as serum miRNA are more resistant to endogenous ribonucleases. In order to study their stability Chen *et al.* (2008) amplified miRNA from lung carcinoma A549 cells with or without RNase A digestion using RT-PCR and reported that more than half of the molecules remained intact after 3 hrs of exposure to RNase A. Furthermore, effect of harsh conditions like low/high pH, boiling, extended storage, freeze-thaw cycle was also studied and no significant difference was observed between treated and non-treated serum. Even DNase-1 did not affect the levels of serum mi-RNA detected by qRT-PCR. Similar results were reported by Li *et al.* (2011) who evaluated the stability of miRNAs from three different sources, cultured liver cancer Huh-7 cell line, clinical liver cancer, and serum under different experimental conditions. In this study liver cancer related miRNAs were found to be extremely stable and resistant to destruction in harsh environmental conditions. Recent studies have found that extracellular miRNAs are associated with microvesicles and exosomes leading to the dominant model that miRNAs are released from cells in membrane-bound vesicles, which protect them from blood RNase activity. The mechanism underlying the unexpected stability of cell-free miRNAs in the RNase-rich environment of blood was stududied by Arroyo *et al.* (2011). They carried out differential centrifugation and size-exclusion chromatography to characterize circulating miRNA complexes in human plasma and serum. It was found, that the majority of circulating miRNAs cofractionated with protein complexes rather than with vesicles. miRNAs were also sensitive to protease treatment of plasma, suggesting that protein complexes protect circulating miRNAs from plasma RNases. Further characterization revealed that Argonaute-2 (Ago2), the key effector protein of miRNA-mediated silencing, was present in human plasma and eluted with plasma miRNAs in size-exclusion chromatography. Furthermore, immunoprecipitation assay suggested that vesicle-encapsulated miRNAs represent only a minor portion of circulating miRNAs. On the basis of these findings it can be concluded that most of the serum miRNA are protected by protein complexes from plasma RNases. mi-RNA Expression profile has been studied in different cancers like breast cancer (Heneghan *et al.*, 2010; Wang *et al.*, 2010), gastric cancer, ovarian cancer, pancreatic cancer etc. Zhang *et al.* (2010) studied expression of miRNA in sera of 290 ESCC patients and 140 age- and sex-matched controls. Solexa sequencing technology was used for an initial screen of miRNAs in serum samples from 141 patients and 40 controls followed by quantitative reverse-transcription PCR (RT-qPCR) to confirm the concentrations of selected miRNAs in serum samples from 149 patients and 100 controls. By Solexa sequencing marked upregulation of 25 serum miRNAs in ESCC patients was observed while RT-qPCR analysis identified a profile of 7 serum miRNAs (miR-10a, miR-22, miR-100, miR-148b, miR-223, miR-133a, and miR-127-3p) as ESCC biomarkers.

Lawrie *et al.* (2008) were the first to discover tumor specific deregulation of circulating miRNAs. Their study demonstrated that miRNA-21 is highly abundant in the sera of diffuse large B-cell lymphoma patients. miRNA profiling of leukemia patients has shown circulating miRNA-92a to be considerably downregulated in the case of malignancy (Tanaka *et al.*, 2009). In 2008, Mitchell *et al.*, reported that miRNAs derived from epithelial tumors are also rapidly released into the blood stream (Mitchell *et al.*, 2008). They used a mouse model to show that human miRNAs can be detected in the blood of mice after prostate cancer xenograft transplantation. The amount of human miRNAs was correlated with the xenograft tumor mass. These results clearly demonstrated that tumor-derived miRNAs can enter the circulation even when originating from epithelial cancers. Additionally, Mitchell *et al.* (2008) found circulating miRNA-141 to be significantly elevated in sera of metastatic prostate cancer when compared to those of healthy controls. Ng and colleagues employed quantitative polymerase chain reaction (qPCR) to analyze miRNA profiles in colon cancer cells, the corresponding adjacent normal colonic tissue and plasma of patients and healthy controls (Ng *et al.*, 2009; Schetter *et al.*, 2009): In this study, five miRNAs were found to be significantly overexpressed in the tumor cells as well as more abundant in the plasma samples of tumor patients compared to those of healthy volunteers (Table 10.1). miRNA-92 and miRNA-17-3p were confirmed as diagnostic markers for colon cancer in an independent validation study (Ng *et al.*, 2009). Both miRNAs belong to the miRNA-17-92 gene cluster, which is supposed to be involved in cancer pathogenesis (He at al. 2009).

Circulating miRNAs in Esophageal Cancer

The performance of circulating miRNAs as diagnostic markers has been compared to establish blood based markers for ESCC by Zhang *et al.* (2010). They investigated the serum miRNA profile in ESCC patients using Solexa sequencing technology verification was carried out using hydrolysis probe-based stem-loop quantitative reverse-transcription PCR assay. The results demonstrated marked upregulation of 25 serum miRNAs in ESCC patients compared with controls. RT-qPCR analysis identified a profile of 7 serum miRNAs (miR-10a, miR-22, miR-100, miR-148b, miR-223, miR-133a, and miR-127-3p) as ESCC biomarkers. More number of such studies validating the potential of circulating miRNAs as markers for diagnosis/prognosis/monitoring response to therapy is warranted for early screening and better management of this dreadful disease.

Conclusion

Aberrant expression of miRNAs in esophageal cancer and their presence in detectable levels in body fluids provides great hope for early diagnosis and improved monitoring of esophageal cancer. The advent of high throughput approaches for miRNA profiling and simple and widely used arrays for quantification and validation of miRNA biomarkers. miRNAs might turn out to be more efficient biomarkers as compared to the proteins which in order to be established as biomarker candidates need to surpass the hurdle of antibody generation. However, the functional roles of miRNAs in tumor development and progression need to be unravelled in order to exploit the blood based mina biomarkers to predict clinical behaviour and/or monitor therapeutic response. Moreover, larger sample sets including long term clinical data will be required for in-depth future studies. Further standardization of strategies applied in isolation, quantification and normalization of miRNAs are warranted before translating them as biomarkers into the clinics.

References

Akagi I, Miyashita M, Ishibashi O *et al.* (2011). Relationship between altered expression levels of MIR21, MIR143, MIR145, and MIR205 and clinicopathologic features of esophageal squamous cell carcinoma. Dis Esophagus doi: 10.1111/j.1442-2050.2011.01177.x.

Ambros V (1989). A hierarchy of regulatory genes controls a larva regulatory specificity, the notion that target-site recogni- to-adult developmental switch in *C. elegans*. Cell 57: 49-57.

Andre F, Schartz NE, Movassagh M, Flament C, Pautier P, Morice P, Pomel C, Lhomme C, Escudier B, Le Chevalier T, Tursz T, Amigorena S, Raposo G, Angevin E, Zitvogel L (2002). Malignant effusions and immunogenic tumour-derived exosomes. Lancet 360: 295-305.

Arroyoa JD, Chevilleta JR, Kroha EM *et al.* (2011). Argonaute2 complexes carry a population of circulating microRNAs independent of vesicles in human plasma. PNAS. doi: 10.1073/pnas.1019055108.

Bansal A, Lee IH, Hong X *et al.* (2011). Feasibility of MicroRNAs as Biomarkers for Barrett's Esophagus Progression: A Pilot Cross Sectional, Phase 2 Biomarker Study. Am J Gastroenterol 106: 1055-1063.

Bartel DP (2004). MicroRNAs: genomics, biogenesis, mechanism, and function. Cell 116: 281-297.

Berezikov E, Guryev V, van de Belt J *et al.* (2005). Phylogenetic shadowing and computational identification of human microRNA genes. Cell 120: 21-24.

Boult JK, Taniere P, Hallissey MT *et al.* (2008). Oesophageal adenocarcinoma is associated with a deregulation in the MYC/MAX/MAD network. Br J Cancer 98: 1985-92.

Caby MP, Lankar D, Vincendeau-Scherrer C *et al.* (2005). Exosomal-like vesicles are present in human blood plasma. Int Immunol 17: 879-887.

Calin GA, Dumitru CD, Shimiju M *et al.* (2002). Frequent deletions and downregulation of micro-RNA genes miR15 and miR16 at 13q14 in chronic lymphocytic leukemia. PNAS 99: 15524-15529.

Calin GA, Sevignani C, Dumitru CD *et al.* (2004). Human microRNA genes are frequently located at fragile sites and genomic regions involved in cancers. PNAS 101: 2999-3004.

Calin GA, Croce CM (2006). MicroRNA signatures in human cancers. Nat Rev Cancer 6: 857-866.

Castoldi M, Schmidt S, Benes V *et al.* (2006). A sensitive array for microRNA expression profiling (miChip). based on locked nucleic acids (LNA). RNA 12: 913-920.

Chen X, Ba Y, Ma L *et al.* (2008). Characterization of microRNAs in serum: a novel class of biomarkers for diagnosis of cancer and other diseases, Cell Res 18: 997-1006.

Chen X, Guo X, Zhang H *et al.* (2009). Role of miR-143 targeting KRAS in colorectal tumorigenesis. Oncogene 28: 1385-1392.

Chen ZL, Zhao XH, Wang JW *et al.* (2011). microRNA-92a promotes lymph node metastasis of human esophageal squamous cell carcinoma via E-cadherin. J Biol Chem 286: 10725-10734.

Cimmino A, Calin GA, Fabbri M *et al.* (2005). miR-15 and miR-16 induce apoptosis by targeting BCL2. Proc Natl Acad Sci USA 102: 13944–13949.

Ding D, Chen Z, Zhao X *et al.* (2011). miR-29c Induces Cell Cycle Arrest in Esophageal Squamous Cell Carcinoma by Modulating Cyclin E expression. Carcinogenesis doi: 10.1093/carcin/bgr078.

Enzinger PC, Mayer RJ (2003). Esophageal cancer. N Engl J Med 349: 2241-2252.

Escola JM, Kleijmeer MJ, Stoorvogel W *et al.* (1998). Selective enrichment of tetraspan proteins on the internal vesicles of multivesicular endosomes and on exosomes secreted by human Blymphocytes. J Biol Chem 273: 20121-20127.

Fassan M, Volinia S, Palatini J *et al.* (2010). MicroRNA expression profiling in human Barrett's carcinogenesis. Int J Cancer 129: 1661-1670.

Feber A, Xi L, Luketich JD *et al.* (2008). MicroRNA expression profiles of esophageal cancer. J Thorac Cardiovasc Surg 135: 255-260.

Felli N, Fontana L, Pelosi E *et al.* (2005). MicroRNAs 221 and 222 inhibit normal erythropoiesis and erythroleukemic cell growth via kit receptor down-modulation. Proc Natl Acad Sci USA 102: 18081-18086.

Gajalakshmi V, Swaminathan R, Shanta V (2001). An Independent Survey to Asses Completeness of Registration: Population Based Cancer Registry, Chennai, India. Asian Pac J Cancer Prev 2: 179-183.

Gilad S, Meiri E, Yogev Y *et al.* (2008). Serum microRNAs are promising novel biomarkers. PLoS ONE 3: e3148.

Guo Y, Chen Z, Zhang L *et al.* (2008). Distinctive microRNA profiles relating to patient survival in esophageal squamous cell carcinoma. Cancer Res 68: 26-33.

Gupta D, Boffetta P, Gaborieau V *et al.* (2001). Risk factors of lung cancer in Chandigarh, India. Indian J Med Res 113: 142-150.

Hammond SM (2006). MicroRNAs as oncogenes. Curr Opin Genet Dev 16: 4-9.

Hamano R, Miyata H, Yamasaki M *et al.* (2011). Overexpression of miR-200c Induces Chemoresistance in Esophageal Cancers Mediated Through Activation of the Akt Signaling Pathway. Clin Cancer Res 17: 3029-3038.

Heneghan HM, Miller N, Lowery AJ *et al.* (2010). Circulating microRNAs as novel minimally invasive biomarkers for breast cancer. Ann Surg 251: 499-505.

Hayashita Y, Osada H, Tatematsu Y *et al.* (2005). A polycistronic microRNA cluster, miR-17–92, is overexpressed in human lung cancers and enhances cell proliferation. Cancer Res 65: 9628–9632.

He L, Thomson JM, Hemann MT *et al.* (2005). A microRNA polycistron as a potential human oncogene. Nature 435: 828–833.

Headrick JR, Nichols FC, Miller DL *et al.* (2002). High-grade esophageal dysplasia: long-term survival and quality of life after esophagectomy. Ann Thorac Surg 73: 1697-1703.

Hiyoshi Y, Kamohara H, Karashima R *et al.* (2009). MicroRNA-21 Regulates the proliferation and invasion in Esophageal Squamous Cell Carcinoma. Clin Cancer Res 15: 1915-1922.

Ho AS, Huang X, Cao H *et al.* (2010). Circulating miR-210 as a Novel Hypoxia Marker in Pancreatic Cancer. Transl Oncol 3: 109-113.

Hong L, Han Y, Zhang H *et al.* (2010). The prognostic and chemotherapeutic value of miR-296 in esophageal squamous cell carcinoma. Ann Surg 251: 1056-1063.

Hu Y, Correa A M, Hoque A *et al.* (2010). Prognostic significance of differentially expressed miRNAs in esophageal cancer. Int J Cancer 128: 132–143.

Hummel R, Hussey DJ, Michael MZ *et al.* (2011). MiRNAs and their association with locoregional staging and survival following surgery for esophageal carcinoma. Ann Surg Oncol 18: 253-260.

Hummel R, Watson DI, Smith C *et al.* (2011). Mir-148a improves response to chemotherapy in sensitive and resistant oesophageal adenocarcinoma and squamous cell carcinoma cells.J Gastrointest Surg 15: 429-438.

Ji X, Takahashi R, Hiura Y *et al.* (2009). Plasma miR-208 as a biomarker of myocardial injury. Clin Chem 55: 1944-1949.

Johnson SM, Grosshans H, Shingara J *et al.* (2005). RAS is regulated by the let7 microRNA family. Cell 120: 635–647.

Kan T, Meltzer SJ (2009). MicroRNAs in Barrett's esophagus and esophageal adenocarcinoma. Curr Opin Pharmacol 9: 727-732.

Kano M, Seki N, Kikkawa N *et al.* (2010). miR-145, miR-133a and miR-133b: Tumor-suppressive miRNAs target FSCN1 in esophageal squamous cell carcinoma. Int J Cancer 127: 2804-2814.

Kim VN, Nam JW (2006). Genomics of microRNA. Trends Genet 22: 165-173.

Kimura S, Naganuma S, Susuki D *et al.* (2010). Expression of microRNAs in squamous cell carcinoma of human head and neck and the esophagus: miR-205 and miR-21 are specific markers for HNSCC and ESCC. Oncol Rep 23: 1625-1633.

Landis SH, Murray T, Bolden S, Wingo PA (1999). Cancer statistics. CA- Cancer J Clin 49: 8-31.

Lawrie CH, Gal S, Dunlop HM *et al.* (2008). Detection of elevated levels of tumour-associated microRNAs in serum of patients with diffuse large B-cell lymphoma. Br J Haematol 141: 672-675.

Lee KH, Goan YG, Hsiao M *et al.* (2009). MicroRNA-373 (miR-373). post-transcriptionally regulates large tumor suppressor, homolog 2 (LATS2). and stimulates proliferation in human esophageal cancer. Exp Cell Res 315: 2529-2538.

Lee RC, Feinbaum RL, Ambros V (1993). The C. elegans heterochronic gene lin-4 encodes small RNAs with antisense complementarity to lin-14. Cell 75: 843-854.

Lewis BP, Burge CB, Bartel DP (2005). Conserved seed pairing, often flanked by adenosines, indicates that thousands of human genes are microRNA targets. Cell 120: 15-20.

Li X, Lin R, Li J (2011). Epigenetic Silencing of MicroRNA-375 Regulates PDK1 Expression in Esophageal Cancer. Dig Dis Sci 56: 2849-2856.

Li Y, Jiang Z, Xu L *et al.* (2011). Stability analysis of liver cancer-related microRNAs. Acta Biochim Biophys Sin (Shanghai). 43: 69-78.

Liu CG, Calin GA, Meloon B *et al.* (2004). An oligonucleotide microchip for genome-wide microRNA profiling in human and mouse tissues. Proc Natl Acad Sci USA 101: 9740-9744.

Liu Q, Lv GD, Qin X *et al.* (2011). Role of microRNA let-7 and effect to HMGA2 in esophageal squamous cell carcinoma. Mol Biol Rep 39: 1239-1246.

Lu J, Getz G, Miska EA *et al.* (2005). MicroRNA expression profiles classify human cancers. Nature 435: 834-838.

Mathe EA, Nguyen GH, Bowman ED *et al.* (2009). MicroRNA expression in squamous cell carcinoma and adenocarcinoma of the esophagus: associations with survival. Clin Cancer Res 15: 6192-6200.

Maru DM, Singh RR, Hannah C *et al.* (2009). MicroRNA-196a is a potential marker of progression during Barrett's metaplasia-dysplasia-invasive adenocarcinoma sequence in esophagus. Am J Pathol 174: 1940-1948.

Matsushima K, Isomoto H, Yamaguchi N *et al.* (2011). MiRNA-205 modulates cellular invasion and migration via regulating zinc finger E-box binding homeobox 2 expression in esophageal squamous cell carcinoma cells. J Transl Med 9: 30.

Matsushim K, Isomoto H, Kohno S *et al.* (2010). MicroRNAs and Esophageal Squamous Cell Carcinoma. Digestion 82: 138-144.

Meng F, Henson R, Lang M *et al.* (2006). Involvement of human micro-RNA in growth and response to chemotherapy in human cholangiocarcinoma cell lines. Gastroenterology 130: 2113-2129.

Mitchell PS, Parkin RK, Kroh EM *et al.* (2008). Circulating microRNAs as stable blood-based markers for cancer detection. Proc Natl Acad Sci USA 105: 10513-10518.

Mori Y, Ishiguro H, Kuwabara Y *et al.* (2009). MicroRNA-21 induces cell proliferation and invasion in esophageal squamous cell carcinoma.Mol Med Report 2: 235-239.

Ng EK, Chong WW, Jin H *et al.* (2009). Differential expression of microRNAs in plasma of patients with colorectal cancer: a potential marker for colorectal cancer screening. Gut doi: 10.1136/gut.2008.167817.

O'Donnell KA, Wentzel EA, Zeller KI *et al.* (2005). c-Myc-regulated microRNAs modulate E2F1 expression. Nature 435: 839–843.

Ogawa R, Ishiguro H, Kuwabara Y *et al.* (2009). Expression profiling of micro-RNAs in human esophageal squamous cell carcinoma using RT-PCR. Med Mol Morphol 42: 102-109.

Papadopoulos GL, Reczko M, Simossis VA *et al.* (2009). The database of experimentally supported targets: a functional update of TarBase. Nucleic Acids Res 37: D155–D158.

Parkin DM, Moss SM (2000). Lung cancer screening: improved survival but no reduction in deaths–the role of "overdiagnosis". Cancer 89: 2369-2376.

Rosenfeld N, Aharonov R, Meiri E *et al.* (2008). MicroRNAs accurately identify cancer tissue origin. Nat Biotechnol 26: 462-469.

Raposo G, Nijman HW, Stoorvogel W *et al.* (1996). B lymphocytes secrete antigen-presenting vesicles. J Exp Med 183: 1161-1172.

Rodriguez A, Griffiths-Jones S, Ashurst JL *et al.* (2004). Identification of mammalian microRNA host genes and transcription units. Genome Res 14: 1902-1910.

Reed CE (1999). Surgical management of esophageal carcinoma.Oncologist 4: 95-105.

Schetter AJ, Harris CC (2009). Plasma microRNAs: a potential biomarker for colorectal cancer? Gut 58: 1318-1319.

Taylor DD, Gercel-Taylor C (2008). MicroRNA signatures of tumor-derived exosomes as diagnostic biomarkers of ovarian cancer. Gynecol Oncol 110: 13-21.

Tanaka M, Oikawa K, Takanashi M *et al.* (2009). Down-regulation of miR-92 in human plasma is a novel marker for acute leukemia patients. PLoS ONE 4: e5532.

Thery C, Regnault A, Garin J *et al.* (1999). Molecular characterization of dendritic cell-derived exosomes. Selective accumulation of the heat shock protein hsc73. J Cell Biol 147: 599-610.

Tian Y, Luo A, Cai Y *et al.* (2010). MicroRNA-10b promotes migration and invasion through KLF4 in human esophageal cancer cell lines. J Biol Chem 285: 7986-7994.

Valadi H, Ekstrom K, Bossios A *et al.* (2007). Exosome mediated transfer of mRNAs and microRNAs is a novel mechanism of genetic exchange between cells. Nat Cell Biol 9: 654-659.

Volinia S, Calin GA, Liu CG *et al.* (2006). A microRNA expression signature of human solid tumors defines cancer gene targets. Proc Natl Acad Sci USA 103: 2257-2261.

Wang F, Zheng Z, Guo J *et al.* (2010). Correlation and quantitation of microRNA aberrant expression in tissues and sera from patients with breast tumor. Gynecol Oncol 119: 586-593.

Wijnhoven BP, Hussey DJ, Watson DI *et al.* (2010). MicroRNA profiling of Barrett's oesophagus and oesophageal adenocarcinoma. Br J Surg 97: 853-861.

Wu BL, Xu LY, Du ZP *et al.* (2011). MiRNA profile in esophageal squamous cell carcinoma: Downregulation of miR-143 and miR-145. World J Gastroenterol 17: 79-88.

Yang H, Gu J, Wang KK *et al.* (2009). MicroRNA expression signatures in Barrett's esophagus and esophageal adenocarcinoma. Clin Cancer Res 15: 5744-5752.

Yeole BB, Kumar AV (2004). Population-based survival from cancers having a poor prognosis in Mumbai (Bombay), India. Asian Pac J Cancer Prev 5: 175-182.

Yuan Y, Zeng ZY, Liu XH *et al.* (2011). MicroRNA-203 inhibits cell proliferation by repressing ΔNp63 expression in human esophageal squamous cell carcinoma. BMC Cancer 11: 57.

Zhang C, Wang C, Chen X *et al.* (2010). Expression Profile of MicroRNAs in Serum: A Fingerprint for Esophageal Squamous Cell Carcinoma. Clin Chem 56: 1871-1879.

Zhou SL, Wang LD (2010). Circulating microRNAs: Novel biomarkers for esophageal cancer. World J Gastroenterol 16: 2348-2354.

2014, Advances in Biochemistry and Biotechnology Volume 2
Edited by: Dr. Biplab Sarkar and Dr. Chiranjib Chakraborty
Published by: DAYA PUBLISHING HOUSE

Pages 183-197

11

Creation of Synthetic Cell: from the Concept of Life to Revisiting the Origin of Life

Jogeswar Satchidananda Purohit[1,2]*, Biplab Sarkar[2],
Madan Mohan Chaturvedi[3] and Pragnya Panda[2]

[1]*Department of Zoology, Smt. C.H.M. College (University of Mumbai),*
Ulhasnagar, Thane, Maharashtra, India
[2]*School of Biotechnology, KIIT University, Bhubaneswar, Orissa, India*
[3]*Department of Zoology, University of Delhi, North Campus, Delhi, India*

ABSTRACT

Understanding the misty of life has remained an unanswerable question since time eternal. Scientists have taken reductionist approach to unravel the characteristics of life. However, recently Craig Venter and his coworkers have reported the creation of the first living cell, whose parent was a computer. The cell was named as synthetic cell. In order to create the synthetic cell, Craig Venter group first determined the minimal genes required for the simplest free living organism.

* *Corresponding author.* E-mail: sachin.jogesh@gmail.com; jspurohit@zoology.du.ac.in

The genome map of the Mycoplasma cell was created and accordingly the entire genome was chemically synthesized. This digitized genome sequence was then transplanted into a *Mycoplasma capricolum* recipient cell to create new synthetic cell that was controlled by the synthetic chromosome. The cell showed all characteristics of living cell and was capable of continuous self replication. The Craig Venter groups have further proposed the synthesis of designer eukaryotic organisms within the next decade.

Creation of the synthetic cells has depicted many unanswered questions regarding origin of life in the universe. At the same time it has show the way for many new schools of thoughts in the concept of origin of species. In addition to the DNA and RNA world, it can now be again hypothesized that life could also have reached earth in some simpler forms from some other planet or even universe.

Here, the process of creation of synthetic cell by Craig Venter's group is discussed. The chapter further includes the proposed future and consequences of synthetic cells. The misery of origin of species and the other schools of thought and reevaluation and arguments regarding origin of species is also included in the chapter.

Keywords: Life, Synthetic cell, Origin of life, Mycoplasma mycoides.

Understanding Life: Ehe Early Days

What is life? To a good extent this question still continues to be a mystery of science and as of today, a definitive answer to this word 'life' remains elusive. This very basic question can be referred even to way back in 1944, when 'Erwin Schrodinger' wrote the famous book entitled **"What Is Life"** to create common understanding on the subject (Schrodinger 1944). The book was based on a course of public lectures delivered by Schrodinger in February 1943, under the auspices of the Dublin Institute for Advanced Studies at Trinity College, Dublin. At that time DNA was not yet accepted as the carrier of hereditary information, which only was the case after the Hershey-Chase's experiment (Hershey *et al.*, 1952). The audiences in the lecture were warned "that the subject-matter was a difficult one." Schrodinger's lecture focused on one important question: "how can the events in space and time which takes place within the spatial boundary of a living organism can be accounted by physics and chemistry?"

Schrodinger introduced life in the idea of an "aperiodic crystal" that contained genetic information in its configuration of covalent chemical bonds. An aperiodic crystal is intermediate between crystalline and amorphous compounds. The hypothesis of aperiodic crystal originated from the fact that Schrodinger believed the genetic material to be a molecule which unlike a true crystal does not repeat itself nor is it a viscous liquid like an amorphous compound. This is essential here to mention that till then the genetic material was not discovered. In the 1950s, Schrodinger's hypothesis stimulated enthusiasm for discovering the genetic molecule. Francis Crick, co-discoverer of the structure of DNA, credited Schrodinger's book with presenting an early theoretical description of how the storage of genetic information would work, and acknowledged the book as a source of inspiration for his initial research. Now we know that inside the cell the DNA exists in the form which is neither crystalline nor amorphous and is called as a semi-crystalline state which was hypothesized by Schrodinger when its existence was yet to be discovered.

According to Schrodinger, life works on an "order-from-disorder" principle. For example diffusion, which can be modeled as a highly ordered process, is caused by random movement of atoms or molecules. The master code of a living organism has to consist of atoms. The main principle involved with "order-from-disorder" is the second law of thermodynamics, according to which entropy only increases. Schrodinger explained that living matter evades the decay to thermo-dynamical equilibrium by feeding on negative entropy. However, Schrodinger's explanations were based on hypothesis and mathematical calculations and it lacked experimental evidences from biology.

Schrodinger's Paradox

The hypothesis made by Schrodinger about life is not valid and true in total. In a world governed by the second law of thermodynamics, all closed systems are expected to approach a state of maximum disorder. In contrast, life approaches and maintains a highly ordered state, which seems to violate the second law. The solution to this paradox is that life is not a closed system, rather an open system. The increase of order inside an organism is more than paid for by an increase in disorder outside this organism. By this mechanism, the second law is obeyed, and life maintains a high order state, which it sustains by causing a net increase in disorder in the Universe (Schneider *et al.,* 2005).

Characteristics of Living Organisms: The Present Day Understanding

One hundred and fifty years of rigorous investigations round the globe have brought us to a better understanding of what constitutes all living organisms, but the why and how of life it-self remain elusive. Life is defined as an open thermodynamic system performing basic life process called metabolism and is subject to Darwinian evolution. However, a concise and discrete definition of life remains obscure. Rather, it was easier to define organisms possessing life. The living organisms are distinguished from nonliving organisms as they possess dome unique characteristics which are as follows: (Koshland, 2002)

1. Living things are organized into units called cells
2. They use energy from their environment
3. They respond to stimuli
4. They are subject to grow and evolve.
5. They are capable of reproduction
6. They contain genetic information

However, there are arguments in support and against the above mentioned characteristics also. Sometimes living organisms do not show all these characteristics, at the same time nonliving things also show some of the above mentioned characteristics. Hence, a true definition of life is still debatable and the knowhow of life also remains elusive.

Understanding Life: Reductionist Approach

Scientists have of-late taken reductionist approach for understanding life. A reductionist approach is nothing but fractionation or simplification of a complex entity. For example if you are asked to answer the question "what is life", you will approach the problem in the following way. Since, cell is the structural and functional unit of life, and cell is living, you would choose to analyze a cell. Immediately, you will break open the cell and see. I mean to say scientifically you will fractionate the cell into organelles, membrane and non membrane components. Further fractionation will lead to simpler components like protein, carbohydrate, lipid, nucleic acid and water etc. Successive fractionation will lead to handful of elements like C, H, N, O, P etc. So, here it can be mentioned that life is basically composed of these handful of simplest components, which can be precisely estimated and characterized. However, if I ask you here a very simple and interesting question: GIVE ME MY CELL BACK? Mixing all these components together will not by any means give the living cell back. So by adopting reductionist approach though it is possible to know the composition of life, reductionist approach by any means does not help in understanding how to create life.

However, Craig Venter (Box 11.1) and his group of scientists had a big hypothesis in mind. "Can a complete genetic system be reproduced by chemical synthesis starting with only the digitized DNA sequence contained in a computer"? In a simpler version the question can be like this: "can we create even a bacterial cell whose parent is a computer". In 2010, they chemically synthesized the entire genome of a simple bacterium named *Mycoplasma mycoides* and transplanted this chemically synthesized genome to *Mycoplasma capricolum* to create first synthetic cell (Gibson *et al.*, 2010).

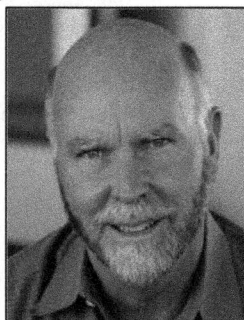

Box 11.1

Dr. J.G. Venter, designer of synthetic cell: Dr. John Craig Venter is an American biologist and entrepreneur. He was instrumental for his role in sequencing the human genome and for his role in creating the first cell with a synthetic genome in 2010. Venter founded Celera Genomics, The Institute for Genomic Research and the J. Craig Venter Institute, now working in the field of synthetic life. He was listed on *Time* magazine's 2007 and 2008 Time 100 list of the most influential people in the world. In 2010, the British magazine New Statesman listed Craig Venter at 14th in the list of "The World's 50 Most Influential Figures 2010".

Journey Towards Creation of the Synthetic Cell

It is known that in case of higher eukaryotes, the genome contains plenty of redundant and junk DNA. The actual euchromatic regions account for only 5-7 per cent of the total genome. The genome becomes smaller as we move down to simpler organisms like bacteria, because the amount of junk DNA also decreases drastically. The Venter group, by virtue of their 15 years of genome sequencing research had known that *Mycoplasma genitalium* possessed the smallest complement of genes of any known free living organism. Further, for this organism also, out of its 485 genes, about 100 genes were dispensable, when disrupted one at a time (Glass *et al.*, 2006). However, since it was a slow growing organism, a related fast growing organism *Mycoplasma mycoides* was chosen for the synthetic cell experiments. The synthetic cell was created in three broad stages: 1. Chemical synthesis of the *Mycoplasma mycoides* genome. 2. Assembly and propagation in yeast. 3. Transplantation to *Mycoplasma capricolum* (Gibson *et al.*, 2010).

Chemical Synthesis of the *Mycoplasma mycoides* Genome

The entire genome of the *Mycoplasma mycoides* was approximately 1.08 Mbp in size. Since, the entire genome could not be chemically synthesized at-a-stretch, as a single piece, it was synthesized in pieces. The entire genome was divided into 1078 overlapping cassettes. Each cassette was 1080 bp long with 80 bp overlapping sequences (Figure 11.1). At both the ends of each cassette a *Not*I cleavage

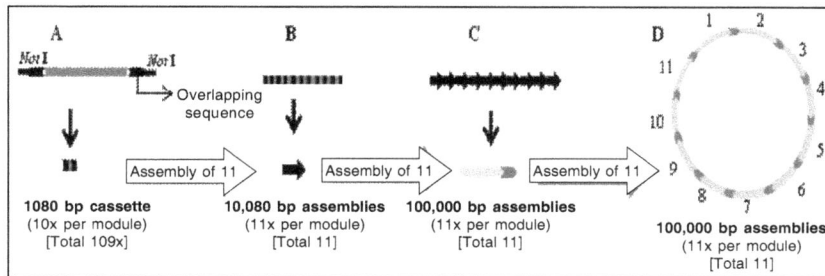

Figure 11.1: A Hierarchical Strategy for Assembly of the Synthetic Genome.
The genome of *Mycoplasma mycoides* was approximately 1.08 Mbp in size. It was divided into 1078 number of overlapping cassettes. Each cassette was 1080 bp in length and was chemically synthesized. These cassettes were then assembled in three stages to give rise to the entire synthetic genome. **A.** 1080 bp long cassette was flanked by 80 bp of overlapping sequence needed for joining with the next sequence. At both ends it had a *Not*I restriction site needed for ligation. **B.** These 1080 bp cassettes 10 in numbers were assembled to give rise to the 10 kb assembly. **C.** 11 of these 10 kb assemblies (as produced in B) joined to give rise to the 100 kb assembly. **D.** 11 of the 100 kb assemblies (as produced in C) joined to give rise to the entire synthetic genome.

site (GCGGCCGC) was included, which was necessary for successive ligation of the cassettes for formation of higher assembly. Out of the 1078 cassettes few cassettes (about 4 of them) were inserted with some watermark sequences [Watermark sequence 1 (1246bp), 2 (1081bp), 3 (1109bp), 4 (1222bp)]. These watermark sequences were inserted in places where insertion of additional sequence would not interfere with viability of the cell. The watermark sequences contained a new DNA code for writing words, sentences and numbers, a web address to send emails, the names of 46 authors related to the research and other key contributors and three famous quotations related to creation of life. The watermark sequences were used to distinguish between synthetic genome and natural genomes of *Mycoplasma mycoides*. A hierarchical strategy was designed to assemble the genome in three stages by transformation and homologous recombination in yeast and bacteria (Figure 11.1). The detailed process is described below and represented in a separate cartoon representation (Figure 11.2).

Assembly of 10-kb Synthetic Intermediates

All the overlapping cassettes (1078 in numbers) representing the entire genome of *M. mycoides* were first chemically synthesized using DNA synthesizer and their sequences were verified by DNA sequencing that there was no unusual mutations entrapped. Then the cassettes DNA were pooled in a set of 10, so as to generate 108 sets. Each pooled set of cassette DNA was then mixed with a yeast/ *Escherichia coli* shuttle vector, termed pCC1BAC-LCYEAST. The shuttle vector contained a histidine selectable marker, a centromere, and an origin of replication and was able to propagate in *E. coli* as well as in *yeast*. The vector had overlapping sequence for the first cassette at one end and the last cassette at the other end. The pool of DNA cassettes and the vector DNA were transformed to yeast spheroplast. Due to presence of overlapping sequences the cassettes joined among themselves (recombine among themselves) and ligated with the vector to give a 10 kb fragment in yeast. However,

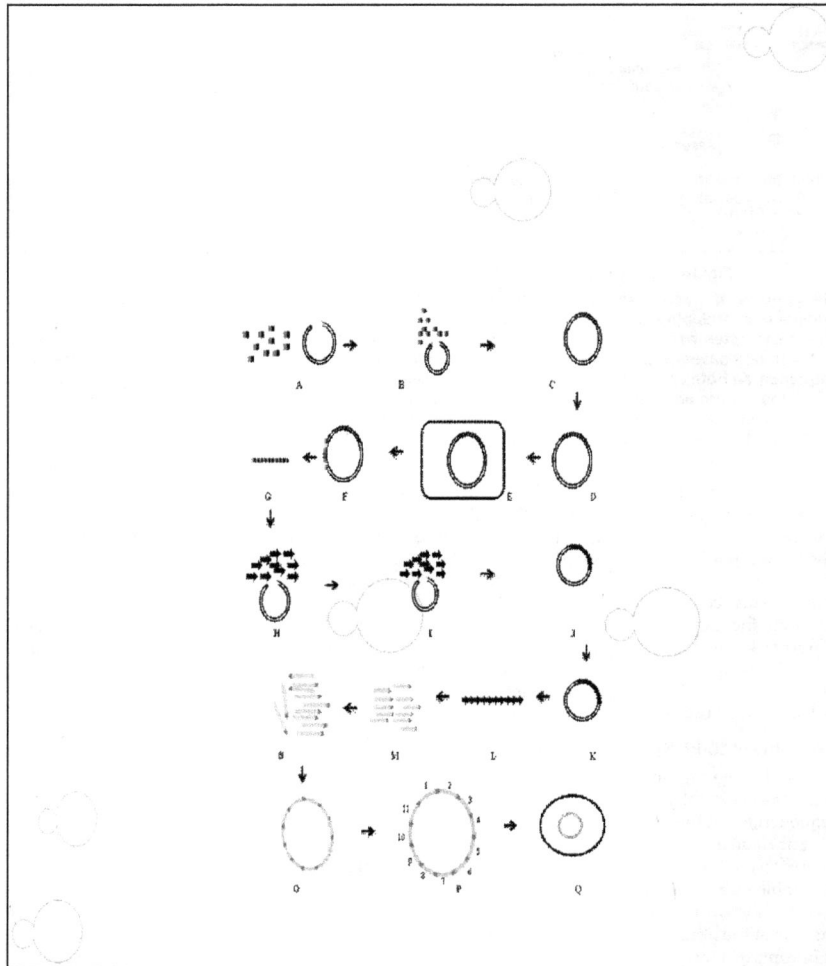

Figure 11.2: Cartoon Representation of the Detailed Process Involved in Making of the Synthetic Genome.

The entire genome of *Mycoplasma mycoides* (approximately 1.08 Mbp in size), was divided into 1078 number of overlapping cassettes. Each cassette was 1080 bp in length and was chemically synthesized. A. Each cassette had 80 bp overlapping sequence to the next cassette and was flanked by a *Not*I restriction site. 10 of such cassettes were mixed with a yeast/ *Escherichia coli* shuttle vector. B. The mixture was transformed to yeast protoplasts. C. The cassettes recombine *in vivo* and with the shuttle vector to give rise to the 10 kb assembly. D. Plasmid vectors containing inserts were isolated. E. The vectors containing inserts were transformed to *E. coli*. F. plasmids were isolated from the bacterial colonies. G. The isolated vectors were digested to release the fragments and right sized fragments were purified following gel electrophoresis. These right fragments were the 10 kb assemblies. H. 10 kb assemblies in a set of 11 were mixed with BAC based vector. I. They were transformed to yeast spheroplast. J. the BAC vector and the 10 kb inserts recombined *in vivo* to give rise to 100 kb assembly vector ligation products. K. The plasmids were isolated. L. The vector inserts were separated by restriction digestion and right sized fragments were selected following gel electrophoresis. M. 100 kb assemblies in a set of 11 were transformed to yeast spheroplast. N. These assemblies were transformed to yeast spheroplast. O. The 100 kb fragments recombined *in vivo* to give rise to the synthetic genome. P. The synthetic genome was isolated from yeast cells. Q. The synthetic genome was then transformed to *M. capricolum* cells to generate *Mycoplasma mycoides* JCVI-syn1.0 cells.

during the process, ligation products less than 10 fragments were also likely to be obtained. Hence, yeast colonies were picked, DNA was isolated from them and again the plasmid DNA was transformed to *E. coli* and screened for the 10kb assembly which was selected. It was expected by rule of probability that by screening every 10 yeast colony one correct 10-kb insert could be obtained.

Assembly of 100 kb Synthetic Intermediates

Positive clones containing the correct 10 kb assembly were grown in suitable medium and DNA was isolated. The 10 kb cassette containing vector assemblies were again pooled in a set of 10. The pooled DNA was digested with *Not*I to separate the insert and vector. 10kb inserts were separated out following gel electrophoresis. These 10 kb inserts were then mixed with the second stage vector (BAC based) and were transformed to yeast for *in vivo* recombination and generation of 100 kb intermediates. However, *E. coli* based screening was not possible in this step due to the larger size of the insert; instead the screening was performed by direct DNA isolation from yeast followed by multiplex PCR to amplify all the 11 assembly cassettes.

Assembly of the Complete Genome

All the 11 circular plasmids were isolated from yeast and were digested with *Not*I to release the inserts. The inserts were pooled and were again transformed to yeast spheroplast for complete assembly of the genome. Here, additional vector sequence was not needed as these sequences were already present in the complete genome. The screening of the right clones was done as above by multiplex PCR.

Transplantation of the Synthetic Genome

The synthetic genome was transplanted to *M. capricolum* recipient cells. The positive colonies were selected by blue white selection on X-gal plates. These cells were called as synthetic cells and were named as *Mycoplasma mycoides* JCVI-syn1.0.

Characterization of the Synthetic Cell

Presence of the watermark sequences in the synthetic cell genome, which could only be amplified by PCR amplification from the synthetic cell and not from the natural cells, was one of the distinguishing features between the synthetic cell and natural cell of *Mycoplasma mycoides*. The cells with only the synthetic genome were also self-replicating and capable of logarithmic growth similar to natural cells. Scanning and transmission electron micrographs (EMs) of *M. mycoides* JCVI-syn1.0 cells showed small, ovoid cells surrounded by cytoplasmic membranes. Proteomic analysis of the *M. mycoides* JCVI-syn1.0 and the wild-type control (YCpMmyc1.1) by two-dimensional gel electrophoresis revealed almost identical patterns of protein spots. These observations suggested the identities and uniqueness of the synthetic cell.

The present work revolutionized the principle for production of cells based on computer designed genomes. The Venter group described it to be a 'synthetic cell' even though the cytoplasm of the recipient cell was not synthetic. According to their discussion, phenotypic effects of the recipient cytoplasm are diluted with protein turnover and as cells carrying only the transplanted genome replicate. Following transplantation and replication on a plate to form a colony, progeny will not contain any protein molecules that were present in the original recipient cell. Rather they will be translated fresh being governed by the synthetic genomic DNA.

Advantages and Future Perspectives of the Created Synthetic Cells

In few public addresses Dr. Venter has set some targets regarding advances in the synthetic cell research, which are as follows (Box 11.2):

Any already sequenced viral genome can be made today, within next ten years synthetic designer virus will be available, bacteria will be available within next two years, and single cell eukaryotes within 10 years.

According to the Venter group, the future perspective of these synthetic organisms will be immense and hard to envision fully. They hope that the creation of a synthetic cell will lead to new applications and products in the field like bio-fuels, vaccines and food. It could yield bacteria capable of cleaning up oil spills or toxic waste, or creating medicines and clean fuels. Scientists of the Craig Venter group

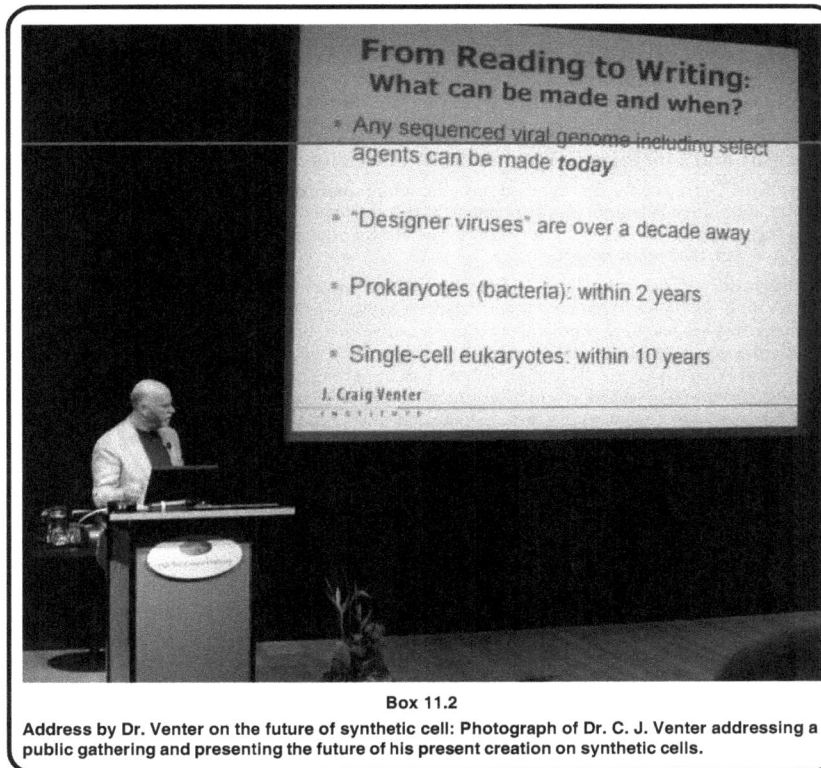

Box 11.2

Address by Dr. Venter on the future of synthetic cell: Photograph of Dr. C. J. Venter addressing a public gathering and presenting the future of his present creation on synthetic cells.

are trying to convert wastewater into drinking water and are exploring the ways the synthetic cell can remove hazardous chemical spills. Synthetic Genomics, Craig Venter's company, is said to have a contract with bio-fuel company Exxon to generate bio-fuels from algae. They are already in the process to create an organism that will translate carbon dioxide into clean fuel. They aim to build an entire algae genome to make super-productive organisms. The synthetic cell advancement could lead to the synthesis of algae cells that produce more plant oils than nature-made algae, boosting the per-acre bio-fuel yield. This will definitely result in cheaper oil. In future they propose that designer bacteria and eukaryotic cells can be produced with minimal genes essential for the survival of the organism and other genes designed for production of some products. So, living cells could be made as a factory for production of medicine, food or can even be used for gene transfer etc. Varying genetic parameters in genome will lead into development of medicines which will be much effective and cheaper also.

Importance of Synthetic Cell on Disease Control and Management

With the creation of synthetic cells, the branches of cell engineering and therapy will meet new directions. Now synthetic cells can be created with minimal genes and they can be used as factories for production of medicines, antibiotics, interferons and hormones. Scientists are also hopeful of generating synthetic blood and organs which will be self customized depending on the genome of an individual and the organ will perfectly suit the individual negating any chance of graft rejection.

Concerns and Bioethics Related to Synthetic Cells

As scientists create the first synthetic cell, the future safety of synthetic biology will depend on sound science. Immediately after announcement from Craig Venter's synthetic cell, President of America called for an urgent study to identify appropriate ethical boundaries and minimize possible risks associated with the breakthrough.

In his address he stated, 'The new "synthetic biology" epitomized by the Venter Institute's work in essence the ability to design new genetic code on computers and then "download" it into living organisms heralds a new era of potentially transformative technology innovation. But the technology also raises serious ethical and safety concerns: Is it right and proper to meddle with the fundamental basis of life? What happens if the technology gets into the wrong hands? And what might occur when synthetic life meets the natural world? The ethics in particular surrounding synthetic biology are far from clear; the ability to custom-design the genetic code that resides in and defines all living organisms challenges our very notions of what is right and what is acceptable. But in placing ethics so high up the agenda, my fear is that more immediate safety issues might end up being overlooked' (Published in American news paper).

The concerns are also posed from other group of scientists. Glenn McGee, founder of the American Journal of Bioethics stated that "We have now accomplished the last piece on the list that was required to do what ethicists called 'playing God". What that literally means is the capacity to be a creator. It is believed that the production of new synthetic bacteria poses potential environmental hazards as we don't know how these organisms will behave in the environment and it can be said that we are releasing new kinds of pollution into the environment.

Just consider the realities of introducing non-indigenous species into an ecosystem. It might not have any effect also. Yet there are also examples such as the Brown Tree Snake in Guam. Shortly after World War II, this brown Tree-snake was accidentally transported from South Pacific to Guam, probably as a stowaway in ship cargo. As a result of abnormally abundant prey resources on Guam and the absence of natural predators and other population controls, brown Tree-snake populations reached unprecedented numbers. Snakes caused the extirpation of most of the native forest vertebrate species and affected private, commercial, and military activities widespread loss of domestic birds and pets; and considerable emotional trauma to the native residents of Guam.

But a man-made species would not just be foreign to an island, region or state but to the *planet itself*. It would truly be an **"alien,"** and it's entirely possible that scientists wouldn't know precisely how it would interact in the environment. There can be also other concerns like bioterrorism and ecosystem destruction also.

There are some schools of thoughts who are asking for complete ban on this technology. Their logic is that the results of the experiment will fuel inventions of such dangerous weapons which will prove hazardous for our species. And they ask for ban on this technology to avoid its use in weapons. Their protest is parallel to the voices raised over the use of nuclear power.

Reaction and Views of Scientists about Synthetic Cell

"To my mind Craig has somewhat overplayed the importance of this," said David Baltimore, a leading geneticist at Caltech. Dr. Baltimore described the result as "a technical tour de force" but not breakthrough science, but just a matter of scale…. "He has not created life, only mimicked it," Dr. Baltimore said (The New York Times).

David Deamer, professor of biomolecular engineering, University of California, Santa Cruz, stated to Nature News that "Now that it has been demonstrated that how to reassemble a microbial genome, it may be possible to answer one of the great remaining questions of biology: how did life begin? Using the tools of synthetic biology, perhaps DNA and proteins can be discarded – RNA itself can act both as a genetic molecule and as a catalyst. If a synthetic RNA can be designed to catalyse its own reproduction within an artificial membrane, we really will have created life in the laboratory, perhaps resembling the first forms of life on Earth nearly four billion years ago."

Beyond Synthetic Cell

Indeed the time has now reached with the advancement of synthetic cell; the mystery of origin of life and its concepts have to be reevaluated. The question can we create life and how life originated in earth go side by side. We would rather state here that these two questions are synonymous. However, many theories are put forwarded relating to the origin of life.

During 1922, Oparin had the opinion that there is no fundamental difference between a living organism and lifeless matter. Life probably originated from nonliving matter. He postulated that the infant Earth had a strong reducing atmosphere, containing methane, ammonia, hydrogen, and water vapor, which were the raw materials for the evolution of life. From here emerged the simple organic substances which remained dissolved in the hot soup. These basic organic chemicals formed into microscopic localized systems which were the possible precursors of the cell from which primitive living things could have developed. These organic compounds in solution might have spontaneously formed droplets and layers. Oparin hypothesized that these *coacervates* might have formed in the Earth's primordial ocean and subject to a selection process leading eventually to life (Oparin L 1922).

The experimental proof of Oparin's hypothesis was given by Miller and Urey (Miller 1953). They investigated whether chemical self-organization would have been possible on the early earth. They recreated the reducing atmospheric semblance of the primitive earth in a sealed glass apparatus. It was filled with methane, ammonia and hydrogen gases, and water representing the atmosphere which scientists thought had then existed. A spark discharge device simulated lightning while a heated coil kept the water bubbling. Within few days a reddish precipitate began to stain the glass which on analysis, was found to be rich in amino acids. Sugars, liquids, were also formed. Nucleic acids were not formed by the reaction. Nevertheless, the common 20 amino acids were formed, though in various concentrations. At that time, the outcome of this experiment was considered the most stunning evidence that the prerequisite organic material for building the bricks of life could originate from natural atmospheric interaction with sea water, producing the 'primordial soup'.

In 2008, a group of scientists examined 11 vials left over from Miller's experiments of the early 1950s. Miller had also performed more experiments, including one with conditions similar to those of volcanic eruptions. This experiment had a nozzle spraying a jet of steam at the spark discharge. By using high-performance liquid chromatography and mass spectrometry, the group found more organic molecules than Miller had. Interestingly, they found that the volcano-like experiment had produced the most organic molecules, 22 amino acids, 5 amines and many hydroxylated molecules, which could have been formed by hydroxyl radicals produced by the electrified steam. The group suggested that volcanic island systems became rich in organic molecules in this way, and that the presence of carbonyl sulfide there could have helped these molecules form peptides (Johnson *et al.*, 2008).

However, there is nothing much in terms of experimental evidence to prove origin of life in earth. Further, since peptides cannot act as genetic material the origin of the first polymer for life is still debatable. In this regard nucleic acids are better options as they act as genetic material. While a school of thought debate that DNA emerged in the primordial soup as the first polymer for life, a parallel school belief that RNA was the first polymer which emerged and led to origin of life in earth. The argument for the first school of thought is due to the fact that excluding some viruses (which are living or nonliving is still a controversy) DNA is the genetic material for all known living organisms. The argument for the second school of thought is also known as RNA world (Gilbert 1986; Gesteland *et al.*, 2006) and can be postulated as follows.

1. RNA can act as genetic material (at least in some viruses) and can give rise to RNA, DNA and protein by different cellular processes.
2. In contrast to DNA, the *de novo* synthesis of RNA is possible
3. RNA also can act as enzyme (example ribozyme)

Dyson believed simultaneous origin of RNA and proteins and has proposed a possible sequence for biological evolution and RNA (Dyson 1985). (1) RNA was present in primitive cells. (2) RNA binding to amino acids aided with polymerization of amino acids and specific binding of RNA to catalytic sites permitted structural precision. (3) RNA complexed to amino acids became tRNA. (4) RNA complexed to catalytic sites becomes ribosomal RNA. (5) Catalytic sites evolved using transfer RNA instead of amino acids for recognition. (6) Recognition unit(s) from ribosomal RNA was removed and became messenger RNA. This is one possible pathway of molecular evolution in the latter stages.

The Connecting Link between Origin of Genetic Material and Life Forms are Missing

There is nothing beyond chemical origin of life as proved by Miller and Urey and origin of life. How did the RNA organized itself with a membrane and it gave rise to living cell is a mystery. There is also no clear-cut evidence for other complex life forms and most of the successive developments and evolution are only hypothesis based.

However, in the hunt of finding a connecting link between origin of genetic material and the cell, Dr. Jack W. Szostak and his groups had a simple hypothesis: How simple can a cell be and still be considered as living? The answer depends on what we consider to be the essential properties of life. An operational approach focuses on identifying simple cellular systems that are both autonomously replicating and subject to Darwinian evolution. His group thus imagined creating simplest living cells; he termed it as **protocell** (Szostak *et al.,* 2001).

His group imagined the protocell to be a collection of molecules that is simple enough to be formed by self-assembly, yet sufficiently complex to take on the essential properties of a living organism.

Designing the Protocell

A protocell would consist of two basic but independent components; the genetic material and the three dimensional structure in which it would reside. Taking into consideration the RNA world hypothesis, his group imagined the genetic material to be RNA. The primordial cells lacking protein synthesis use RNA both as the repository of 'genetic' information and as enzymes that catalyze metabolism. Such a RNA molecule performing both types of function was termed as RNA replicase. For performing both the above mentioned reactions it was imagined that definitely the replicase would consist of two RNA molecules, one will act as the genetic material template and the other RNA would act as the RNA polymerase to copy the above genetic material.

Further, for effective availability of the replicase to the RNA genome a compartmentalization was required, in which they would interact as well as co-evolve. Since, all known cells use membranes composed of amphipathic lipids as their compartment-defining barriers, the easiest way to construct the simple protocell was to surround it with a lipid membrane.

So they designed the simple protocell consisting of an RNA replicase replicating inside a replicating membrane vesicle. Both these components were self-assembling; the catalytically active structure of the replicase would form spontaneously as a consequence of its nucleotide sequence, while membrane vesicles assembled spontaneously as a result of interactions between the lipid molecules. As RNA molecules can become spontaneously encapsulated in vesicles as they form, the protocell as a whole could self-assemble. With compartmentalization, the replicase component was also inevitably subject to, variation, natural selection and thus Darwinian evolution.

From Protocell to Living Cell

The next question was how they can design correct living cells with all cellular functions. A simple example would be a ribozyme that synthesizes amphipathic lipids and so enables the membrane to grow. The membrane and the genome would then be coupled, and the 'organism' as a whole could evolve. Early attempts to derive an RNA replicase from the natural group-I self-splicing introns produced ribozymes that could direct the assembly of oligonucleotide substrates on a template, and even the assembly of full-length RNA strands complementary to the ribozyme itself (Doudna *et al.,* 1989; Green *et al.,* 1992). Successively by *in vivo* selection even RNA ligases could be generated experimentally. Derivatives of this ribozyme were subsequently shown to act as primitive polymerases capable of template-directed extension of a 'primer' strand of RNA complexed to the RNA template, using nucleoside triphosphates as substrates (Ekland *et al.,* 1996; Ball 2005).

Similarly, the membrane component was also investigated. Many bilayer-membrane vesicles, depending on their composition and environment, can exhibit complex morphological changes such as growth, fusion, fission, budding, internal vesicle assembly and vesicle-surface interactions. The rich dynamic properties of these vesicles provide interesting models of how primitive cellular replication might have occurred in response to purely physical and chemical forces (Hanczyc *et al.,* 2003).

Origin of Life: Different Schools of Thoughts but Still a Mystery

The RNA world hypothesis is not accepted fully in the scientific world and is argued in multiple facets. The first argument comes from the fact that RNA itself is unstable in water and is susceptible to rapid hydrolysis. In contrast DNA is relatively stable in water. Since, all hypotheses converge to a point that life originated in water, it is argued that RNA would not have been the first molecule to emerge and DNA could be the first polymer to emerge.

Even a school of scientists believe that life might not have originated in water. According to Philip Ball where there is water, there is life. NASA seems determined to follow the water. But is it right to see water as the sole medium for extraterrestrial life (Ball 2005)? Further, it has been pointed out that water is generally not a good solvent for doing organic chemistry- which is, in the end what life is all about. Water is rather reactive, tending to split apart the bonds that link the building blocks of life. It breaks peptide bond and bonds in RNA. The structure of RNA screams "I did not arise in water" (Benner *et al.,* 1988). According to Jack W. Szostak, water is really a noxious, toxic, corrosive and generally lethal environment for life. In fact given the well known properties of water one might almost be tempted to say that it's a miracle that life ever began in such a solvent! Rather it can be stated that probably life originated in close association to water (Szostak *et al.,* 2001).

Fitting Synthetic Cell and Origin of Life to the Same Box and Looking Beyond

With the creation of synthetic cells arising from synthetic DNA and on the other hand not having a proper clue regarding RNA world, the time has now arrived to reinvestigate the origin of species concept. We ask a very general question that with the validation of UFO and aliens in the present era and probable hypothesis of existence of life forms also in Mars or other planets we need to again look back at the same question that probably life did not originate in earth but it reached earth in some primitive form. We further argue that why nature will invest energy in originating life in different planets and galaxies rather will consider about their dispersal from a single origin. However, this hypothesis is premature at the moment due to lack of solid evidences. Nevertheless, creation of synthetic cells is a new step towards understanding the origin of life and the other mysteries of life.

The authors thank Prof. K.Muralidhar, University of Delhi and Prof. P. Balram, IISc Bangalore for their valuable suggestions. The authors are also thankful to Dr. S. Garg, Dr. R. K. Mishra and Dr. S.M. Pandey, Smt. C.H.M. College for their discussions and suggestions and help in making the models.

References

Ball P (2005). Water and life: seeking the solution. Nature 436: 1084-1085.

Benner S, Ellington AD (1988). Interpreting the behavior of enzymes: purpose or pedigree? CRC Crit Rev Biochem 23: 369-426.

Doudna JA, Szostak JW (1989). RNA-catalysed synthesis of complementary-strand RNA. Nature 339: 519-522.

Dyson F (1985). Origin of Life, Cambridge University Press, Cambridge, UK.

Ekland EH, Bartel DP (1996). RNA-catalysed RNA polymerization using nucleoside triphosphates. Nature 382: 373-376.

Gesteland RF, Cech T, Atkins JF (2006). The RNA world: the nature of modern RNA suggests a prebiotic RNA world. Plainview, N.Y: Cold Spring Harbor Laboratory Press ISBN 0-87969-739-3.

Gibson DG, Glass JI, Lartigue C *et al.* (2010). Creation of a bacterial cell controlled by a chemically synthesized genome. Science 329: 52-56.

Gilbert W (1986). The origin of life: The RNA World. Nature 319: 618.

Glass JI, Assad-Garcia N, Alperovich N *et al.* (2006). Essential genes of a minimal bacterium. Proc Natl Acad Sci USA 103: 425-430.

Green R, Szostak JW (1992). Selection of a ribozyme that functions as a superior template in a self-copying reaction. Science 258: 1910-1915.

Hanczyc M M, Fujikawa SM, Szostak JW (2003). Experimental Models of Primitive Cellular Compartments: Encapsulation, Growth, and Division. Science 302: 618-622.

Hershey AD, Chase M (1952). Independent functions of viral protein and nucleic acid in growth of bacteriophage. J Gen Physiol 36: 39-56.

Johnson AP, Cleaves HJ, Dworkin JP *et al.* (2008). The Miller volcanic spark discharge experiment. Science 322: 404.

Koshland DE Jr (2002). Special essay. The seven pillars of life. Science 295: 2215-2216.

Lazcano A, Bada JL (2003). The 1953 Stanley L Miller Experiment: Fifty Years of Prebiotic Organic Chemistry. Origins Life Evol Bios 33: 235–242.

Miller SL (1953). A production of amino acids under possible primitive earth conditions. Science 117: 528-529.

Miller SL, Urey HC (1959). Organic Compound Synthesis on the Primitive Earth. Science 130: 245.

Oparin AI, (1924). The Origin of Life. Moscow: Moscow Worker publisher (in Russian). English translation: Oparin A I, (1968). The Origin and Development of Life. (NASA TTF-488). Washington: D.C.L GPO.

Schneider ED, Sagan D (2005). Into the cool: Energy Flow, Thermodynomics and life. The University of Chicago Press.

Schrodinger E (1944). *What is Life? The Physical Aspect of the Living Cell*, Cambridge: Cambridge University Press.

Szostak JW, Bartel DP, Luisi PL *et al.* (2001). Synthesizing life. Nature 409: 387-390.

2014, Advances in Biochemistry and Biotechnology Volume 2

Pages 199-208

Edited by: Dr. Biplab Sarkar and Dr. Chiranjib Chakraborty

Published by: DAYA PUBLISHING HOUSE

12

Synthesis, Characterization, Application and Toxicological Aspects of Silver Nanoparticle

Biplab Sarkar[1], U.K. Maurya[1]*, Subendu Sarkar[2] and Surya Prakash Netam[3]

[1]*National Institute of Abiotic Stress Management, Malegaon, Baramati – 413 115 Pune, Maharashtra*
[2]*Calcutta National Medical College, 32 Gorachand Road, Kolkata – 700 014, West Bengal*
[3]*KIIT School of Biotech, KIIT University, Patia, Bhubaneswar – 751 024, Odisha*

ABSTRACT

Silver is a noble metal since time immemorial and has been used as an antibacterial agents before antibiotics came into picture. Nanosilver which is a nanoform of silver is more antimicrobial than original silver and is effective against a series of microbes including AIDS. Silver nanoparticles can be synthesized by top down and bottom up process using chemical reduction, ultrasonic, electron irradiation, thermal decomposition and green synthesis methods.It can be characterized using TEM-EDX, SEM, UV-VIS, XRD, AFM, FTIR and DLS techniques. Silver nanoparticle is showing its antimicrobial impact against almost all organisms and can be used as a potential

* *Corresponding author.* E-mail: uk_maurya63@yahoo.co.in

.

alternative of antibiotics and best therapeutics against multidrug resistant microbes. For its antimicrobial activity, it is used in shocks, utensils, bandages, food packaging and many other industries and become very useful for quality control and export of living material. Though it is commercially very successful, yet reports are deciphered regarding its toxicological impacts on *in vivo and in vitro* system which will stop the indiscriminate usage of these nanomaterials, and only dose dependant applications can be permitted.

Introduction

Nanotechnology can be explained as the upcoming scientific and technological tools involves in design, manufacturing, characterization, and application of devices by modifying its shape, size and composition at the nanoscale. Nanoparticle can be referred as small size particles within the range of 1 to 100 nm, and would exhibit different properties and behaviour in relation to bulk materials. Some properties are important at the nano level as it increases the surface area to volume ratio which can alter its mechanical, thermal and catalytic behavior. Nanoparticles may be classified as organic and inorganic nanoparticles. Chitosan, Polystrene Carbon nanoparticles are the examples of organic nanoparticles while inorganic nanoparticles include silver, gold, ferrous oxide, zinc oxide, titanium dioxide etc. The application and popularity of nanotechnology is spearheading promptly both in public and private regime and is projecting a n exponential growth for near future. Above all, nanomaterials will grab greatest percent of the global nanotechnology market by 2013.

Silver

Silver (Ag) is a noble metal positioned as the 47th element of periodic table alongwith an atomic weight of 108. It is also a representative of the heaviest metals like lead, cadmium, and gold. Silver possessed a background of minimum toxic features against animals, and it was applied as a life saving drug over 6000 years(Hongbao et al.2007). It is attributed with higher thermal, electrical conductivity, optical reflectivity and lower contact resistance. Silver nitrate works as the template for synthesizing several silver compounds and also a potential antimicrobial agent. Silver has also been applied as a contact substance in electric and electronic industries, and recently also in the manufacturing of contact tips or coatings (G³uchowski *et al.,* 2008).

Silver Nanoparticle (AgNP)

Silver nanoparticle is colloid form of metal silver which exhibits significant differences in properties in comparison to metal silver.

Silver Nanoparticle Synthesis

There are two methods to the synthesis of nanoparticle, namely the bottom up and the top down approach. In the top down approach, scientists try to formulate nanoparticles by breaking larger forms. The bottom up approach is a process that builds larger and more complex systems by adding and stabilizing molecular structure with precise control.

Method for Synthesis

A variety of preparatory routes have been reported for silver nanoparticles. Some of the methods have been described under following heads:

Chemical Reduction Method

This method for the synthesis of nanosilver is very popular. In this method, silver nitrate solution is applied as a precursor. Sodium boro hydrate solution, hydrazine hydrates solution and sodium citrate solution can be utilized as reducing agents. For this synthesis, two stabilizing agents, *i.e.* Sodium Dodecyl Sulphate (SDS) and sodium citrate (SC) were incorporated by Guzman *et al.,* 2008. This synthesis was reported to be carried out with the option of adding 1 ml of 5mM $AgNO_3$ to 4 ml of Poly Acrylic Acid (10 per cent W/V) and 2ml of aqueous solution of trisodium citrate followed by the addition of 6ml of 25mM sodium dodecyl sulphate. The mixture was stirred for 10 minutes and thereafter 4ml of ammonium hydroxide (25 per cent W/V) was added under constant stirring of further 10 minutes. After that, 10mM sodium borohydrate was added drop wise till the appearance of brownish colour.

Ultrasonic Method

The basis of utilizing ultrasonic treatment on chemical reactions is to initiate or accelerate difficult new reactions. The reaction rate can be increased along with sonic amplitude. Impacts of stirring, temperature, concentration, and reaction time can mobilize the synthesis, shape, size and morphology of the nanosilver structures.

Electron Irradiation Method

Bogle *et al*. (2006) invented a synthetic method for nanosilver on the basis of electron irradiation. In his innovation, silver nanoparticles had been prepared by irradiating solutions, mixing $AgNO_3$ and Polyvinyl Alcohol (PVA) in multiple ratios with 6 MeV electrons at room temperature. This method is precise, single step, easy and required about 10 minutes for conversion of colour.

Thermal Decomposition Process

Silver nanoparticle had been synthesized with the reaction of silver nitrate and sodium oleate in water. The developed nanoparticles were monodispersed when high temperature was applied on reaction mixture.

Green Synthesis Method

Now-a-days, green synthesis is popular as it is ecofriendly, nonhazardous and does not require any extra chemicals and stabilizing agent (Naveen *et al.,* 2010; Safaepour *et al.,* 2009). Green sources including plant, microbial and organic materials can be used as reducing agents (Sharma *et al.,* 2009, Bar *et al.,* 2009). Biosynthesis of silver nanoparticles can be performed using phyto-extracts including leaves after washing and removing the dust and thoroughly dried to remove any trace of water. The leaf broth will be prepared by taking 4-8gms in 100ml water and heating it at 55 °C for 30minutes and the leaf extract will be collected by decanting. 2ml of leaf extract will be added to 20ml of 1mM aqueous solution of $AgNO_3$. The reaction mixture will be kept at room temperature for 24 hours until the conversion of colour into yellowish-brown. This process will be standardized according to plant and microbial varieties.

Characterization

Characterization of silver nanoparticle is important to prove and confirm its nanoscale nature and to understand its behavior. Characterization can significantly throw light on different parameters like shape, size, morphology, crystal nature etc. of different nanostructures. There are several routes to characterize nanoparticles. Some of them are represented here:

UV-VIS Spectrophotometer

UV-visible spectroscopy is another most widely used tools for evaluating primary characterization and stability of many nanomaterials including nanosilver. The absorption spectrum of the pale yellow-brown silver colloids prepared by hydrazine reduction showed a surface plasmon absorption band at 418 nm indicating the presence of spherical or roughly spherical Ag nanoparticle (Guzmán *et al.,* 2009). Saxena *et al.* (2010) reported the UV-VIS absorption spectrum of silver nanoparticles prepared from onion extract remained close to 413 nm throughout the reaction period. It suggests that the nanoparticles were dispersed in the aqueous solution without aggregation. A strong, but broad, surface plasmon peak located at 430, 419 and 420 nm was studied for nanosilver synthesized using microorganisms like *Klebsiella pneumoniae, Escherichia coli* and *Enterobacterioacae.*

Scanning Electron Microscope (SEM)

The SEM applies beam of high-energy electrons to generate multiple signals on upper surface of solid specimens. These signals unleash the information about external morphology texture, chemical structure and orientation of the nanomaterials. This instrument is very important to evaluate 2D image of different nanostructured materials. The EDX attachment with SEM exhibit crystalline structure of nanoparticle. SEM images shown that high density nanosilver synthesized by *Trianthema decandra* extract had a particle size between 25-50 nm and a cubic in structure (Geethalakshmi and Sarada, 2010). Sudhalakshmi *et al.* (2011) observed that SEM analysis of nanosilver prepared using *Cleome viscosa* elicited uniformity in distribution on cell surface. The SEM image of silver nanoparticle synthesized from papaya extract has shown high density silver nanoparticles (Jain *et al.,* 2009).

Transmission Electron Microscope (HR-TEM) and EDX Analysis

TEM is one the best method to evaluate shape and size of nanoparticle. High resolution TEM helps to study elemental composition other than shape, and size and of nanosilver. Liu *et al.* (2007) synthesized silver nanoparticles by the addition of silver nitrate solution and ammonia gas and characterized in TEM. Saifuddin *et al.* (2009) synthesized silver nanoparticles using s of bacterial strain with microwave irradiation and also studied its nature under TEM. The morphology of these nanoparticles varied from spherical to hexagonal, triangular etc. in the size range of 5–50 nm. They also observed stabilization property of the silver nanoparticles by a capping agent. Mallikarjuna *et al.* (2011) described that the TEM image of silver nanoparticles derived from Ocimum leaf extract was morphologically spherical and were surrounded by a faint thin layer of other materials, which was capping organic material from Ocimum leaf broth. The obtained nanoparticles were in the range of sizes 3–20 nm. The TEM analyses of the silver nanoparticles are generally carried out by drop coating of silver nanoparticle solution on carbon coated copper grids. The samples will be dried and kept under vacuum in desiccators before loading them onto a specimen holder.

X-ray Diffractometer (XRD)

X-ray diffraction elucidates detailed crystallographic structure and chemical composition of natural, and synthesized materials. It can determine the status of orientation, shape, size, and internal modification in crystal. A rapid and easy method for synthesis of AgNP was used by aqueous gaseous phase reaction between silver nitrate and ammonia by Liu *et al.,* 2007. The XRD pattern of prepared nanoparticle showed diffraction peaks at 2è =38.2, 44.4, 64.6, 77.5, 81.7, which can be indexed to (111), (200), (311) and (222) planes of pure silver. It confirmed the presence of silver as elemental metal in nanoparticles solution. The biosynthesised nano silver by using *Trianthema decandra* root extract exhibited three intense peaks in the whole spectrum of 2è value ranging from 10 to 80. The typical XRD pattern elucidated the fact that sample contains a mixed phase (cubic and hexagonal) structures of silver nanoparticles (Geethalakshmi and Sarada,2010).Barud *et al.* (2008)synthesized silver nanoparticles applying bacterial cellulose membrane. Their XRD results showed peaks at 38.3 and 44.5 and confirmed the cubic phase of silver. Sun and Xia (2002) innovated a shape controlled silver nanoparticle synthesis. Their XRD showed peaks at 111 and 200 which depicted the FCC structure of the synthesized nanosilver.

Fourier Transforms Infrared Spectroscopy (FTIR)

FTIR is an unique superior spectroscopic technique which utilizes infra red sources and superior than conventional infra red spectroscopy in the parameters like sensitivity, speed, mechanical simplicity, and calibration. This machine can be used for samples of all nature including nanomaterials. It identifies chemical bonding pattern and its alterations within interacting molecule in nanoformulations. Mallikarjuna *et al.* (2011) synthesized silver nanoparticles applying ocimum leaf extract and conducted their FTIR characterization. The results reported the fact that the band of FTIR spectrum of silver nanoparticles can be obtained at 3419 cm^{-1} corresponds to O-H stretching H-bonded alcohols and phenols. The peak can also be obtained at 2923 cm^{-1} corresponds to O-H stretch carboxylic acids. Katumba *et al.* (2008) described a characteristic bonding pattern in the C–SiO$_2$ samples where he identified three distinct absorption bands. The major band was marked at approximately 1,050 cm^{-1} which narrated s stretching vibrations of Si–O–Si or Si–O–X, where X cited ethoxy groups bonded to silicon.

Atomic Force Microscopy (AFM)

AFM is a kind of scanning probe microscope which can take images of conducting, semi-conducting and other surfaces like ceramics, polymers, composites, glass and also 3D based biological samples. It can assist to catch images of morphological details in various nanomaterials like silver. Hemath *et al.* (2010) reported nanosilver synthesis using filamentous fungus *penicillium* sp. AFM characterization of synthesized nanosilver showed trends of agglomeration. The topographical pattern of irregular silver nanoparticles and its agglomeration was clearly projected. The particle size of the silver nanoparticles was detected in the range between 52-104nm.Fe *et al.* (2008) prepared silver nanoparticles by applying femtosecond laser ablation in water. Images of AFM analysis described the particles as spherical. The diameter of bright and dark particles were near to 120 nm and 35 nm respectively. The aggregation of particles was evaluated by absorption spectrum. The peak of the spectrum had a red-shift which implied the growth of particles.The broadening pattern of the spectrum predicted the fact that particles distribution was becoming wider.

Dynamic Light Scattering (DLS)

Dynamic light scattering (also known as photon correlation spectroscopy or quasi elastic light scattering) determines the size of particles in nano suspensions from a few nanometers to a few micrometers. It is an advantageous tools which takes automatic, minimum time, carries medium developmental cost, auto correction facility and not functions on the basis of concentration. Roh *et al.* (2009) reported the ecotoxicity of silver nanoparticle. Size of their prepared AgNP was evaluated by DLS method which showed the presence of nanosilver between 14-20 nm. Biologically synthesized silver nanoparticle applying onion extract exhibited average mean size of 33.6 nm by DLS (Saxena *et al.,* 2010). Ruparelia *et al.* (2008) studied the strain specificity of nanosilver. The DLS results elucidated a size range of 12–21 nm and 41–82 nm, respectively at DI water and in nutrient media.

Applications

Silver nanoparticles have received wide attention from scientific and industrial community because of their widespread application in easy, cheap and noble technology developement. Nanosilver can be applicable in diversified sectors, like medicine and diagnostics, drug delivery and therapeutics, textiles, energy (production, catalysis, storage), electronics (chips, screens), optics,), food (additives, packaging), cosmetics (skin lotions and sun screens), materials (lubricants, abrasives, paints, tires, sports ware), remediation (pollution absorption, water filtering and disinfection,. These variety of applications can be enumerated under following heads-

Drug Delivery and Therapeutics

Silver nanoparticles are known for their antimicrobial potential against many common and fatal microbials like viruses, including hepatitis B, respiratory syncytial virus, herpes simplex virus type 1, and monkey pox virus etc.Silver nanoparticles are having therapeutic potential in the recovery of multiple diseases, like retinal neovascularization, and acquired immunodeficiency syndrome (AIDS) etc. It can also exhibit antitumor property. Results of microbiological studies described that interaction of nanosilver with molecules of an extracellular lipoprotein matrix increases the permeability of the plasma membrane of microbial cells and eventually causes their death. Silver nanoparticle fulfills almost all the criteria necessary to be a good vehicle for drug delivery as it is biocompatible, biodegradable non-antigenic, amendable to chemical modifications, encapsulate efficiently to administer as well as release to targeted site etc. It can uncouple respiratory electron transport from oxidative phosphorylation which inhibits enzymes activity of respiratory chain or intermediates with membrane permeability to protons and phosphates (Duran *et al.*, 2010).

Medicine and Diagnostics

Multifunctional nanosilver emerges with multifarious opportunities in medical arena like drug delivery, intra cellular imaging, biomedical diagnostics and therapeutics because of their small sizes and unique set of properties. Colloidal nanosilver are applicable in various biomedical tools because of their enhanced resonance, scattering properties as well as strong raman scattering which assists in photo thermal therapy, optical imaging and probe designing (Lansdown, 2006 and Lee *et al.*, 2005).Like silver, nano silver has a strong antibacterial effects on wide range of microbes *e.g.*, viruses, bacteria, fungi (Chen *et al.*, 2003, Prashanth *et al.*, 2011). It is widely associated to develope devices for sterilized materials in hospitals, medical catheters, surgical instruments, contraceptive devices, wound dressings, artificial teeth etc. It is observed that smaller nanosilver are more lethal due to its high surface area to volume ratio (Guzman *et al.*, 2008).

Catalyst

Another important application of nanosilver is its activity as a catalyst (Jiang *et al.*, 2003). Silver nanoparticles when immobilized on silica spheres have been tested positive for their role as catalyst. Catalysis of dyes was selected as it is handy to detect colour conversion when dyes are reduced. In the absence of nanosilver, sample exhibited very little or no reduction of the dyes.

Textiles

Nanosilver have also been attached with textile product to inhibit bacterial proliferation. Application of nanosilver in textiles are another commercial applications to improve the quality and sterility of the products which includes anti-bacterial clothes, wound dressings materials etc. Gupta *et al.* (2008) examined the antibacterial potency of nanosilver-loaded poly (acrylamide-co-itaconic acid)-grafted cotton fabric. He recommended it as an efficacious process for antibacterial fabrics. The uniform distribution of narrow dispersed nanosilver is a value addition. Antibacterial impact was evaluated against *Staphylococcus aureus* on textile fabrics. The results exhibited a significant antibacterial activity against *S. aureus* that on cotton fabrics impregnated with nanosilver coating.

Paints and other Public Usages

Nanosilver mixed paints have been developed by many corporates and have been reported to have good antibacterial activity (Kumar *et al.,* 2008)**.** As nanopaints are antimicrobials, they are more durable, which are required for all sky scrapers. Silver nano coated tiles are encased in cinema hall, metro station, shopping mail for sterile,long lasting protection of these building of public use. Silver nano coated refrigerators, washing machine,water filter are also very popular domestic candidate for customers.

Toxicological Aspects

Though silver nanoparticle has vast commercial market covering all spheres of life, reports are also coming regarding its fatal, toxicological consequences. Researcher has examined on different *in vivo or in vitro* systems and obtained significant alterations on toxicological markers. Braydich-et al.,(2005) depicted that the toxicity of nanosilver is greater than bulk form and silver is comparatively more toxic than other heavy metals when exists in nano form. *In vitro* studies described that nanosilver is toxic to mammalian liver cells (Hussain *et al.,* 2003), stem cells (Braydich *et al.,* 2005) and even brain cells (Hussain, *et al.,* 2006). Trop *et al.* (2006) examined the absorption of nanosilver (15 nm) from a burn wound dressing. A burn patient received an *acticoat* wound dressing, which was replaced in every 4 and 6 days of post injury. Though wounds healed rapidly, grey discoloration of skin and variation in lip colour (to pale blue) was seen (termed argyria), as a toxic effect.

Skin discoloration is happened as a consequence from silver deposition on skin. Lee *et al.* (2007) conducted a trial, and characterized the transport of single silver NPs (5–46 nm) into zebra fish embryos and evaluated their impacts on early embryonic stages of development. They depicted that the Ag-NPs became trapped inside chorion pore canals (CPCs) and the inner mass of the embryos showed restricted diffusion. These data highlighted the occurrence of silver NPs inside embryos at each developmental stage and deformed, and dead zebra fish was marked. The group interpreted that toxicity and impairments observed in zebra fish were highly dose dependant. Takenaka *et al.* (2001) estimated the pulmonary retention and tissue distribution of inhaled silver particulates and was deciphered that silver was detected within the lungs immediately after exposure. Tian *et al.* (2007) applied a mouse model with thermal injury to examine the wound-healing capabilities of a particulate silver-containing wound dressing. The healing of burn wounds was much quicker when treated with nanosilver (14 nm) as compare to silver sulfadiazine (a standard burn treatment).

Rahman *et al.* (2009) studied the impacts of nanosilver (25 nm) on gene expression status in different regions of mouse brain. The particles were administered via an intraperitoneal injection to adult male mice at multiple doses (exceptionally high) for 24 hours. Alterations in the expression level of genes were seen in the definite experimental organs. Analysis of these changes explained the fact that silver NPs may initiate neurotoxicity by stimulating oxidative stress and altered gene expression which finally leads to apoptosis. Kim *et al.* (2007) further described the toxicity and tissue specific distribution of nanosilver during oral delivery. The silver content of a number of organs like blood, brain, liver, kidneys, lungs, and testes was evaluated as very high level.

Conclusion

Silver nanoparticle and its functions as antimicrobial were explored at a juncture when scientific communities were investigating for an alternative to antibiotics, as multidrug resistance problem became acute. Broad based inhibitory role against major pathogens including virus, bacteria, fungi etc. has widen the scope of its commercial applicability in all sphere of life which will be disseminated more in forthcoming days. Till date, only few entrepreneurial products has been launched in the market by embedding silver nano which will be enhanced in multiple proportions in near future. But applicable dose, toxicity assessment as well as conservation of utility bacteria within the community will be a matter of concern.

References

Bar H, Bhui DK, Gobinda P (2009). Green synthesis of silver nanoparticles using seed extract of Jatropha curcas. Coll Surf A: Physicochem Eng Aspects 348: 212-216.

Barud HS, Barrios C, Regiani T (2008). Self-supported silver nanoparticles containing bacterial cellulose membranes. Mater Sci Eng C 28: 515–518.

Bogle KA, Dhole SD, Bhoraskar VN (2006). Silver nanoparticles: synthesis and size control by electron irradiation. Nanotechnology 17: 3204-3208.

Braydich L, Hussain S, Schlager JJ (2005). In vitro cytotoxicity of nanoparticles in mammalian germline stem cells. Toxicol Sci 88: 412-419.

Chen Y, Wang L, Jiang S (2003). Study on novel antibacterial polymer materials (I). preparation of zeolite antibacterial agents and antibacterial polymer composite and their antibacterial properties. J Polymer Mater 20: 279–284.

Duran N, Marcato PD, Conti RD (2010). Potential Use of Silver Nanoparticles on Pathogenic Bacteria, their Toxicity and Possible Mechanisms of Action. J Braz Chem. Soc 21: 949-959.

Fei B, Xin-Zheng Z, Zhen-Hua W (2008). Preparation and Size Characterization of Silver Nanoparticles Produced by Femtosecond Laser Ablation in Water. Chin Phys Lett 25: 4463.

Geethalakshmi R, Sarada DVL (2010). Synthesis of plant-mediated silver nanoparticles using Trianthema decandra extract and evaluation of their anti microbial activities. Int J Eng Sci Technol 2: 970-975.

G³uchowski W., Rdzawski Z. (2008). Stabilization of mechanical properties in silver alloys by addition of lanthanides. Jr of Achievements in Materials and Manufacturing Engineering, Vol 30 (2), 129-134p.

Gupta P, Bajpai M, Bajpa SK (2008). Investigation of Antibacterial Properties of Silver Nanoparticle-loaded Poly (acrylamide-co-itaconic acid)-Grafted Cotton Fabri. J Cotton Sci 12: 280–286.

Guzman, M. G., Dille J. and Godet S (2008). World Acad. Sci. Eng. Technol.,43, 357-364.

Guzman MG, Dille J, Godet S (2009). Synthesis of silver nanoparticles by chemical reduction method and their antibacterial activity. Int J Chem Biol Eng 2: 104-111.

Hemath Naveen K.S., Gaurav Kumar, Karthik L., Bhaskara Rao KV (2010).Extracellular biosynthesis of silver nanoparticles using the filamentous fungus Penicillium sp. Archives of Applied Science Research, 2 (6): 161-167.

Hongbao M, Deng-Nan H, Shen C (2007). Colloidal Silver. Journal of American Science 3: 74-77.

Hussain SM, Hess KL, Gearhart JM (2003). *In vitro* toxicity of nanoparticles in BRL 3A rat liver cells. Toxicology 19: 975-983.

Hussain SM, Javorina MK, Schrand AM (2006). The interaction of manganese nanoparticles with PC-12 cells induces dopamine depletion. Toxicol Sci 92: 456-463.

Jiang J, Bosnick K, Maillard M (2003). Single molecule Raman spectroscopy at the junctions of large Ag nanocrystals. J Phys Chem B107: 9964–9972.

Jain D, Daima HK, Kachhwaha S (2009). Synthesis of plant-mediated silver nanoparticles using papaya fruit extract and evaluation of their anti microbial activities. Dig J Nanomater Bios 4: 557-563.

Katumba G, Mwakikunga BW and Mothibinyane TR (2008). FTIR and Raman spectroscopy of carbon nanoparticles in SiO2,ZnO and NiO matrices.Nanoscale research letters,3: 421-426.

Kim JS, Kuk E, Yu KN *et al.* (2007). Antimicrobial effects of silver nanoparticles. Nanomedicine: Nanotechnology, Biology, and Medicine 3: 95-101.

Kumar A, Vemula PK, Ajayan PM *et al.* (2008). Silver-nanoparticle-embedded antimicrobial paints based on vegetable oil. Nat mat 20: 1-6.

Lansdown AB (2006). Silver in health care: antimicrobial effects and safety in use. Curr Probl Dermatol 33: 17-34.

Lee D, Cohen RE, Rubner MF (2005). Antibacterial properties of Ag nanoparticle loaded multilayers and formation of magnetically directed antibacterial microparticles. Langmuir 21: 9651-9659.

Lee KJ, Nallathamby PD, Browning LM *et al.* (2007). *In vivo* imaging of transport and biocompatibility of single silver nanoparticles in early development of zebrafish embryos. Am Chem Soc 1: 133-143.

Liu C, Yang X, Yuan H *et al.* (2007). Preparation of Silver Nanoparticle and Its Application to the Determination of ct-DNA.Sensors 7: 708-718.

Mallikarjuna K, Narasimha G, Dillip GR (2011). Green synthesis of silver nanoparticles using ocimum leaf extract and their characterization. Dig J Nanomater Bios 6: 181 – 186.

Naveen KSH, Kumar G, Karthik L (2010). Extracellular biosynthesis of silver nanoparticles using the filamentous fungus *Penicillium* sp. Arch Appl Sci Res 2161-167.

Prashanth S, Menaka I, Muthezhilan R *et al.* (2011). Synthesis of plant-mediated silver nano particles using medicinal plant extract and evaluation of its anti microbial activities. Int J Eng Sci Technol 3: 6235-6250.

Rahman MF, Wang J, Patterson TA, Saini UT, Robinson BL, Newport GD, *et al.* (2009). Expression of genes related to oxi-dative stress in the mouse brain after exposure to silver-25 nanoparticles. Toxicol Lett 187: 15–21.

Roh JY, Sim SJ, Ji J (2009). Ecotoxicity of Silver Nanoparticles on the Soil Nematode Caenorhabditis elegans Using Functional Ecotoxicogenomics. Environ Sci Technol 43: 3933–3940.

Ruparelia JP, Chatterjee AK, Duttagupta SP (2008). Strain specificity in antimicrobial activity of silver and copper nanoparticles. Acta Biomater 4: 707-716.

Safaepour M, Shahverdi AR, Shahverdi HR (2009). Green Synthesis of Small Silver Nanoparticles Using Geraniol and Its Cytotoxicity against Fibrosarcoma-Wehi 164, AJMB 1: 111-115.

Saifuddin N, Wong CW, Nuryasumira AA (2009). Rapid Biosynthesis of Silver Nanoparticles Using Culture Supernatant of Bacteria with Microwave Irradiation. E-J Chem 6: 61-70.

Saxena A, Tripathi RM, Singh RP (2010). Biological Synthesis of Silver nanoparticles by using onion (allium cepa). extract and their antibacterial activity. Dig J Nanomater Bios 5: 427-432.

Sharma VK, Yngard RA, Lin Y (2009). Silver nanoparticles: Green synthesis and their antimicrobial activities. Adv Colloid Interface Sci 145: 83–96.

Sudhalakshmi GY, Banu F, Ezhilarasan (2011). Green Synthesis of Silver Nanoparticles from Cleome Viscosa: Synthesis and Antimicrobial Activity. International Conference on Bioscience, Biochemistry and Bioinformatics IPCBEE 5: 334-337.

Sun Y, Xia Y (2002). Shape-Controlled Synthesis of Gold and Silver Nanoparticles.Science 298: 2176-2179.

Takenaka S, Karg E, Roth C (2001). Pulmonary and systemic distribution of inhaled ultrafine silver particles in rats. Environ Health Perspect 109: 547–551.

Tian J, Wong KK, Ho CM (2007). Topical delivery of silver nanoparticles promotes wound healing. ChemMed Chem 2: 129–136.

Trop M, Novak M, Rodl S (2006). Silver coated dressing acticoat caused raised liver enzymes and argyria-like symptoms in burn patient. J Traum Inj Infect Crit Care 60: 648-652.

2014, Advances in Biochemistry and Biotechnology Volume 2   Pages 209-224
Edited by: Dr. Biplab Sarkar and Dr. Chiranjib Chakraborty
Published by: DAYA PUBLISHING HOUSE

13

Cell Free DNA

Dibyajyoti Banerjee[1]*, Kirtimaan Syal[1, 2] and Rajasri Bhattacharyya[1]

[1]Department of Experimental Medicine and Biotechnology,
Postgraduate Institute of Medical Education and Research, Chandigarh – 160 012, India
[2]Current: Molecular Biophysics Unit, Indian Institute of Science, Bangalore – 560 012, Karnataka, India

ABSTRACT

From the time, DNA is discovered; its functions have been variably speculated. In late 1900s, DNA double helix structure and its function as predominant genetic material is realized. So, the DNA located inside the cell, is credited with the role of genetic coding and inheritance. In 1940s, cell free (cf) DNA has been discovered. But, role and significance of cfDNA is still the matter of inquisitivity. In this article, we have discussed the historical perspective of cfDNA, its sources, sequential analysis and methods of quantification, with special emphasis on clinical significance of cfDNA and its potential as biomarker in various pathological conditions. We have also attempted to develop a working hypothesis about biological function of cfDNA

Keywords: Cell-free DNA, Biomarker, Malignancy, Gene.

---

* *Corresponding author.* E-mail: cdibyajyoti5200@yahoo.co.in

DNA: A Historical Perspective

Friedrich Meischer discovered DNA for the first time in 1869. He isolated DNA from leukocytes of pus cells and called it nuclein. Interestingly, he also believed that proteins are the molecules responsible for heredity. In 1920s and 1940s, Griffith's transformation results and experiments by Oswald Avery, Maclyn McCarty and Colin MacLeod, lead to the discard of belief that protein is a hereditary material (Ghose, 2004). Through their experiments, role of DNA as genetic material is deciphered. Rosalind Elsie Franklin and Maurice Hugh Frederick Wilkins are credited for the X-ray diffraction images of DNA which led to discovery of DNA double helix. A-DNA and B-DNA nomenclature has been given in accordance with the notations given by her to diffraction patterns. The structure of DNA has been worked out by James Watson and Francis Crick in 1953. The Nobel Prize has been awarded to them along with Maurice Wilkins in 1962 (Arnott, 2006). Unfortunately, Rosalind Franklin died in 1958 and Nobel Prize cannot be given posthumously. We recommend readers to go through this historical paper for an elaborate discussion of these historical aspects (Watson *et al.*, 1953). Today, role of DNA as genetic material has been fully accepted. This has laid the foundation stone of Biotechnology.

Variability in functions, forms and locations of DNA are still the matter of considerable current interest. In this article, cell-free DNA, which is one of the highly primed targets of today's scientific community, has been discussed. Its unique location, unknown function and potential to be developed as biomarker, make it a fascinating topic of discussion (Table 13.1).

Table 13.1: Historical Landmarks for cfDNA.

1948	Discovery of cell-free DNA (in blood)	(Stroun, Anker *et al.*, 1987)
1953	Double Helix structural model for DNA	(Watson and Crick, 1953)
1958	Central Dogma of life	(Ghose, 2004)
1960s	Circulating DNA and cancer: correlation	(Bendich, Wilczok *et al.*, 1965)
1970s	Detection of high levels in patients with several degenerative diseases and leukemia, biomarker potential in cancer, development of methods for determining cfDNA in samples	(Leon, Shapiro *et al.*, 1977)
1980s	Evidence of similar characteristics between circulating DNA and tumor DNA in cancer patients, biomarker potential related investigations	(Stroun, Anker *et al.*, 1989)
1990s	Evidence of further tumor-related genetic alterations in circulating DNA, presence of fetal DNA in plasma of pregnant women, plasma DNA chimerism after transplantation	(Lo, Tein *et al.*, 1998)
2000s	cfDNA in diagnosis and prognosis of numerous other diseases like trauma, heart infarction, stroke etc.), characterization of cfDNA, Development of more efficient methods for qualitative and quantitative detection	(Rainer, Wong *et al.*, 2003; Kamat, Baldwin *et al.*, 2010)
2010 and onwards	Oncogenic transformation of cultured cells by circulating DNA, Understanding the role of cfDNA study of distinguished markers present in cfDNA	(Jung, Fleischhacker *et al.*, 2010; Kamat, Baldwin *et al.*, 2010)

Nuclear DNA

In eukaryotes, a considerable amount of DNA is present in the nucleus rapped with histone proteins that transcribes and is responsible for the heredity. In last few decades, understanding of its function has been revolutionary. Today, we can manipulate nuclear DNA, modulate its expression, and thus alter its function. Nuclear DNA, in most cases, is passed sexually rather than maternally.

Thus, nuclear DNA is not an exact replication of the DNA of the individual's one parent, but rather a mixing of their both maternal and paternal parent's nuclear DNA. It consists of most of the coding regions essential for running and maintaining cellular systems. Any mutation in the essential region may lead to the genetic disease that may be inheritable. Today it is proved beyond any doubt that mutation or polymorphism in nuclear DNA is linked with many common diseases. Diabetes mellitus, coronary artery disease, obesity, cancer and many others can be added in the list. Nuclear DNA is the most common DNA used in forensic examinations. Epigenetic studies have further added a new unexplored chapter in it on which extensive research is going on.

Discovery of Cell-Free DNA

Cell-free DNA (cell-free DNA) is the extracellular DNA present in various biological fluids like blood, urine, pleural fluid etc. The presence of cell-free DNA has been first elucidated in 1947 even before the discovery of double helix model for DNA by Watson and Crick. The cell-free DNAs are mostly double-stranded molecules with molecular weights in the wide range of 6.6 kDa to 777.8 kDa. The cell-free DNA fragments apparently circulate as nucleoprotein complexes; however, in healthy individuals, the main part of cell-free DNA has been found to be adsorbed on the surface of blood cells (Stroun et al., 1987; Jahr et al., 2001; Skvortsova et al., 2006). In 1965, for the first time, it is held as a factor responsible for oncogenesis (Bendich et al., 1965). In mid 1960s and early 1970s, many studies indicated high levels of cell-free DNA in patients with systemic lupus erythematosus, rheumatoid arthritis, leukemia, and other diseases. In earlier times, cell-free DNA has been presumed to be present only in pathogenic manifestations. At that time, low cell-free DNA levels in the plasma of healthy people could not be reliably detected because of the lack of methods having high analytical sensitivity. However, the development of sophisticated techniques such as PCR and assays with fluorescent dyes, have resulted in the detection of cell-free DNA in healthy people as well. Now, its presence in healthy individuals is well evident and it can be detected in plasma or serum samples of not only in patients suffering from cancer or other destructive diseases but also in healthy individuals (Steinman, 1975). The major historical landmarks about cfDNA are summarized in Table 13.1.

Still, its importance and role are largely unknown. It has been found that cell-free DNA concentration varies with tumor stage and treatment (Leon et al., 1977). It has been advocated that levels of circulating DNA can help in diagnosis and indicate prognosis of various diseases. The diagnostic potential of measuring cell-free DNA is becoming increasingly recognized as a tool in the management of patients in various dynamic clinical situations such as trauma, stroke, sepsis, pre-eclampsia and cancer. Since it reflects cell necrosis and apoptosis, it can be used to assess the activity and severity of the diseases (Goldshtein et al., 2009) (Table 13.1).

Sources of Cell-Free DNA

(a) Apoptosis and Necrosis

Apoptosis and necrosis are two distinct mechanisms of cell death and are potential sources of cell-free DNA. In apoptosis, DNA degradation involves the cleavage of chromosomal DNA into large fragments of 50–300 kb and subsequently into multiples of nucleosomal units of 180–200 bp, which is a hallmark of apoptosis (Nagata et al., 2003; Holdenrieder et al., 2004). This ladder pattern can be visualized on agarose gel after electrophoresis. In apoptosis, the contents of cells dying by apoptosis are rapidly ingested by professional phagocytes (macrophages and dendritic cells) or neighboring cells (Viorritto et al., 2007) and the DNA is consequently completely digested into nucleotides by DNase II in lysosomes (Nagata et al., 2003; Nagata 2005). Thus it is expected that DNA fragments released by apoptosis are completely removed before they can appear in the circulation (Pisetsky 2004). But, if this engulfment of apoptotic bodies is impaired or cell death is amplified or there is a condition of tissue injury or autoimmunity, cfDNA may appear in plasma (Ren *et al.*, 1998).

Macrophage has also been shown to get involved in the generation of circulating DNA. After massive macrophage apoptosis induced by clodronate liposome treatment in mice, a dramatic increase of circulating DNA occurs. It is observed that intraperitoneal administration of dead, apoptotic or necrotic, Jurkat cells into mice lacking macrophages caused no further increase in the amount of circulating DNA. However, the administration of the same dead cells into normal mice caused an increase in circulating DNA in the blood of the mice and the characteristic ladder pattern could be observed after electrophoresis for both necrotic and apoptotic cells, respectively. This may indicate that necrotic human cells are engulfed by mouse macrophages or that DNA from necrotic cells is cleaved by the same enzymes functioning in apoptosis, thus causing the same ladder pattern as apoptotic cells (Pisetsky, 2004).

In contrast to apoptosis, necrosis causes random, nonspecific, and incomplete digestion of DNA and thus a smear is observed in an electrophoresis gel. If lysis of circulating cells is the origin of circulating DNA, many more dying circulating cells should have been present in the blood since the amount of DNA in the plasma undoubtedly exceeds the amount of such circulating cells, indicating that circulating DNA does not originate from circulating cells dying in the blood. Another interesting hypothesis suggests active secretion of protein-bound DNA into circulation by lymphocytes, although the cellular mechanisms mediating the release are majorly unknown (Anker *et al.*, 1976). So, lysis of T-lymphocytes has been examined, but interestingly it is shown that T-lymphocytes are not the source of circulating DNA (van der Vaart *et al.*, 2008).

(b) Living Cells

The possibility that DNA may be released by living cells has been suggested by a number of reports, (Anker *et al.*, 1999; Stroun *et al.*, 2001; Goebel *et al.*, 2005; Rhodes *et al.*, 2006) but convincing evidence does not exist to prove this hypothesis. Anker *et al.*, realized more than 30 years ago that DNA can be actively released by cells, but the mechanism of this active release process is still not elucidated. Significant lines of evidence to support the hypothesis that living cells release DNA has been highlighted by Chen *et al.* (Chen *et al.*, 2005). Anker *et al.*, in 1975 has reported that human blood lymphocytes actively release double-stranded DNA into their culture medium until a certain concentration is reached, no matter how long the incubation lasts, and that newly synthesized DNA is released preferentially. In the early stages of cancer, when seemingly little cell death is occurring, circulating DNA may already be present in higher than normal levels. As the cancer burden increases, so does cell death, however, the amount of proliferating cancer cells and thus the DNA levels increased significantly because of the increased amount of proliferating cells and not because of the amount of cells that die. So it can be said that lymphocytes are not the only cells that spontaneously release DNA into culture media when stimulated; release may also occur during division of other cell types, which include normal and malignant cells in the body.

(c) Other Sources of Circulating Cell-Free DNA

On the basis of the observations made by Raptis *et al.*, in the early 1980s, an exogenous source of free circulating DNA has been excluded in earlier times (Raptis, 1980). However, these observations have been shown to be wrong by the presence of viral DNA circulating in the plasma of some patients with cancer associated with viral infection, such as nasopharyngeal carcinoma, where Epstein-Barr

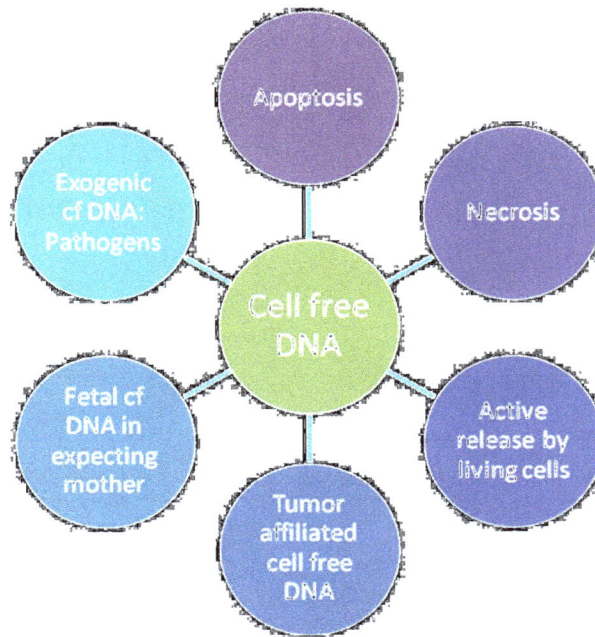

Figure 13.1: Sources of Cell Free DNA.

virus DNA can be detected in 96 per cent of cases, cervical cancer, where human papilloma virus DNA can be detected in 50 per cent of cases, and hepatocellular carcinoma, where hepatitis B virus DNA can be detected (Raptis 1980; Yang *et al.,* 2004). Cells that have lost their nuclei but remain functional undergo a process termed denucleation or terminal differentiation. This may be another source of circulating DNA (Bischoff *et al.,* 2005).

Quantification of cfDNA

Cell-free DNA (cfDNA) can be purified from biological samples by the regular methods of nuclear DNA purification like the phenol chloroform extraction method or the spin column based method (Wang *et al.,* 1995; Di Pietro *et al.,* 2011). There are several kits available for the purpose and there sensitivity and specificity of various methods has been studied for isolation of cfDNA (Sharma *et al.,* 2011). The above reference can also serve the purpose of mass spectrometry (MALDI-TOF MS and ESI-MS) based quantitation of DNA. Since cfDNA is present in much lower concentration in comparison to nuclear DNA, so its quantification is really difficult and adding to it, relative quantification is even more troublesome. Techniques like real time Polymerase Chain Reaction (PCR) and spectrophotometry have been extensively used for this quantification purpose.

Table 13.2: Fluorescent Dyes Available for the Detection of Nucleic Acids (for more details please refer https://www.phenixresearch.com/Images/ TN_FluorecentProbeQuantitation.pdf)

Fluorecent Dyes	Specificity
Hoechst 33258	A-T of dsDNA
Cyanine Dye	dsDNA, some single stranded oligonucleotides
SybrGreen I	dsDNA
PicoGreen	all dsDNA
4', 6-diamidino-2-phenylindole	A-T
RiboGreen	G of all nucleic acids
OliGreen	T of all nucleic acids
Ethidium bromide	dsDNA and RNA

cfDNA can be quantified by using single PCR for each locus by exploring short tandem repeats (STR) for the purpose. The STRs used has minimum of penta- and tetra-nucleotide repeat motifs in an attempt to minimize the stutter effect. The loci include D13S631 (chromosome 13), D18S535 (chromosome 18), D21S11, D21S1411, D21S1414 (chromosome 21) and X22 (pseudo-autosomal region 2 of chromosomes X and Y). All the forward oligonucleotide primers can be labeled at 52 end with a suitable fluorescent dye followed by the amplification of each target STR by PCR. The PCR reaction involves an initial incubation at 94°C for 5 minutes, followed by 25 cycles and then analysis by electrophoresis (Davanos, 2011).

In many conditions like malignancy, DNA integrative index of cfDNA become a crucial parameter and its quantification is highly desirable. The concentration and integrity of free DNA in serum and Cerebral Spinal Fluid (CSF) can be determined by quantitative real-time PCR (qPCR) based on amplification of the ALU gene. Since the annealing sites of ALU115 are within the ALU247 annealing sites and the primer set for ALU115 amplifies both shorter (truncated by apoptosis) and longer DNA fragments (truncated by non-apoptosis), whereas the primer set for the 247-bp amplicon (ALU247) amplifies only longer DNA fragments (non-apoptotic cells release). Thus, the ALU115 qPCR value represents the total amount of free DNA. DNA integrity can be determined by the ratio of longer to shorter DNA fragments (ALU 247/ALU115) (Shi *et al.*, 2011).

A fluorescent dye based method is described in the literature that appears to be much more sensitive is quantification of cfDNA when compared to absorption spectrophotometry based method (Wu *et al.*, 2002). The conventional technique for measuring nucleic acid concentrations involves the determination of absorbance at 260nm (A260). The major disadvantages of the absorbance method includes relative large contribution of nucleotides, single-stranded nucleic acids and proteins to the signal, the inability to distinguish between DNA and RNA, and the relative insensitivity of the assay (an A260 of 0.1 corresponds to a 5 µg/mL dsDNA solution). In recent times, fluorescent dyes like SYBR green have been explored for the purpose of detection of DNA and they shows significant fluorescence advancement only in the presence of dsDNA. It does not show significant fluorescence enhancement in the presence of proteins and allows the detection and quantitation of DNA concentrations as low as 10 ng/mL. In fact, now fluorescence based method has been marketed and manufactured as kits like PicoGreen DNA detection kit (http://probes.invitrogen.com/media/pis/mp07581.pdf). Calf thymus DNA (100 mg/ml) can be used as standard (Wu *et al.*, 2002). The concentration of DNA can be plotted in the standard curve range from 0 to 100ng/ml. Fluorescence intensity can be measured in spectrofluorometer at by taking care of appropriate excitation and emission wavelength that varies in accordance with the fluorescent dye. We recommend readers to go through the following paper for the purpose of in depth details of fluorescent dyes (Cosa, Focsaneanu *et al.*, 2001).

Now, it is possible to quantitate cfDNA omitting steps of DNA isolation using conventional spectroflurimetry using DNA sensitive fluorescent dyes (Goldshtein, Hausmann *et al.*, 2009). Other high end techniques like capillary electrophoresis and DNA flow cytometry can also been employed to quantitate cell-free DNA (Nunez 2001; Chou *et al.*, 2004).

Observation in Pathological Scenario

Patient groups and controls are both required to evaluate the impact of total DNA concentrations under different clinical situations. In serum, gender- and age-dependent cell-free DNA mean concentrations in healthy individuals have been found to be nearly 13ng/ml (Jahr *et al.*, 2001). In healthy individuals, the concentration of circulating DNA is low, as dead cells are efficiently removed from the circulation by phagocytes (Zeerleder *et al.*, 2003). Although detectable amounts of cell-free DNA are constantly present in the plasma of healthy individuals, markedly elevated levels have been reported in cancer, autoimmune disorders, stroke, sepsis, pre- eclampsia and organ transplant rejection (Tong 2006; Swarup *et al.*, 2007). Circulating DNA has a short half-life and is removed mainly by the liver. Excessive accumulation of DNA in the plasma may result from the release of DNA caused by massive cell death, inefficient removal of dying cells or a combination of both (Zeerleder *et al.*, 2003). The current view proposes that, at least in clinical situations, circulating DNA originates from apoptotic or necrotic cells and thus reflects the extent of cellular damage. Supporting this hypothesis, cell-free DNA has frequently been observed with a nucleosomal (150-200 bp in length) or a ladder-like appearance (Jahr *et al.*, 2001; Langford *et al.*, 2007) and it has also been shown to display malignancy-specific genetic and epigenetic characteristics (Gormally *et al.*, 2007).

(a) Malignancy

Presence of double-stranded DNA fragments has been widely reported in considerable quantities in the serum or plasma of cancer patients (Leon *et al.*, 1975; Leon *et al.*, 1977). The quantitation of this free DNA in the serum of patients with various types of cancer and healthy individuals has showed that the DNA concentration in the normal controls has a mean of 13ng/ml, whereas in the cancer patients the mean value is 180ng/ml. Levels of plasma cell-free DNA have been found to be significantly elevated in patients with ovarian cancer, lung cancer and many others in comparison to benign and controls (Chen *et al.*, 1996; Nawroz *et al.*, 1996; Goessl *et al.*, 1998; Kamat *et al.*, 2010; Goto *et al.*, 2011). Although no correlation has been found between circulating DNA levels and the size or location or the primary tumor, significantly higher DNA levels have been reported in the serum of patients with metastasis. Presence of oncogene or tumor suppressor gene mutations that characterize DNA in tumor cells have been also reported in plasma DNA. K-*ras* mutations in the DNA derived from pancreatic tumors have been found in the circulating DNA of the same patients (Sorenson *et al.*, 1994), just as the same microsatellite alterations, detected in head and neck carcinomas, small cell lung carcinomas, or renal carcinomas, could be determined in patients' plasma DNA (Chen *et al.*, 1996; Goessl *et al.*, 1998). Furthermore, tumor-specific epigenetic alterations such as the hypermethylation of sequences in the promoters of tumor suppressor genes can be frequently identified in the plasma DNA of carcinoma patients (Esteller *et al.,* 1999; Wong *et al.,* 1999; Sanchez-Cespedes *et al.,* 2000). These and similar findings indicate that a certain percentage of circulating DNA originates from degenerating tumor cells. Currently it is widely thought that there is a positive correlation of cell-free DNA and malignancy status of an individual and substantial research is being done to evaluate its biomarker potential for the purpose of early diagnosis/screening of malignancies or predicting prognosis of cancer patients.

(b) Bacterial, Parasitic and Viral Infections

Higher levels of host cfDNA have been consistently observed in severe bacteremia. Multiple reports claim that the levels of cell-free plasma DNA can predict the outcome in severe sepsis and septic shock (Rhodes *et al.,* 2006; Saukkonen *et al.,* 2008). One study shows that cfDNA can predict the presence of infection in febrile patients and the potential of cfDNA to predict the outcome in such cases (Moreira *et al.,* 2010). The increased levels of plasma cfDNA concentrations have been reported to be significantly increased in bacteremia patients and it has been shown that non survivor patients express apoptotic DNA fragmentation bands as well. So, it can also be said that apoptosis plays pivotal role in severe bacteremic infection (Huttunen *et al.,* 2011). In bacterial infections, bacterial cell-free DNA can helps bacteria to felicitate spread of resistance genes, thus making really difficult to treat resistant bacterium (de Vries *et al.,* 2011).

In pathogens like parasites capable of causing diseases such as schistosomiasis, have a huge turnover value involving replication, maturation, and death of organisms. These multi-cellular parasites (like Schistosoma) contain DNA copies in stoichiometrical excess over parasite count. Their cell-free DNA can be found in the plasma (Wichmann *et al.,* 2009). Its role is still not understood.

It has been hypothesized that viruses emerge from the population of organisms they infect. Evolution of many viruses has been always linked with the genomic DNA of host and cell-free DNA role can be really significant in this regard.

(c) Degenerative Disease

Degenerative diseases are often related with the quantitative and qualitative measures of cell-free DNA. Conditions like heart failure (HF) and cardiomyopathies are associated with the apoptosis and cell death of both cardiac myocytes and cardiac non-myocytes. In such conditions, DNA fragments released from programmed cell death or acute cellular injury are the main sources of disease-associated elevation of cell-free (cf) DNA. Interestingly, levels of cfDNA have been proposed as a relevant marker of cardiac apoptosis in HF patients that could be affected by the improvement of myocardial performance (Zaravinos *et al.,* 2011). In other degenerative diseases like atherosclerosis, diabetes, eczema, psoriasis and many others, correlation with cell-free DNA has been reported (Marini *et al.,* 2006; Konorova *et al.,* 2009; El Tarhouny *et al.,* 2010).

Biomarker Potential of Cell-free DNA

Cell-free DNA hold strong promises in the area of diagnosis. Researchers have always tried to develop non-invasive procedures for diagnosing diseases. Especially, in diseases like lung cancer, non invasive samples like plasma/Expectorants/or any other, always have been the hot targets for researchers, in order to locate possible biomarkers for screening. Recent interest in the study of circulating cell-free DNA has led to interest in it as a screening tool for lung cancer. As illustrated earlier, the presence of cell-free DNA circulating in plasma or serum has been described in patients with malignant processes as well (Zhang *et al.,* 2010). In diagnosing cancer, DNA integrity index might play an important role. It is represented by the ratio of longer fragments to shorter DNA. In healthy individuals, the main source of free-circulating DNA is apoptotic cells. Apoptotic cells release DNA fragments that are usually 185 to 200 base pair (bp) in length, produced by a programmed enzymatic cleavage process during apoptosis. On the other hand, DNA released from malignant cells varies in size because pathologic cell death *i.e.* in the malignant tumors death does not result only from apoptosis. In such conditions, necrosis and autophagy can also play crucial role in cell death. Tumor necrosis is a frequent event in solid malignancy, and it generates a spectrum of DNA fragments with different strand lengths because of random and incomplete digestion of genomic DNA by a variety of deoxyribonucleases. Therefore, elevated levels of long DNA fragments may be a good marker for detection of malignant tumor DNA in blood (Holdenrieder *et al.,* 2008; Gao *et al.,* 2010).

It also holds excellent promises as biomarker for diagnosis of fetal impairment. Since the discovery of fetal cell-free DNA in pregnant women in 1997 by Lo *et al.,* (Lo *et al.,* 1997), scientific community is trying to explore it as biomarker. Initially, its isolation has been a problem, but now it is resolved by using manual and automated methods (Huang *et al.,* 2008). Cell-free DNA of fetus can be easily isolated from the plasma of the expecting mother. Till now, invasive procedures like amniocentesis have been followed for diagnosing such conditions. Cell-free fetal DNA comprises only 3–6 per cent of the total circulating cell-free DNA, therefore, diagnosis is primarily limited to those caused by paternally inherited sequences and conditions that can be inferred by the unique gene expression patterns in the fetus and placenta. Broadly, it can be exploited in two ways: primarily, high genetic risk families with inheritable monogenic diseases, including sex determination in cases at risk of X-linked diseases and detection of specific paternally inherited single gene disorders; and secondly, routine care offered to all pregnant women, including prenatal screening/diagnosis for aneuploidy, particularly Down syndrome (DS), and diagnosis of Rhesus factor status in RhD negative women (Wright, 2009) could be done without any side effects and harm.

It is possible to find cell-free parasite DNA (CFPD) circulating in plasma, and that this could be used to diagnose schistosomiasis. In contrast to eggs in stool or urine, CFPD would be equally distributed throughout the plasma volume of the patient, resolving the issue of random sampling that spoils clinical sensitivity of classical detection methods. In fact, applicability of these can be understood by the fact that, Schistosoma-specific real-time PCR has already been established and optimized for detection of DNA from large volumes of plasma (Wichmann *et al.,* 2009). This can really help in limiting the occurrence of the disease. We advocate extensive research on other similar important pathogens as well.

Sequencing Data of Cell Free DNA and Significance

As discussed earlier, genomic DNA sequences in cell-free plasma show strong correlation with many types of pathogenic manifestations, where characteristic changes in methylation and acetylation of oncogene DNA regions, presence of various tandem repeats and genes directly involved in pathogenic manifestations are indicative of changes in gene activity.

Cell-free fetal DNA can be distinguished from the maternal DNA in the plasma of pregnant women, by its methylation status. In fetus it can invariably act as non-invasive biomarkers for conditions like aneuploidy and genetic aberrations.

Immune responses have been reported in case of specific bacterial unmethylated CpG DNA and mammalian DNA sequences that include unmethylated CpG sites, as in the case of SLE where unmethylated DNA from peripheral blood monocytes stimulates an autoimmune response (Januchowski *et al.,* 2004).

Also, production and clearance of cell-free DNA from plasma in relation to its methylation status are still poorly understood processes and the matter of inquisitivity. There are reports which suggest abundances of pattern of different DNA sequences in the plasma of healthy individuals (Puszyk *et al.*, 2009). But, relative study in cases of different pathogenic condition is still an ongoing quest. There is still a lot of scope for extensive research in the field of sequential analysis of cell-free DNA. Varieties of computational tools are available for sequence alignment of cfDNA which are currently being used extensively (Fan *et al.*, 2010).

Ageing and Cell-free DNA

Ageing can be defined as an accumulation of damage to molecules, cells and tissues over a lifetime, often leads to frailty and malfunction. Old age is the biggest risk factor for many diseases, including cancer, cardiovascular and neurodegenerative diseases (Heemels, 2010). But tracing of ageing is still not fully feasible and researchers are still looking for specific biomarker for it. Various aging biomarkers presented so far have focused on measuring the indicators or clinical manifestations of systemic low-grade inflammation (Bandeen-Roche *et al.*, 2009; Hsu *et al.*, 2009). But these marker's predictive values have been often compromised due to confounding effects introduced by age- related co-morbidities. Also, multiple biomarkers of ageing and the discovery of new ones are of great importance to better understand the aging process per se as well as its accompanying events. Multiple have assessed cell-free DNA concentrations with regard to age. Zhong *et al.* (Zhong *et al.*, 2007) observed that healthy women over 60 years old have elevated plasma cell-free-DNA levels compared to younger women whereas Wu et al.(Wu *et al.*, 2002) reported that serum cell-free-DNA has a U-shaped age-correlated distribution in women. It has been observed that the highest cell-free-DNA values in women <20 and >70 years of age, whereas the lowest cell-free DNA values have been detected in women aged between 30and 50 years. Interestingly, Wu *et al.* (Wu *et al.*, 2002) observed no age-association for cell-free DNA values in men. In a different study of institutionalized elderly patients, involving both men and women, plasma cell-free DNA levels have been found to be increased in subjects with pathological conditions involving cell death. Also, it has been demonstrated that individuals with increased cell-free DNA levels have reduced short-term survival (Fournie *et al.*, 1993). Still, cell-free DNA is too non specific in discriminating between distinct age-related conditions and due to the interferences due to the other clinical conditions. As discussed earlier necrosis and apoptosis are taken as the main source of cell-free DNA. Also, many other theories advocate other sources of cell-free DNA as well. In old age, other factors also become dominant like the cellular death rate usually increases, while the cellular debris-clearance mechanisms simultaneously decline (Aprahamian *et al.*, 2008). Age-associated oxidative damage can promote endothelial cell injury and inflammatory cell accumulation, thus increasing the levels of cell turnover material in circulation (Jylhava *et al.*, 2011). Thus, increase in cell-free DNA amount in old age is highly expected which has been further supported by multiple clinical evidences.

Hypothesis: About Biological Function of Cell-free DNA

Does cell-free DNA in blood have potential biological implications? Multiple reports indicate its role in metastasis, autoimmunity and cell mediated immune response, and blood flow in microcirculation. Cell culture experiments with plasma from tumor-bearing rats showed that cell-free DNA could be taken up by cells and that DNA has been found to be incorporated into the genome. This effect resulted in the hypothesis of "genometastasis". According to this concept, the formation of metastasis might be generated by the tumor-derived cell-free DNA in blood. It is thought that the oncogenic DNA fractions can be taken up by susceptible cells, for example stem cells, in distant target organs, providing the basis for building metastases. Several types of experimental data appear to support this hypothesis (Garcia-Olmo *et al.*, 2001). It has been shown that the processes of cellular transformation and tumorigenesis in fibroblasts as a consequence of the uptake of oncogene containing DNA (Bergsmedh *et al.*, 2001). A recent investigation showed that tumor-specific methylated DNA fragments can penetrate into cells more efficiently and that they have a higher transformation potential than the corresponding unmethylated DNA fragments (Skvortsova *et al.*, 2008). Chen *et al.*, extended this hypothesis by postulating that the oncogenic DNA would be primarily released by living cancer cells and that it could act like an intrinsic oncovirus (Skvortsova *et al.*, 2008).

In addition, tumor derived cell-free DNA could have biological implications for cancer immunology. It is hypothesized that cell-free DNA binding to cell surface receptors of lymphocytes induces a cell-mediated immune response by forming immune-responding helper-T or killer-T cells. Earlier studies have discussed the endocytosis and degradation of exogenous DNA by white blood cells in relation to a ligand receptor function (Bennett *et al.*, 1985). Cell-free DNA can also, as such, be immunogenic as exposed chromatin with unmethylated CpG sites is known to stimulate autoimmune response (Januchowski *et al.*, 2004). This is a phenomenon often encountered in aged individuals.

It has also been proposed that elevated cell-free DNA concentrations may increase the viscosity of blood and thus be a disadvantage to blood flow in microcirculation (Fournie *et al.*, 1993).

Recently, mode of action of aluminium based adjuvants has been linked with cell-free DNA. Aluminum-based adjuvants are widely implicated in human vaccination, but their mode of action is poorly understood. Marichal *et al.*, has proposed that alum causes cell death and the subsequent release of host cell DNA, which acts as a potent endogenous immunostimulatory signal mediating alum adjuvant activity. They have suggested the host DNA mediated: induction of primary B-cell responses, including IgG1 production, through interferon response factor-3 (Irf3)-independent mechanisms and stimulation of 'canonical' T-helper type-2 (T_H2) responses, associated with IgE isotype switching and peripheral effector responses, through Irf3-dependent mechanisms (Marichal *et al.*, 2011).

Before we come to an end, we propose that cell-free DNA may be present in the exosomes and that can transfer genetic material from one cell to another. This may serve as a novel mechanism for genetic exchange among various cells in-vivo. Exosomes are vesicles of endocytic origin released by many cell types. These vesicles can mediate communication between cells via transfer of RNA and protein which has already been proved (Valadi *et al.*, 2007). We believe that exosomes and cell-free DNA are analogously associated for cell to cell communication. We propose a scientific validation for the above hypothesis.

References

Anker P, Mulcahy H, Chen XQ *et al.* (1999). Detection of circulating tumour DNA in the blood (plasma/serum). of cancer patients. Cancer Metastasis Rev 18: 65-73.

Anker P, Stroun M, Maurice PA (1976). Spontaneous extracellular synthesis of DNA released by human blood lymphocytes. Cancer Res 36: 2832-2839.

Aprahamian T, Takemura Y, Goukassian D *et al.* (2008). Ageing is associated with diminished apoptotic cell clearance *in vivo*. Clin Exp Immunol 152: 448-455.

Arnott S (2006). Historical article: DNA polymorphism and the early history of the double helix. Trends Biochem Sci 31: 349-354.

Bandeen-Roche K, Walston JD, Huang Y *et al.* (2009). Measuring systemic inflammatory regulation in older adults: evidence and utility. Rejuvenation Res 12: 403-410.

Bendich A, Wilczok T, Borenfreund E (1965). Circulating DNA as a Possible Factor in Oncogenesis. Science 148: 374-376.

Bennett RM, Gabor GT, Merritt MM (1985). DNA binding to human leukocytes. Evidence for a receptor-mediated association, internalization, and degradation of DNA. J Clin Invest 76: 2182-2190.

Bergsmedh A, Szeles A, Henriksson M *et al.* (2001). Horizontal transfer of oncogenes by uptake of apoptotic bodies. Proc Natl Acad Sci U S A 98: 6407-6411.

Bischoff FZ, Lewis DE, Simpson JL (2005). Cell-free fetal DNA in maternal blood: kinetics, source and structure. Hum Reprod Update 11: 59-67.

Chen XQ, Stroun M, Magnenat JL *et al.* (1996). Microsatellite alterations in plasma DNA of small cell lung cancer patients. Nat Med 2: 1033-1035.

Chen Z, Fadiel A, Naftolin F *et al.* (2005). Circulation DNA: biological implications for cancer metastasis and immunology. Med Hypotheses 65: 956-961.

Chou JS, Jacobson JD, Patton WC *et al.* (2004). Modified isocratic capillary electrophoresis detection of cell-free DNA in semen. J Assist Reprod Genet 21: 397-400.

Cosa G, Focsaneanu KS, McLean JR *et al.* (2001). Photophysical properties of fluorescent DNA-dyes bound to single- and double-stranded DNA in aqueous buffered solution. Photochem Photobiol 73: 585-599.

Davanos N, Spathas DH (2011). Relative quantitation of cell-free fetal DNA in maternal plasma using autosomal DNA markers. Clin Chim Acta 412: 1539-1543.

de Vries LE, Valles Y, Agerso Y *et al.* (2011). The gut as reservoir of antibiotic resistance: microbial diversity of tetracycline resistance in mother and infant. PLoS One 6: e21644.

Di Pietro F, Ortenzi F, Tilio M *et al.* (2011). Genomic DNA extraction from whole blood stored from 15- to 30-years at -20 degrees C by rapid phenol-chloroform protocol: a useful tool for genetic epidemiology studies. Mol Cell Probes 25: 44-48.

El Tarhouny SA, Hadhoud KM, Ebrahem MM *et al.* (2010). Assessment of cell-free DNA with microvascular complication of type II diabetes mellitus, using PCR and ELISA. Nucleosides Nucleotides Nucleic Acids 29: 228-236.

Esteller M, Sanchez-Cespedes M, Rosell R *et al.* (1999). Detection of aberrant promoter hypermethylation of tumor suppressor genes in serum DNA from non-small cell lung cancer patients. Cancer Res 59: 67-70.

Fan HC, Blumenfeld YJ, Chitkara U *et al.* (2010). Analysis of the size distributions of fetal and maternal cell-free DNA by paired-end sequencing. Clin Chem 56: 1279-1286.

Fournie GJ, Martres F, Pourrat JP *et al.* (1993). Plasma DNA as cell death marker in elderly patients. Gerontology 39: 215-221.

Gao YJ, He YJ, Yang ZL *et al.* (2010). Increased integrity of circulating cell-free DNA in plasma of patients with acute leukemia. Clin Chem Lab Med 48: 1651-1656.

Garcia-Olmo D, Garcia-Olmo DC (2001). Functionality of circulating DNA: the hypothesis of genometastasis. Ann N Y Acad Sci 945: 265-275.

Ghose T (2004). Oswald Avery: the professor, DNA, and the Nobel Prize that eluded him. Can Bull Med Hist 21: 135-144.

Goebel G, Zitt M, Zitt M *et al.* (2005). Circulating nucleic acids in plasma or serum (CNAPS). as prognostic and predictive markers in patients with solid neoplasias. Dis Markers 21: 105-120.

Goessl C, Heicappell R, Munker R *et al.* (1998). Microsatellite analysis of plasma DNA from patients with clear cell renal carcinoma. Cancer Res 58: 4728-4732.

Goldshtein H, Hausmann MJ, Douvdevani A (2009). A rapid direct fluorescent assay for cell-free DNA quantification in biological fluids. Ann Clin Biochem 46: 488-494.

Gormally E, Caboux E, Vineis P *et al.* (2007). Circulating free DNA in plasma or serum as biomarker of carcinogenesis: practical aspects and biological significance. Mutat Res 635: 105-117.

Goto K, Ichinose Y, Ohe Y *et al.* (2011). Epidermal Growth Factor Receptor Mutation Status in Circulating Free DNA in Serum: From IPASS, a Phase III Study of Gefitinib or Carboplatin/Paclitaxel in Non-small Cell Lung Cancer. J Thorac Oncol 7: 115-121.

Heemels MT (2010). Ageing. Nature 464: 503.

Holdenrieder S, Burges A, Reich O *et al.* (2008). DNA integrity in plasma and serum of patients with malignant and benign diseases. Ann N Y Acad Sci 1137: 162-170.

Holdenrieder S, Stieber P (2004). Apoptotic markers in cancer. Clin Biochem 37: 605-617.

Hsu FC, Kritchevsky SB, Liu Y *et al.* (2009). Association between inflammatory components and physical function in the health, aging, and body composition study: a principal component analysis approach. J Gerontol A Biol Sci Med Sci 64: 581-589.

Huang DJ, Mergenthaler-Gatfield S, Hahn S *et al.* (2008). Isolation of cell-free DNA from maternal plasma using manual and automated systems. Methods Mol Biol 444: 203-208.

Huttunen R, Kuparinen T, Jylhava J *et al.* (2011). Fatal outcome in bacteremia is characterized by high plasma cell free DNA concentration and apoptotic DNA fragmentation: a prospective cohort study. PLoS One 6: e21700.

Jahr S, Hentze H, Hardt D *et al.* (2001). DNA fragments in the blood plasma of cancer patients: quantitations and evidence for their origin from apoptotic and necrotic cells. Cancer Res 61: 1659-1665.

Januchowski R, Prokop J, Jagodzinshi PP. *et al.* (2004). Role of epigenetic DNA alterations in the pathogenesis of systemic lupus erythematosus. J Appl Genet 45: 237-248.

Jung K, Fleischhacker M, Rabien A (2010). Cell-free DNA in the blood as a solid tumor biomarker–a critical appraisal of the literature. Clin Chim Acta 411: 1611-1624.

Jylhava J, Kotipelto T, Raitala A *et al.* (2011). Ageing is associated with quantitative and qualitative changes in circulating cell-free DNA: the Vitality 90+ study. Mech Ageing Dev 132: 20-26.

Kamat AA, Baldwin M, Urbauer D *et al.* (2010). Plasma cell-free DNA in ovarian cancer: an independent prognostic biomarker. Cancer 116: 1918-1925.

Konorova IL, Veiko NN, Ershova ES *et al.* (2009). [Haemodynamic role of blood-plasma circulating cell-free DNA and contained therein high-molecular-weight CpG-rich fraction in pathogenesis of arterial hypertension and atherosclerosis obliterans of carotid arteries]. Angiol Sosud Khir 15: 19-28.

Langford MP, Redens TB, Harris NR *et al.* (2007). Plasma levels of cell-free apoptotic DNA ladders and gamma-glutamyltranspeptidase (GGT). in diabetic children. Exp Biol Med (Maywood). 232: 1160-1169.

Leon SA, Green A, Yaros MJ *et al.* (1975). Radioimmunoassay for nanogram quantities of DNA. J Immunol Methods 9: 157-164.

Leon SA, Shapiro B, Sklaroff DM *et al.* (1977). Free DNA in the serum of cancer patients and the effect of therapy. Cancer Res 37: 646-650.

Lo YM, Corbetta N, chamberlain PF *et al.* (1997). Presence of fetal DNA in maternal plasma and serum. Lancet 350: 485-487.

Lo YM, Tein MS, Pang CC *et al.* (1998). Presence of donor-specific DNA in plasma of kidney and liver-transplant recipients. Lancet 351: 1329-1330.

Marichal T, Ohata K, Berdoret D *et al.* (2011). DNA released from dying host cells mediates aluminum adjuvant activity. Nat Med 17: 996-1002.

Marini A, Mirmohammadsadegh A, Nambiar S *et al.* (2006). Epigenetic inactivation of tumor suppressor genes in serum of patients with cutaneous melanoma. J Invest Dermatol 126: 422-431.

Moreira VG, Prieto B, Rodriguez JSM *et al.* (2010). Usefulness of cell-free plasma DNA, procalcitonin and C-reactive protein as markers of infection in febrile patients. Ann Clin Biochem 47: 253-258.

Nagata S (2005). DNA degradation in development and programmed cell death. Annu Rev Immunol 23: 853-875.

Nagata S, Nagase H, Kawane K *et al.* (2003). Degradation of chromosomal DNA during apoptosis. Cell Death Differ 10: 108-116.

Nawroz H, Koch W, Anker P *et al.* (1996). Microsatellite alterations in serum DNA of head and neck cancer patients. Nat Med 2: 1035-1037.

Nunez R (2001). DNA measurement and cell cycle analysis by flow cytometry. Curr Issues Mol Biol 3: 67-70.

Pisetsky DS (2004). The immune response to cell death in SLE. Autoimmun Rev 3: 500-504.

Puszyk WM, Crea F, Old RW *et al.* (2009). Unequal representation of different unique genomic DNA sequences in the cell-free plasma DNA of individual donors. Clin Biochem 42: 736-738.

Rainer TH, Wong LK, Lam W *et al.* (2003). Prognostic use of circulating plasma nucleic acid concentrations in patients with acute stroke. Clin Chem 49: 562-569.

Raptis L, Menard HA (1980). Quantitation and characterization of plasma DNA in normals and patients with systemic lupus erythematosus. J Clin Invest 66: 1391-1399.

Ren Y, Savill J (1998). Apoptosis: the importance of being eaten. Cell Death Differ 5: 563-568.

Rhodes A, Wort SJ, Thomas H *et al.* (2006). Plasma DNA concentration as a predictor of mortality and sepsis in critically ill patients. Crit Care 10: R60.

Sanchez-Cespedes M, Esteller M, Wu L *et al.* (2000). Gene promoter hypermethylation in tumors and serum of head and neck cancer patients. Cancer Res 60: 892-895.

Saukkonen K, Lakkisto P, Pettila V *et al.* (2008). Cell-free plasma DNA as a predictor of outcome in severe sepsis and septic shock. Clin Chem 54: 1000-1007.

Sharma VK, Vouros P, Glick J *et al.* (2011). Mass spectrometric based analysis, characterization and applications of circulating cell free DNA isolated from human body fluids. Int J Mass Spectrom 304: 172-183.

Shi W, Lv C, Qi J *et al.* (2011). Prognostic Value of Free DNA Quantification in Serum and Cerebrospinal Fluid in Glioma Patients. J Mol Neurosci. doi: 10.1007/s12031-011-9617-0.

Skvortsova TE, Rykova EY, Tamkovich SM *et al.* (2006). Cell-free and cell-bound circulating DNA in breast tumours: DNA quantification and analysis of tumour-related gene methylation. Br J Cancer 94: 1492-1495.

Skvortsova TE, Vlassov VV, Laktionov PP. *et al.* (2008). Binding and penetration of methylated DNA into primary and transformed human cells. Ann N Y Acad Sci 1137: 36-40.

Sorenson GD, Pribish DM, Valone FH *et al.* (1994). Soluble normal and mutated DNA sequences from single-copy genes in human blood. Cancer Epidemiol Biomarkers Prev 3: 67-71.

Steinman CR (1975). Free DNA in serum and plasma from normal adults. J Clin Invest 56: 512-515.

Stroun M, Anker P, Lyautey J *et al.* (1987). Isolation and characterization of DNA from the plasma of cancer patients. Eur J Cancer Clin Oncol 23: 707-712.

Stroun M, Anker P, Maurice P *et al.* (1989). Neoplastic characteristics of the DNA found in the plasma of cancer patients. Oncology 46: 318-322.

Stroun M, Lyautey J, Lederrey C *et al.* (2001). About the possible origin and mechanism of circulating DNA apoptosis and active DNA release. Clin Chim Acta 313: 139-142.

Swarup V, Rajeswari MR (2007). Circulating (cell-free). nucleic acids–a promising, non-invasive tool for early detection of several human diseases. FEBS Lett 581: 795-799.

Tong YK, Lo YM (2006). Diagnostic developments involving cell-free (circulating). nucleic acids. Clin Chim Acta 363: 187-196.

Valadi H, Ekstrom K, Bossios A *et al.* (2007). Exosome-mediated transfer of mRNAs and microRNAs is a novel mechanism of genetic exchange between cells. Nat Cell Biol 9: 654-659.

van der Vaart M, Pretorius PJ (2008). Circulating DNA. Its origin and fluctuation. Ann N Y Acad Sci 1137: 18-26.

Viorritto IC, Nikolov NP, Siegel RM *et al.* (2007). Autoimmunity versus tolerance: can dying cells tip the balance? Clin Immunol 122: 125-134.

Wang K, Gan L, Boysen C *et al.* (1995). A microtiter plate-based high-throughput DNA purification method. Anal Biochem 226: 85-90.

Watson JD, Crick FH (1953). Molecular structure of nucleic acids; a structure for deoxyribose nucleic acid. Nature 171: 737-738.

Wichmann D, Panning M, Quack T *et al.* (2009). Diagnosing schistosomiasis by detection of cell-free parasite DNA in human plasma. PLoS Negl Trop Dis 3: e422.

Wong IH, Lo YM, Jhang J *et al.* (1999). Detection of aberrant p16 methylation in the plasma and serum of liver cancer patients. Cancer Res 59: 71-73.

Wright CF, Burton H (2009). The use of cell-free fetal nucleic acids in maternal blood for non-invasive prenatal diagnosis. Hum Reprod Update 15: 139-151.

Wu TL, Zhang D, Chia JH *et al.* (2002). Cell-free DNA: measurement in various carcinomas and establishment of normal reference range. Clin Chim Acta 321: 77-87.

Yang HJ, Liu VW, Tsang PC *et al.* (2004). Quantification of human papillomavirus DNA in the plasma of patients with cervical cancer. Int J Gynecol Cancer 14: 903-910.

Zaravinos A, Tzoras S, Apostolakis S *et al.* (2011). Levosimendan reduces plasma cell-free DNA levels in patients with ischemic cardiomyopathy. J Thromb Thrombolysis 31: 180-187.

Zeerleder S, Zwart B, Wuillemin WA *et al.* (2003). Elevated nucleosome levels in systemic inflammation and sepsis. Crit Care Med 31: 1947-1951.

Zhang R, Shao F, Wu X *et al.* (2010). Value of quantitative analysis of circulating cell free DNA as a screening tool for lung cancer: a meta-analysis. Lung Cancer 69: 225-231.

2014, Advances in Biochemistry and Biotechnology Volume 2

Pages 225-233

Edited by: Dr. Biplab Sarkar and Dr. Chiranjib Chakraborty

Published by: DAYA PUBLISHING HOUSE

14

Point of Care Testing: Beginning of an Era of Near Patient Diagnosis

Dibyajyoti Banerjee[1], Kirtimaan Syal[2],
Nitish Nagpal[1] and Rajasri Bhattacharyya[1]*

[1]*Department of Experimental Medicine and Biotechnology,
Postgraduate Institute of Medical Education and Research, Chandigarh – 160 012, India*
[2]*Molecular Biophysics Unit, Indian Institute of Science, Bangalore – 560 012, Karnataka, India*

ABSTRACT

In-spite of tremendous improvement of laboratory medicine, sample transport requirement in a classical clinical laboratory is a prevalent practice throughout the globe. This can contribute to pre analytical errors for the estimated result. The analytical errors are minimized by available strict quality control measures and also due to advent of automation in such laboratory settings. In a classical clinical laboratory setting the possibility of post analytical errors also exist due to compartmentalization of laboratory patient interface. Along with substantial chance of

* *Corresponding author.* E-mail: dibyajyoti5200@yahoo.co.in

preanalytical and post analytical error the reporting of a classical clinical laboratory is time consuming which can affect therapeutic decision even in emergency settings. To overcome these problems, a new modality of laboratory management is gradually getting available for patient care that aims near patient analysis even at the point of patient care including the bedside of patient. In this review this relatively new concept of point of care diagnosis is introduced for the biological scientists and general readers.

Keywords: POCT, Clinical laboratory, Quality control, Laboratory accreditation.

Introduction

From the inception of laboratory medicine, all the major analysis of vital parameters related to patient care is done in a classical clinical laboratory where sample transport is necessary from the sample collection site. The result of such analysis is possible to be obtained for patient care only after a considerable amount of time. This is mostly due to technical complexities of estimation related to the analysis of parameters requiring high end instruments that are not transportable at bedside of patients. Even automation in a clinical laboratory although aided the robust patient care system to some extent in term of minimizing analytical error but it still requires a classical clinical laboratory set up and currently unable to provide patient support at point of care. Recent biotechnological advancement particularly the advancement of nano biotechnology, development of human sample matrix compatible biosensors and successful application of computer chip technology to biological samples paved the path of analysis of vital parameters at the site of patient care with obtainable quality result within a very short time. This modality of analysis gained wide popularity throughout the globe and is known as "Point of Care" testing or POCT. Point of care testing is currently carried out in all internationally reputed health care organizations. Many world accreditation bodies published standard guidelines for point of care testing. Washington State Clinical Laboratory Advisory Council published standard guidelines for POCT care as early as in the year 2000 which are revised in 2009. The Royal Collage of Pathology guideline for POCT is also available from the year 2004. The popularity of POCT care as a biotechnological contribution of the new millennium to the health care system is mostly due to the fact that it reached the laboratory medicine at the very site of patient care with obtainable quality result at site of minimal sample collection within no time. Establishment of POCT infrastructure in the emergency/ward/OPD/OT etc. also known to reduce the work load of the classical clinical laboratory and so it minimizes amount of sample collection from the patient, sample transport, delay of reporting and undoubtedly gives a different impetus to the laboratory medicine in general and emergency patient care in particular. It is no more a whisper that this modality of incorporation of biotechnological advancement in the patient care system have driven the laboratory medicine from bench to bedside and already saved millions of human life in emergency settings. Therefore, it is definitely need of the hour to develop accredited POCT infrastructure in health care system devoted to the service of the mankind.

Classical Clinical Laboratory

A classical clinical laboratory of recent times receives biological sample of hospitalized patients or collects the sample by trained personnel on its own after receiving such requests from clinicians or patients. Generally the transported or collected biological sample requires some kind of processing. For example we can cite example of requirement of centrifugation of blood, collected in heparin vial to separate the plasma that is subjected to further analysis. The analytical procedure is commonly done in automated instruments using customized kits available for the purpose (Hawker, 2007). Semi-automated and manual methods are still being carried out in many clinical laboratories throughout the globe for the purpose of analysis of biomolecules. The analysis part requires high skilled technical personnel. Then the report of analysis thus obtained is collected by the patient or physician or such report is sent to the health care provider by a standard procedure practiced at a particular health care system. Therefore, sample collection, analysis and reporting are integral component of a classical clinical laboratory set up that requires high end dedicated instruments and high technical competence for successful functioning. Preanalytical, analytical or post analytical errors are accompanied with this kind of laboratory set up that affects the observed results and which in turn interfere with the therapeutic decisions. Although there is a growing trend of awareness of professionalism, quality control and management involvement to make the laboratory services more healthy to patients and health care providers, a substantial time is still required from the point of decision of requirement of a test and obtaining an authenticated report of such analysis in the current set up of functioning of a classical clinical laboratory. Therefore, the data generated in a centralized classical laboratory is not a real time information and is historical in nature (Halpern *et al.,* 1999).

To improve the laboratory clinical interface there is a favorable trend of providing interpretative comments by laboratory medicine specialists (Haeckel and Wosniok, 2009). Since the laboratory medicine specialist has generally no direct control on the data record of admitted patients; quality of interpretative comment of a laboratory medicine expert limits only to empirical reasoning which may not be at per with the personalized patient care. An example will make the above statement clear. Alkaline picrate method based on Jaffe's reaction is popularly employed for serum creatinine estimation which is a vital parameter to understand renal function. Many cephalosporin antibiotics positively interfere in that method and produces non creatinine chromogen resulting in false positive value for creatinine. Any patient who is on cephalosporin antibiotic can show false positive value for serum creatinine in absence of any renal failure. The laboratory physician under whose supervision the analytical tests are performed are normally not in a position to know the drug history of the patient (whose sample is being tested) and the clinicians generally have no control on the method of analysis chosen. Therefore, proper interpretations of such analytical result are not done. In this compartmentalized scenario of clinical laboratory and other management modality of the health care system, which is more apparent in developing nations; the interpretation of clinical laboratory data is difficult and may be even misleading. Despite of the above mentioned problems the concept of a quality classical clinical laboratory is well established since 1920's and in recent days up to 70 per cent of clinical decisions are dependent on functioning of a classical clinical laboratory (Hilborne *et al.,* 2009).

Establishment of a clinical laboratory happened only in modern times after the advent of science in its modern sense (Kricka and Savory, 2011). If the history of modernization of clinical laboratory is considered two points are very apparent (Sunderman FW, 1992).

1. Gradual requirement of small amount of biological sample by development of sensitive clinically relevant laboratory methods.
2. Development of clinical laboratory proficiency testing.

Biomarker researches lead to genesis of various panels of investigations. For existence of such clinically relevant panel of investigation, involvement of the clinical laboratory in patient care is now almost mandatory. The sensitivity, specificity, precision and accuracy of the analytical procedures of a wide range of biomarker analysis gradually improved and practice of laboratory medicine enriched in enormous scale.

The Seeds of Bench at the Bedside

In the early era of medical practice the observations at the site of patient care served for the purpose of patient management. So, the concept of point of care testing is not new. There is evidence in the literature that the mediaeval physicians observed body fluids for diagnosis of clinical condition (Willmott and Arrowsmith 2010). Ants are used in ancient period to know about the sugary urine of diabetes mellitus (Trowell 1982). Urinoscopy (inspection of 24 hour urine by a physician) was also popular for several centuries earlier for diagnosis of diseases (Trowell, 1982). Although such seeds of concept of POCT was present from ancient and mediaeval times its systematic use to serve the mankind happened only after the proper establishment of the classical clinical laboratory.

Technologies that Favored POCT

The advent of nanotechnology has guided the path of successful instrumentation for POCT applications (Chapman 2011). The development of instrumentation for POCT has been driven by medical and organizational needs and involves a wide range of technologies that allow miniaturization of the devices. Mechanisms to facilitate digital signal processing and connectivity are always welcome in a POCT device. Miniaturized hydraulic circuits for fluid handling have been developed. It provides reproducible performance characteristics, particularly when new materials and large-scale manufacturing processes are used (Gouget et al., 2001).

Portable electrowetting based digital microfluidic platform is developed that has the potential to perform polymerase chain reaction or immunoassays in shorter time when compared to the conventional methods (Sista et al., 2008). Simple nucleic acid amplification based tests for HIV detection from biological samples are described that are suitable for near patient testing (Lee et al., 2010). The conventional dipstick assays often done at the bedside of a patient are improved tremendously by improvement of sample binding to the strip matrix and substantial improvement in strip based reactions producing visible colors (Lee and Dineva 2002).

Sophisticated test requiring radioisotope detection from breath is possible to perform at point of care utilizing improved infrared spectrophotometer near patient care (Opekun et al., 2005). This test has the implications for development of non-invasive diagnostics at point of care in days to come. New developments in POCT technology is a wide concern broadly in three areas: connectivity, test menu expansion, and noninvasiveness. Connectivity for POCT devices has evolved from point-of-service workstations to standardize POCT data transmission protocols for remote roaming wireless connectivity with automatic data capture. POCT test menus are expected to expand further, with more of coagulation testing, chemistries, infection screening and also on-site drug screening, intra-operative hormone levels, and microchip DNA diagnostics (Bissell, 2001).

POCT devices commonly use biosensor based detection systems. According to the IUPAC definition, a biosensor is an analytical device for the detection of analytes that combines a biological component with a physicochemical-detector component. This is generally performed by the use of miniaturized analysis systems. The biological samples (like whole blood etc.) are immobilized on a solid-state surface, which, in turn, interacts with the analyte. These interactions are detected by using either electrochemical or optical methods. In case of optical detection a significant role is often played by fluorescence or reflection spectroscopy. Miniaturized spectrophotometers are available that are commonly used for oximetry at point of care. The instruments and corresponding parameters relevant to POCT are extensively reviewed recently (Nichols 2007; Luppa *et al.*, 2011).

Quality Control aspects of POCT

With growing miniaturization of a wide range of POCT infrastructure applicable for a wide range of clinically relevant parameters quality control aspects of POCT are gaining considerable current interest. It is no more a whisper that quality POCT must control every aspect of the test and testing process which can affect the ultimate test result. Philosophy of laboratory quality control is very similar to industrial quality requirements and POCT can be viewed like any manufacturing business where the product being produced is the test result that is communicated to the end user. Use of industrial management techniques has been suggested to be applied to POCT to isolate and reduce the sources of testing error. Data management is fundamental to maintain quality of any diagnostic testing and in case of POCT any deviation from above principle is not advisable. Proper analysis of POCT data can show quality trends before they affect the test result. More recent POCT devices have computerized data capture or storage functions that can collect the critical information at the time the test is performed followed by transmission of that data to a POCT data manager or hospital information system (Nichols, 2003).

It is widely accepted that centralized laboratory (or the classical clinical laboratory) offers high-quality results, as guaranteed by the use of regulated quality management programs by specially trained staff dedicated for the purpose. POCT is commonly performed by clinical staff at the indoor or emergency settings. POCT has the advantage of shortening the turnaround time, which potentially benefits the patient if a quality test result, is obtained that is reasonable to take a clinical decision. However, the clinical laboratory testing expertise and expertise in traditional quality control aspect of clinical staff is limited throughout the globe when compared to the central laboratory staff. Therefore, POCT is currently not in a position to replace the centralized laboratory service (Schimke 2009). But the quality of POCT devices available so far has attained sufficient quality reasonable to be used at clinical settings by health care providers. This is more apparent for point of care estimation of vital parameters. The various kinds of errors that occur at POCT settings are attempted to be quantified (Auxter, 1998). Therefore, it is expected that in future further studies will be designed with the objectives to design measures to correct those errors.

Many home testing devices, when used in hospitals, physicians' chamber, and mobile nursing practices, have presented technical issues that are not predictable from the experience of its use by general public. These problems may arise from the way the devices are used, the patient population, and even differences in sample type. Thus, to get an usable information at point of care, management of POCT in the health-care environment requires interdisciplinary cooperation of clinical nursing staff, physicians and laboratory staff (Nichols and Poe, 1999).

Creating an interdisciplinary POCT committee is critical for successful management. Every discipline through its expertise and common goal to provide quality patient care contributes to the success of the POCT program. It is proved beyond any doubt that the development of a comprehensive Quality Assurance program ensures accurate results in POCT that are reliable by end users. The quality of POCT improves significantly if such testing is performed by trained personnel. Continuous quality improvement diminishes the POCT programmes potential for undesirable outcomes related to patient care. Improved data management is necessary with the increased demands for point-of-care tests (Humbertson, 2001).

For the purpose of proper quality assurance POCT is currently regulated by several guidelines of the respected professional bodies or known expert in the field (Carlson 1996; Briggs, Guthrie *et al.*, 2008). Analogous to centralized laboratory accreditation POCT third party accreditation services are available with the aim of overall improvement of near patient testing (Bennett, Cervantes *et al.*, 2000). It is needless to emphasize that strict adherence to the regulatory guidelines in time being forced is one of the cornerstone of achieving improved quality in POCT(Anderson, 2001). There is also evidence in the literature that improved nations are continuously improving in regulatory compliance for POCT and strictly adhering to quality control practices (Ehrmeyer and Laessig, 2009).On the other hand there is also evidence in the literature about non practicing of good laboratory and quality control practices in many clinical settings which definitely improves with quality assurance and staff training (Hortas, Montiel *et al.*, 2001).

Cost Effectiveness of POCT Approach

The studies reporting cost effectiveness of POCT approach are less and the overall data available on the subject is limited (Hobbs, Delaney *et al.*, 1997; Price 2001). Some studies report blatantly that POCT is not cost effective. Since POCT requires less amount of biological materials the cost of analysis requiring biological materials as reagents are expected to be substantially reduced in POCT when compared with its centralized laboratory counterpart. This is definitely evident in coagulation studies (Despotis *et al.*, 1994). On the other hand for popular POCT by patients or health care providers is shown to be costly compared to a corresponding classical laboratory testing (Grieve *et al.*, 1999). Recently it is also observed that statistical significant cost difference between POCT and central laboratory testing does not exist for multiple popular parameters (Laurence *et al.*, 2010).

It is generally thought that unit costs for a few test results generated by POCT are likely to cost more than those produced by the central laboratory (Ehrmeyer and Laessig 1999). The above idea is strengthened by a few observations that recorded only analysis cost of a few POCT and compared with the cost of those tests in a classical clinical laboratory (Greendyke 1992; Lee-Lewandrowski *et al.*, 1994; Winkelman *et al.*, 1994). Real cost comparisons are truly difficult because they must evaluate the entire testing process, from ordering through recording. Particularly in such comparisons the comparative outcome analysis, sample transport cost, sample processing cost etc. of the both the testing modes is absolutely necessary to arrive at a reasonable conclusion. One such study that analyses more than true analysis cost of both the modalities observes that POCT approach is cost effective (Bailey *et al.*, 1997). There is every chance that with future improvement of POCT technology the cost effectiveness of POCT will increase further.

POCT Informatics

Managing patient test data and documenting regulatory compliance for tests performed at the point of care have traditionally been significant problems. In many situations, manual record-keeping has proven entirely inadequate for maintaining the integrity of the patient medical record or for providing an audit trail for quality assurance activities. Starting in the 1990s, a number of companies began to develop and market point-of-care data management systems. Over time, these data management systems have become increasingly sophisticated. It is now possible to interface multiple point-of-care devices from different manufacturers to a central data manager that is bidirectionally interfaced to the laboratory and hospital information systems. Despite these advances, many challenges remain. True real-time point-of-care "connectivity" across an entire institution has yet to be achieved, and there is still no satisfactory solution for manually performed visually read tests, some of which are commonly performed at the point of care. In the future, wireless point-of-care connectivity solutions hold great promise, but these technologies are yet to be fully developed (Kim and Lewandrowski, 2009).

Health informatics on POCT devices used within the home environment will need to process data quickly in order to underpin service provision. However, owing to insufficient medical expertise at the point of use, a bottleneck in service-provision is likely to occur. Data will, therefore, need to be transferred to an external location where advice may be obtained from health professionals who must then contact the user (Adeogun *et al.*, 2010). The developing telemedicine approach may be a solution of the above scenario by which the generated data may be transferred electronically from point of care at real time to a distant place to an expert who has the capacity to interpret the data and take appropriate measures (Eren *et al.*, 2008). Many POCT systems available throughout the globe is equipped with comprehensive data management system with an option of connectivity through world wide web and a central computer making the telemedicine approach a real possibility in days to come (Blick, 2001).

For effective inpatient POCT services health professionals like nursing staff is trained today in various aspects of POCT informatics and the subject is even included in academic curriculum of health professionals (Curran, 2008).

Research and Future Directions

POCT is one of the most recent fields that have attracted considerable current interest to a wide range of researchers spanning over various disciplines of Life Science and Medical Science. Already there is a journal dedicated to report various aspects of POCT (http://journals.lww.com/poctjournal/ pages/aboutthejournal.aspx). Many other periodicals concerned with laboratory medicine or clinical medicine or biomedical engineering started publishing articles related to near patient testing. The number of articles reporting various aspect of POCT is increasing at a tremendous rate.

It is widely recognized that future growth of POCT is dependent of three factors. They are wireless connectivity of various POCT devices, POCT clinical management software development for therapeutic interventions and design of molecular applications for POCT (Kiechle, 2008). At present a number of researchers from various disciplines are engaged in such research.

In this era of rapidly developing biomarkers, newly developed suitable biomarkers are being tried for POCT application. Appropriate biomarkers are now attempted to be developed keeping near patient testing application in mind. Clinical outcome analysis and cost-effectiveness analysis are other two vital areas of research that is expected to influence POCT in future.

Conclusion

POCT is a modality of patient care service that is recently getting popular among patients and health care providers. The aim of near patient testing technology is not to replace or to stop centralized hospital laboratory service. It should be judiciously used along with the available central laboratory service for the benefit of the patients. With the development of accurate, precise, sensitive and specific POCT modalities some laboratory tests may become obsolete. Therefore, with the continuous development of knowledge pool by biomedical research throughout the globe, both POCT and laboratory testing should modify its services in a manner that renders the best clinical outcome to the majority of patients.

References

Adeogun O, Tiwari A, Alcock JR (2010). Informatics-based product-service systems for point-of-care devices. CIRP-JMST 3: 107-115.

Anderson M (2001). POCT regulatory compliance: what is it and how does it impact you? Crit Care Nurs Q 24: 1-6.

Auxter S (1998). Clin Lab News 24: 20–22.

Bailey TM, Topham TM, Wantz S et al. (1997). Laboratory process improvement through point-of-care testing. Jt Comm J Qual Improv 23: 362-380.

Bennett J, Cervantes C, Pachecho S (2000). Point-of-care testing: inspection preparedness. Perfusion 15: 137-142.

Bissell M (2001). Point-of-Care Testing at the Millennium. Crit Care Nurs Q 24: 39-43.

Blick KE (2001). The essential role of information management in point-of-care/critical care testing. Clin Chim Acta 307: 159-168.

Briggs C, Guthrie D, Hyde K et al. (2008). Guidelines for point-of-care testing: haematology. Br J Haematol 142: 904-915.

Carlson DA (1996). Point of care testing: regulation and accreditation. Clin Lab Sci 9: 298-302.

Chapman WH, Joshi K, Chang Y-L at al. (2011). Nanocharacterization of carbon nanotube biosensors for point-of-care diagnostics. Microsc Microanal 17: 1554-1555.

Curran CR (2008). Faculty Development Initiatives for the Integration of Informatics Competencies and Point-of-Care Technologies in Undergraduate Nursing Education. Nurs Clin North Am 43: 523-533.

Despotis GJ, Grishaber JE, Goodnough LT et al. (1994). The effect of an intraoperative treatment algorithm on physicians' transfusion practice in cardiac surgery. Transfusion 34: 290-296.

Ehrmeyer SS, Laessig RH (1999). Point-of-care testing: Implementation and practice of cost-effective total quality management. Accreditation and Quality Assurance: Journal for Quality, Comparability and Reliability in Chemical Measurement 4: 419-422.

Ehrmeyer SS, Laessig RH (2009). Regulatory compliance for point-of-care testing: 2009 United States perspective. Clin Lab Med 29: 463-478.

Eren A, Subasi A, Coskun O (2008). A decision support system for telemedicine through the mobile telecommunications platform. J Med Syst 32: 31-35.

Gouget B, Barclay J, Rakotoambinina B (2001). Impact of emerging technologies and regulations on the role of POCT. Clin Chim Acta 307: 235-240.

Greendyke RM (1992). Cost analysis. Bedside blood glucose testing. Am J Clin Pathol 97: 106-107.

Grieve R, Beech R, Vincent J et al. (1999). Near patient testing in diabetes clinics: appraising the costs and outcomes. Health Technol Assess 3: 1-74.

Haeckel R, Wosniok W (2009). Quantity quotient reporting. A proposal for a standardized presentation of laboratory results. Clin Chem Lab Med 47: 1203-1206.

Halpern NA, Brentjens T (1999). Point of care testing informatics: The critical care-hospital interface. Crit Care Clin 15: 577-591.

Hawker CD (2007). Laboratory Automation: Total and Subtotal. Clin Lab Med 27: 749-770.

Hilborne LH, Lubin IM, Scheuner MT (2009). The beginning of the second decade of the era of patient safety: Implications and roles for the clinical laboratory and laboratory professionals. Clin Chim Acta 404: 24-27.

Hobbs FD, Delaney BC, Fitzmaurice DA *et al.* (1997). A review of near patient testing in primary care. Health Technol Assess 1: 1-229.

Hortas ML, Montiel N, Redondo M *et al.* (2001). Quality assurance of point-of-care testing in the Costa del Sol Healthcare Area (Marbella, Spain). Clin Chim Acta 307: 113-118.

Humbertson SK (2001). Management of a point-of-care programme. Organization, quality assurance, and data management. Clin Lab Med 21: 255-268.

Kiechle FL (2008). Point-of-Care Testing: 3 New Developments Needed for Future Growth. Point of Care 7: 97-99.

Kim JY, Lewandrowski K (2009). Point-of-Care Testing Informatics. Clin Lab Med 29: 449-461.

Kricka LJ, Savory J (2011). International Year of Chemistry 2011: A Guide to the History of Clinical Chemistry. Clin Chem 57: 1118-1126.

Laurence C, Moss J, Briggs NE *et al.* (2010). The cost-effectiveness of point of care testing in a general practice setting: results from a randomised controlled trial. BMC Health Services Research 10: 165.

Lee-Lewandrowski E, Laposata M, Eschenbach K *et al.* (1994). Utilization and cost analysis of bedside capillary glucose testing in a large teaching hospital: implications for managing point of care testing. Am J Med 97: 222-230.

Lee HH, Dineva MA, Chua YL *et al.* (2010). Simple amplification-based assay: A nucleic acid-based point-of-care platform for HIV-1 testing. J Infect Dis 201: S65-S71.

Lee HH, Dineva MA (2002). Improved detection signal and capture in dipstick assay . International patent WO 2002/004667. Diagnostics for the Real World, assignee.

Luppa PB, Muller C, Schlichtiger A *et al.* (2011). Point-of-care testing (POCT): Current techniques and future perspectives. TrAC Trends in Analytical Chemistry 30: 887-898.

Nichols JH (2003). Quality in point-of-care testing. Expert Rev Mol Diagn 3: 563-572.

Nichols JH (2007). Point of care testing. Clin Lab Med 27: 893-908.

Nichols JH, Poe SS (1999). Quality assurance, practical management, and outcomes of point-of-care testing: laboratory perspectives, Part I. Clin Lab Manage Rev 13: 341-350.

Opekun AR, Gotschall AB, Abdalla N *et al.* (2005). Improved infrared spectrophotometer for point-of-care patient 13C-urea breath testing in the primary care setting. Clin Biochem 38: 731-734.

Price CP (2001). Point of care testing. BMJ 322: 1285-1288.

Schimke I (2009). Quality and timeliness in medical laboratory testing. Anal Bioanal Chem 393: 1499-1504.

Sista R, Hua Z, Thwar P *et al.* (2008). Development of a digital microfluidic platform for point of care testing. Lab Chip 8: 2091-2104.

Sunderman FW Sr (1992). The history of proficiency testing/quality control. Clin Chem 38: 1205-1209.

Trowell HC (1982). Ants distinguish diabetes mellitus from diabetes insipidus. British Med J 285: 217.

Willmott C, Arrowsmith JE (2010). Point-of-care testing. Surgery (Oxford). 28: 159-160.

Winkelman JW, Wybenga DR, Tanasijevic MJ (1994). The fiscal consequences of central vs distributed testing of glucose. Clin Chem 40: 1628-1630.

2014, Advances in Biochemistry and Biotechnology Volume 2   *Pages 235-241*

Edited by: Dr. Biplab Sarkar and Dr. Chiranjib Chakraborty

Published by: DAYA PUBLISHING HOUSE

15

Kisspeptin in Fish

Ashis Saha, S.C. Rath and S.S. Giri

Central Institute of Freshwater Aquaculture, Bhubaneswar, Orissa, India

ABSTRACT

Kisspeptins are a family of structurally related peptides, encoded by the *KISS1/Kiss1* gene, that act through binding and subsequent activation of the G protein-coupled receptor GPR54. The initial product of the *Kiss1* gene is a 145-amino-acid peptide. This peptide is cleaved into a 54-amino-acid peptide known as kisspeptin-54. Shorter peptides (kisspeptin- 10, -13, and -14) that share a common RFamidated motif with kisspeptin-54 also exist. In fish two distinct genes encoding kisspeptins (kiss1 and kiss2), whereas in mammals mostly one gene encode kisspeptin. The structural organization of both kiss1 and kiss2 genes is similar, containing two coding exons, with the exon 2 coding for the kisspeptin-10 sequence (*i.e.*, YNWNSFGLRY for kiss1 and FNFNPFGLRF for kiss2). Kisspeptins influence gonadotropin release in fish. In those species with two kiss genes, different potencies of kiss1- or kiss2-derived peptides are observed, but their relative potency depends on the species. Kisspeptin is also having role in photoperiodic control of reproduction.

Reproduction is an indispensable function for the perpetuation of the species and, as such, is under the control of a sophisticated network of regulatory signals. While different reproductive strategies have been co-opted during evolution, in mammals and other species the above regulatory factors mainly originate and/or integrate at the so-called hypothalamic-pituitary-gonadal (HPG) axis. The function of this neurohormonal system relies primarily on the dynamic interaction of three major groups of signals arising from 1) the hypothalamus which synthesize and release the decapeptide, gonadotropin-releasing hormone (GnRH); 2) the anterior pituitary, where gonadotropes, secrete the gonado-tropins, luteinizing hormone (LH), and follicle-stimulating hormone (FSH); and 3) the gonads that, in addition to generating gametes, are responsible for the synthesis and release of sex steroid and peptide hormones. These major components of the HPG axis are connected via feed-forward loops whereby GnRH stimulates the secretion of gonadotropins and these, in turn, promote gonadal maturation and function.

Recently, our knowledge about the neuroendocrine pathways responsible for the control of GnRH secretion has enriched significantly. Neuronal transmitters like glutamate and norepinephrine act as major excitatory signals, and GABA and endogenous opioids as key inhibitory factors. Yet, GABA can also directly excite GnRH neurons under specific conditions (Herbison and Moenter 2011), thus illustrating the complexity of the system. More recent evidence suggested the involvement of other factors, such as members of the RF-amide superfamily, which include not only kisspeptins but also gonadotropin-inhibiting hormone (GnIH), and its orthologs, RF-releasing peptides (RFRP) (Navarro *et al.*, 2006; Clarke *et al.*, 2009; Smith and Clarke 2010); metabolic neuropeptides, such as neuropeptide Y (NPY) and nesfatin-1 (Garcia-Galiano *et al.*, 2010, Pralong FP 2010); and tachykinins, including neurokinin B (NKB) (Lehman *et al.*, 2010).

The Kiss System

A major advance in our understanding of the neuronal mechanisms controlling GnRH secretion, and therefore gonadal function, came with the identification of the physiological roles of kisspeptins and their receptor, GPR54. Kisspeptins are a family of structurally related peptides, encoded by the *KISS1/Kiss1* gene, that act through binding and subsequent activation of the G protein-coupled receptor GPR54. The *Kiss1* gene was so named in part because it was cloned in Hershey, Pennsylvania, a city known for its chocolate kisses (Lee *et al.*, 1996.). The initial product of the *Kiss1* gene is a 145-amino-acid peptide. This peptide is cleaved into a 54-amino-acid peptide known as kisspeptin-54. Shorter peptides (kisspeptin- 10, -13, and -14) that share a common RFamidated motif with kisspeptin-54 also exist.

Kiss in Fish

Contrary to mammals where, with the exception of the platypus (monotreme), only one gene coding for the kisspeptin is present, while two distinct genes encoding kisspeptins (kiss1 and kiss2), is present in fish (Um *et al.*, 2010;Zohar *et al.*, 2010),. The first reports of cloning of kiss genes in fish (zebrafish *Danio rerio*) were published in 2008 (Aerle *et al.*, 2008). Besides this, it has been identified in medaka *Oryzias latipes* (Kanda *et al.*, 2008; Kitahash *et al.*, 2009), goldfish *Carassius auratus* (Li *et al.*, 2009), sea bass *Dicentrarchus labrax* (Felip *et al.*, 2009), orange-spotted grouper *Epinephelus coioides* (Shi *et al.*, 2010), grass puffer *Takifugu niphobles* (Shahjahan *et al.*, 2010), chub mackerel *Scomber japonicas* (Selvaraj *et al.*, 2010) and striped bass *Morone saxatilis* (Zmora *et al.*, 2011). All of these teleost species possess the kiss2 gene, while there is also evidence that the kiss1 gene is present in the genomes of zebrafish, medaka, sea bass, goldfish and chub mackerel. In several fish species, such as tiger puffer *Takifugu rubripes*, green puffer *Tetraodon nigroviridis*, and stickleback *Gasterosteus aculeatus*, lack the kiss1 gene and possess only kiss2 (Yang *et al.*, 2010). On the other hand, there is also evidence that both kiss1 and kiss2 genes are present in cartilaginous fish such as the elephant shark *Callorhinchus milii* (Chondrichthye) and in the sea lamprey *Petromyzon marinus* (Agnatha). Genome and cDNA analyses of the kisspeptin genes have revealed that the structural organization of both kiss1 and kiss2 genes is similar, containing two coding exons, with the exon 2 coding for the kisspeptin-10 sequence (*i.e.*, YNWNSFGLRY for kiss1 and FNFNPFGLRF for kiss2) (Felip *et al.*, 2009; Kitahash *et al.*, 2009; Yang *et al.*, 2010; Zohar *et al.*, 2010)].

Kisspeptin act through binding of its receptor GPR54. Parhar *et al.* (2004) isolated GPR54 cDNA from Nile tilapia *Oreochromis niloticus* (L.), which was the first report on the presence of fish kisspeptin receptors. Thereafter, fish *kissr* genes have been isolated in several species, such as cobia *Rachycentron canadum* (L.) (Mohamed *et al.*, 2007), flathead mullet *Mugil cephalus* L. (Nocillado *et al.*, 2007), Senegalese sole *Solea senegalensis* Kaup (Mechaly *et al.*, 2009), *D. rerio* (Biran *et al.*, 2008) and *C. auratus* (Li *et al.*, 2009). Two distinct subtypes of kisspeptin receptors have been found in *D. rerio* (Biran *et al.*, 2008), *O. latipes* (Lee *et al.*, 2009) and *C. auratus* (Li *et al.*, 2009).

Tissue Distribution and Expression of Kisspeptins and Gpr54 in Fish

In fish, expression of the genes encoding kisspeptins and their receptors have been found in different brain areas, namely in the hypothalamus, telencephalon, thalamus, mid brain tegumentum, olfactory bulbs and tracts, optic tectum, optic nerves, medulla oblongata, cerebellum and pituitary. The expression of these genes has been also reported in other tissues including ovary, testes, heart, muscle, stomach, intestine, liver, spleen, kidney, adipose tissue, pancreas, gills, eye and skin, to a variable extent depending on the fish species and gene [Oakley *et al.*, 2009]. The first evidence of the expression of a non-mammalian gpr54 in GnRH neurons of the brain of a cichlid fish, the tilapia (Oreochromis niloticus), suggesting a potential anatomical association of gpr54 with the GnRH system [Parhar *et al.*, 2004]. Thereafter, two distinct kisspeptin receptor transcripts (gpr54-1b and gpr54-2b) have been isolated in a variety of fish species and its expression examined by quantitative PCR. The detection of gpr54-1b and gpr54-2b mRNAs in brain and gonads at different reproductive stages reinforces their potential reproductive role, although their functional relevance may vary among gender and species (Akazome *et al.*, 2010, Oakley *et al.*, 2009).

Kisspeptin Signaling Pathways

Generally mammalian kiss receptor Gpr54 activated by its ligand through activation of protein kinase (PKC) pathway (Ohtaki *et al.*, 2001; Moon *et al.*, 2009). However, no activation of the cAMP/ Protein kinase A (PKA) pathway has been described for mammalian Gpr54s (Castellano *et al.*, 2006,. Kotani *et al.*, 2001).

The functionality and ligand specificity of the kiss/gpr54 system has been analyzed in very few fish species containing a duplicated kiss system, namely zebrafish (Biran *et al.*, 2008, Lee *et al.*, 2009), goldfish (Li *et al.*, 2009) and European sea bass ; and in one species, orange spotted grouper, with a single kiss/gpr54 pair (Shi *et al.*, 2010). All the fish gpr54 functionally tested were able to activate luciferase expression driven by a SRE promoter, indicating that, as it is the case in mammals, activation of PKCMAPKs is involved as signaling pathway. Whereas it has been reported that mammalian Gpr54s do not activate the cAMP/PKA signaling pathway, even when transfected in heterologous cell lines where this pathway is functional, the same does not stand for fish receptors. The ability to activate this pathway has been tested in gpr54 receptors of some fish species, by measuring CRE-driven luciferase activity. In sea bass, goldfish and zebrafish, gpr54-1b elicits stronger activation of the cAMP/PKA pathway than gpr54-2b. But in orange spotted grouper, where only the gpr54-2b receptor has been studied, no signaling through the PKA pathway was observed.

However, differences have been observed depending on the receptor-ligand combination, for activating the PKC-MAPK route, it has observe that gpr54-1b is more efficiently activated by kiss1–10 than by kiss2–10 in zebrafish (Lee *et al.*, 2009) and sea bass, while the opposite occurs for goldfish gpr54-1b (Li *et al.*, 2009). However, gpr54-2b is preferably activated by kiss1–10 in goldfish, but similarly activated by kiss1–10 or kiss2–10 in zebrafish and sea bass. In the orange spotted grouper, which only harbors a kiss2/grp54-2b ligand-receptor pair, human kiss1–10 was as effective as the homologous grouper kiss2–10 in activating the gpr54-2b receptor (Shi *et al.*, 2010).

Regulation of Kisspeptin

Sex steroid can play an important regulatory role of the kisspeptin system in non-mammals. In medaka ovariectomy significantly reduced the number of kiss1 neurons in the NVT compared to control but treatment with estradiol (E2) completely reversed this effect, so it is suggested that these neurons could be involved in the positive feedback control of the brain–pituitary–gonadal axis (Grone *et al.*, 2010). In juvenile zebrafish, E2 treatment caused an increase in the number of kiss2 neurons in the hypothalamus. It also caused a significant increase of brain kiss1 mRNA, although of lower magnitude than kiss2 responses. E2 treatment also increase the expression of gpr54-2b, but not gpr54-1b in zebrafish (Servili *et al.*, 2011)]. In the orange-spotted grouper, both kiss2 and gpr54-2b expression decreased in the first week after 17 α-methyltestosterone implantation, but kiss2 increased in the fourth week coinciding with a significant increase of gnrh1 in the hypothalamus. Apart from sex steroids, various metabolic regulators such as leptin, ghrelin, NPY, insulin-like growth factor I and insulin also influence, either directly or indirectly, the expression of Kiss1.

Biological Effects

The biological effects of kisspeptin have been studied after systemic administration of kiss-10 in some fish species. The expression of gnrh genes in the brain and of gonadotropin subunits in the hypophysis and gonadotropin levels in blood has been measured. In early-mid pubertal fathead minnow, kiss1–10 injection showed an increase in the expression of gpr54-2b and gnrh3 (likely to be the hypophysiotropic form) in the brain, but not of gnrh2. However, injections of kiss1–10 and kiss2–10 in sexually mature female zebrafish did not show any expression variation in gnrh3 (hypophysiotropic form) or gnrh2 (Kitahashi *et al.*, 2009). In orange spotted grouper, whose genome contains only kiss2, the administration of the kiss2–10 peptide in sexually mature females elicit an increase in hypothalamic expression of gnrh1(probably the hypophysiotropic form in this species) but not of gnrh3 (Shi *et al.*, 2010).

In female zebrafish, kiss2–10 was significantly more potent than kiss1–10 for inducing the expression of the fsh-β and lh-β subunits in the pituitary (Kitahashi *et al.*, 2009). In female orange spotted grouper, kiss2–10 injection also caused an increase in fsh-β expression, but had no effect on expression of the lh-β gene (Shi *et al.*, 2010). Administration of kisspeptin in the European sea bass and goldfish also having some response in gonadotropin levels in blood. In sea bass, kiss2–10 was more potent than kiss1–10 in inducing LH and FSH release in pre-pubertal fish, and LH secretion in pubertal males (Felip *et al.*, 2009). On the other hand, kiss1–10 administration in goldfish significantly increased blood LH levels in a dose dependent manner, while kiss2–10 showed no effect (Li *et al.*, 2009). All together, these data conclusively demonstrate that kisspeptins influence gonadotropin release in fish. In those species with two kiss genes, different potencies of kiss1- or kiss2-derived peptides are observed, but their relative potency depends on the species.

Relation with Photoperiodism

The environment plays an important role in the regulation of reproduction in many animals, including fish. Among various components of the environment, annual changes in the duration of the solar day or photoperiod is the primary and regular variable that alone or in combination with water temperature or other environmental factor(s) drives the sexual periodicity in most fish species. In mammals the photoperiodic control of reproduction involves direct or indirect modulation of the kisspeptin system. But information in this area in fish is very scanty. It has been reported that long-day photoperiods, which inhibit the onset of puberty, also inhibit kisspeptin receptor expression in tilapia (Martinez-Chavez *et al.*, 2008). Long photoperiods (stimulatory to reproduction) induced higher number of NVT kiss1 neurons than short photoperiods (inhibitory to reproduction) in medaka (Kanda *et al.*, 2008). Like many other organisms, zebrafish modulate their reproductive activity photoperiodically by the nocturnal release of melatonin. In zebrafish, melatonin increase the level of kiss1, kiss2, gnrh3 genes in the brain, and lh-β in the pituitary (Carnevali *et al.*, 2011). So it is suggested that melatonin may act as a signal mechanism to trigger reproductive capacity in teleosts, by activating a cascade involving kisspeptin pathways which, in turn, stimulate hypothalamic GnRH neurons to switch on the gonadotropic axis, thus supporting the hypothesis that the photoperiod, via melatonin, modulates kiss1 neurons to drive reproductive axis.

In general, kisspeptin is a peptide with a diverse and multifunctional nature, involving varied whole body physiological systems and acting at all levels of the reproductive axis–brain, pituitary, gonad, and accessory organs. Kisspeptin exercises a crucial role in stimulating GnRH, relaying steroid hormone negative and positive feedback signals to GnRH neurons, serving as a gatekeeper to the onset of puberty, and relaying photoperiodic information. Most of the research has been done in mammalian system. Few sporadic information are available in fish system but systematic research in the regulation of fish reproduction are yet to be carried out. This research expects a new horizon to further streamline the captive induce breeding and seed production of commercially important fin fishes.

References

Akazome Y, Kanda S, Okubo K, Oka Y (2010). Functional and evolutionary insights into vertebrate kisspeptin systems from studies of fish brain. J Fish Biol 76: 161–182.

Biran J, Ben-Dor S, Levavi-Sivan B (2008). Molecular identification and functional characterization of the kisspeptin/kisspeptin receptor system in lower vertebrates, Biol Reprod 79: 776–786.

Carnevali O, Gioacchini F, Maradonna I, Olivotto B, Migliarini (2011). Melatonin induces follicle maturation in *Danio rerio*, PLoS ONE 6 (5). e19978.

Castellano JM, Navarro VM, Fernandez-Fernandez R, Castano JP, Malagon MM, Aguilar E, Dieguez C, Magni P, Pinilla L, Tena-Sempere M (2006). Ontogeny and mechanisms of action for the stimulatory effect of kisspeptin on gonadotropin-releasing hormone system of the rat. Mol Cell Endocrinol 257–258: 75–83.

Clarke IJ, Qi Y, Puspita SI, Smith JT (2009). Evidence that RF-amide related peptides are inhibitors of reproduction in mammals. Front Neuroendocrinol 30: 371–378.

Felip A, Zanuy S, Pineda R, Pinilla L, Carrillo M, Tena-Sempere M, Gomez A (2009). Evidence for two distinct KiSS genes in non-placental vertebrates that encode kisspeptins with different gonadotropin-releasing activities in fish and mammals. Mol Cell Endocrinol: 312 61–71.

Garcia-Galiano D, Navarro VM, Roa J, Ruiz-Pino F, Sanchez-Garrido MA, Pineda R, Castellano JM, Romero M, Aguilar E, Gaytan F, Dieguez C, Pinilla L, Tena-Sempere M (2010). The anorexigenic neuropeptide, nesfatin-1, is indispensable for normal puberty onset in the female rat. *J Neurosci* 30: 7783–7792.

Grone BP, Maruska KP, Korzan WJ, Fernald RD (2010). Social status regulates kisspeptin receptor mRNA in the brain of *Astatotilapia burtoni*. Gen Comp Endocrinol 169: 98–107.

Herbison AE, Moenter SM (2011). Depolarising and hyperpolarising actions of GABA(A). receptor activation on gonadotrophin-releasing hormone neurones: towards an emerging consensus. J Neuroendocrinol 23: 557–569.

Kitahashi T, Ogawa S, Parhar IS (2009). Cloning and expression of kiss2 in the zebrafish and medaka, Endocrinol 150: 821–831.

Kotani M, Detheux M, Vandenbogaerde A, Communi D, Vanderwinden JM, Poul Le E, Brezillon S, Tyldesley R, Suarez-Huerta N, Vandeput F, Blanpain C, Schiffmann SN, Vassart G, Parmentier M (2001). The metastasis suppressor gene KiSS-1 encodes kisspeptins, the natural ligands of the orphan G proteincoupled receptor GPR54. J Biol Chem 276: 34631–34636.

Lee JH, Miele ME, Hicks DJ, Phillips KK, Trent JM (1996). *KiSS-1*, a novel human malignant melanoma metastasis-suppressor gene. J Natl Cancer Inst 88: 1731–37.

Lee YR, Tsunekawa K, Moon MJ, Um HN, Hwang JI, Osugi T, Otaki N, Sunakawa Y, Kim K, Vaudry H, Kwon HB, Seong JY, Tsutsui K (2009). Molecular evolution of multiple forms of kisspeptins and GPR54 receptors in vertebrates. Endocrinol 150: 2837–2846.

Lehman MN, Coolen LM, Goodman RL (2010). Minireview: kisspeptin/neurokinin B/dynorphin (KNDy). cells of the arcuate nucleus: a central node in the control of gonadotropin- releasing hormone secretion. Endocrinology 151: 3479–3489.

Li S, Zhang Y, Liu Y, Huang X, Huang W, Lu D, Zhu P, Shi Y, Cheng CH, Liu X, Lin H (2009). Structural and functional multiplicity of the kisspeptin/GPR54 system in goldfish (*Carassius auratus*). J Endocrinol 201: 407–418.

Martinez-Chavez CC, Minghetti M, Migaud H (2008). GPR54 and rGnRH I gene expression during the onset of puberty in *Nile tilapia*. Gen Comp Endocrinol 156: 224–233.

Muir AI, Chamberlain L, Elshourbagy NA, Michalovich D, Moore DJ, Calamari A, Szekeres PG, Sarau HM, Chambers JK, Murdock P, Steplewski K, Shabon U, Miller JE, Middleton SE, Darker JG, Larminie CGC, Wilson S, Bergsma DJ, Emson P, Faull R, Philpott KL, Harrison DC (2001). AXOR12, a novel human G protein-coupled receptor, activated by the peptide KiSS-1. J Biol Chem 276: 28969–28975.

Navarro VM, Fernandez-Fernandez R, Nogueiras R, Vigo E, Tovar S, Chartrel N, Le Marec O, Leprince J, Aguilar E, Pinilla L, Dieguez C, Vaudry H, Tena-Sempere M. (2006). Novel role of 26RFa, a hypothalamic RFamide orexigenic peptide, as putative regulator of the gonadotropic axis. J Physiol 573: 237–249.

Oakley AE, Clifton DK, Steiner RA (2009). Kisspeptin signaling in the brain. Endocrinol Rev 30: 713–743.

Parhar IS, Ogawa S, Sakuma Y (2004). Laser-captured single digoxigenin-labeled neurons of gonadotropin-releasing hormone types reveal a novel G proteincoupled receptor (Gpr54). during maturation in cichlid fish. Endocrinol 145: 3613–3618.

Pralong FP (2010). Insulin and NPY pathways and the control of GnRH function and puberty onset. Mol Cell Endocrinol 324: 82–86.

S. Kanda, Y. Akazome, T. Matsunaga, N. Yamamoto, S. Yamada, H. Tsukamura, K. Maeda, Y. Oka (2008). Identification of KiSS-1 product kisspeptin and steroidsensitive sexually dimorphic kisspeptin neurons in medaka (*Oryzias latipes*). Endocrinology 149: 2467–2476.

Selvaraj S, Kitano H, Fujinaga Y, Ohga H, Yoneda M, Yamaguchi A, Shimizu A, Matsuyama M (2010). Molecular characterization, tissue distribution, and mRNA expression profiles of two Kiss genes in the adult male and female chub mackerel (*Scomber japonicus*). during different gonadal stages. Gen Comp Endocrinol 169: 28–38.

Servili A, Page Le Y, Leprince J, Caraty A, Escobar S, Parhar IS, Seong JY, Vaudry H, Kah O (2011). Organization of two independent kisspeptin systems derived from evolutionary-ancient kiss genes in the brain of zebrafish. Endocrinol 152: 1527–1540.

Shahjahan M, Motohashi E, Doi H Ando H (2010). Elevation of Kiss2 and its receptor gene expression in the brain and pituitary of grass puffer during the spawning season. Gen Comp Endocrinol 169: 48–57.

Shi Y, Zhang Y, Li S, Liu Q, Lu D, Liu M, Z Meng, Cheng CHK, Liu X, Lin H (2010). Molecular identification of the Kiss2/Kiss1ra system and its potential function during 17alpha-methyltestosterone-induced sex reversal in the orangespotted grouper, *Epinephelus coioides*. Biol Reprod 83: 63–74.

Smith JT, Clarke IJ (2010). Gonadotropin inhibitory hormone function in mammals. Trends Endocrinol Metab 21: 255–260.

Um HN, Han JM, Hwang JI, Hong SI, Vaudry H, Seong JY (2010)Molecular coevolution of kisspeptins and their receptors from fish to mammals. Ann. N Y Acad Sci 1200: 67–74.

Van Aerle R, Kille P, Lange A, Tyler CR (2008). Evidence for the existence of a functional Kiss1/Kiss1 receptor pathway in fish, Peptides 29: 57–64.

Yang B, Jiang Q, Chan T, Ko W K, Wong AO (2010). Goldfish kisspeptin: molecular cloning, tissue distribution of transcript expression, and stimulatory effects on prolactin, growth hormone and luteinizing hormone secretion and gene expression via direct actions at the pituitary level. Gen Comp Endocrinol 165: 60–71.

Zmora N, Stubblefield J, Zulperi Z, Klenke U, Zohar Y (2011). Kisspeptinphotoperiodic/gonadal steroid relationships in the brain of two perciforms, the striped and hybrid basses. Indian J Sci Technol 4: 10–11.

Zohar Y, Munoz-Cueto JA, Elizur A, Kah O (2010). Neuroendocrinology of reproduction in teleost fish. Gen Comp Endocrinol 165: 438–455.

Contents of Previous Volume

Index

Color Type	Area of Biotech
Red	Health, Medical, Diagnostics
Yellow	Food Biotechnology, Nutrition Science
Blue	Aquaculture, Coastal and Marine Biotech
Green	Agricultural, Environmental Biotechnology – Biofuels, Biofertilizers, Bioremediation, Geomicrobiology
Brown	Arid Zone and Desert Biotechnology
Dark	Bioterrorism, Biowarfare, Biocrimes, Anticrop warfare
Purple	Patents, Publications, Inventions, IPRs
White	Patents, Publications, Inventions, IPRs(White)
Gold	Bioinformatics, Nanobiotechnology
Grey	

Figure 1.1: Colours of Biotechnology. (Page-3)

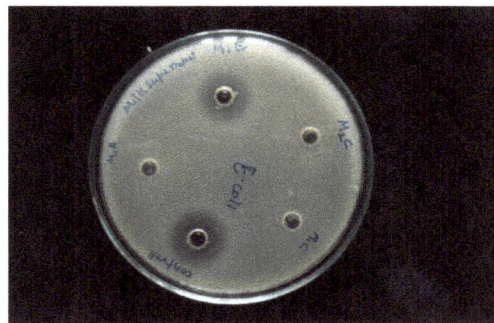

Figure 2.1: Antimicrobial Peptides Produced by *Lactobacillus* sp. Isolated from Indigenous Fermented Product of Orissa Showing Zone of Inhibition Against *E. coli*. (Page-10)

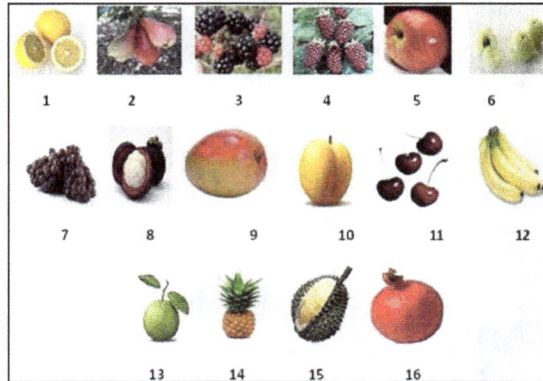

Figure 7.1

1: Citrus fruits; 2: Malay apple; 3: Blackberry; 4: Dessert date; 5: Apple; 6: Indian gooseberry; 7: Grapes; 8: Mangosteen; 9: Mango 10: Apricot; 11: Cherry; 12: Banana; 13: Guava; 14: Pineapple; 15: Durian; 16: Pomegranate: (Page-107)

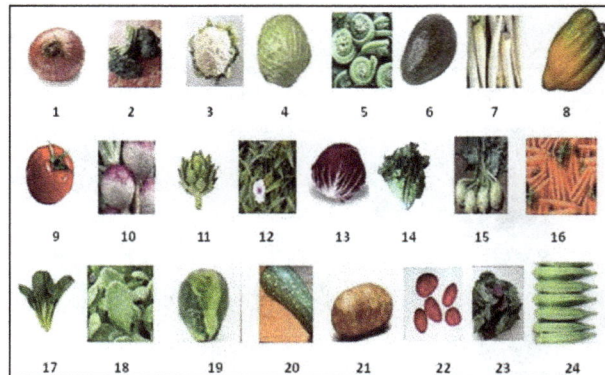

Figure 7.2

1: Onion; 2: Broccoli; 3: Cauliflower; 4: Cabbage; 5: Fiddle head; 6: Avocado; 7: Daikon; 8: Winter squash; 9: Tomato; 10: Turnip; 11: Artichoke; 12: Water cress; 13: Radicchio; 14: Lettuce; 15: Kohlrabi; 16: Carrot; 17: Komatsuna; 18: Salt bush; 19: Brussels sprout; 20: Zucchini; 21: Potato; 22: Ulluco; 23: Spinach; 24: Okra. (Page-107)

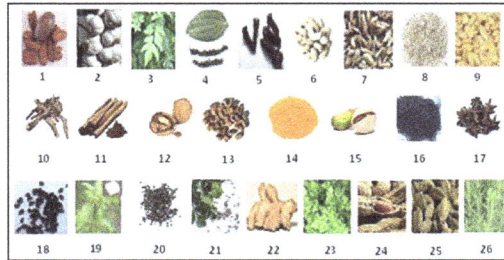

Figure 7.3

1: Pecan; 2: Garlic; 3: Curry leaves; 4: Black pepper; 5: Clove; 6: Cashew nut; 7: Fennel; 8: Sesame seed; 9: Flax seed; 10: Licorice; 11: Cinnamon; 12: Walnut; 13: Fenugreek; 14: Turmeric; 15: Pistachio; 16: Mustard; 17: Star anise; 18: Kalonji; 19: Camphor; 20: Black mustard; 21: Coriander; 22: Ginger; 23: Parsley; 24: Peanut; 25: Cardamom; 26: Rosemary. (Page-108)

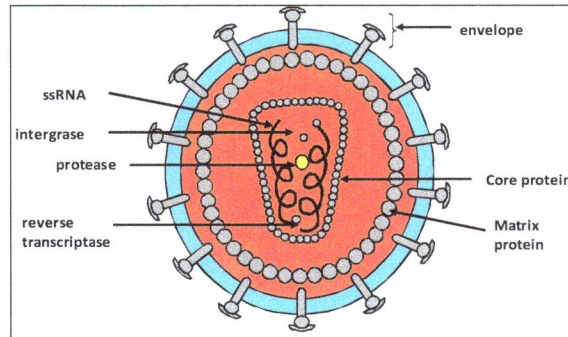

Figure 7.5: Structure of HIV-1 Virion. (Page-131)

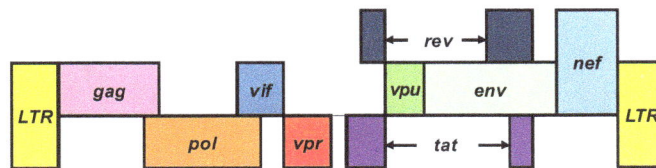

Figure 7.6: Genetic Organization of HIV-1. (Page-131)

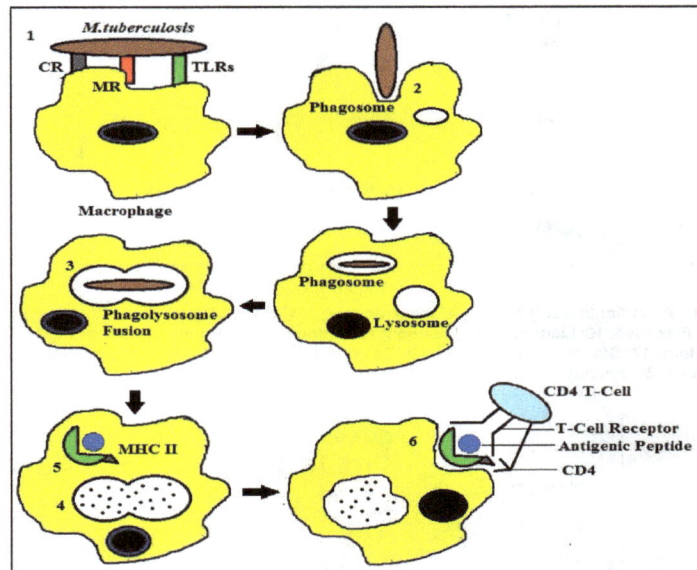

Figure 9.1 (1) Antigen interacts with macrophage receptors (2) Engulfment of antigen by phagosome (3) Fusion of phagosome and lysosome *i.e.* phagolysosome (4) Antigen processed to peptides in phagolysosome (5) Peptides bind to MHC II (6) Phagolysosome fuse with plasma membrane. Peptide MHC II complex is presented to CD4 helper T cell. (Page-147)

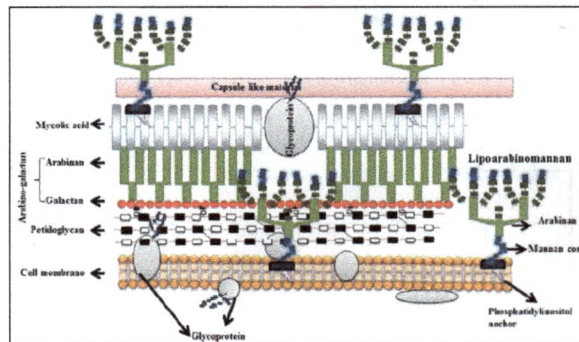

Figure 9.2: Schematic Diagram of Cell Wall of *Mycobacterium tuberculosis*. (Page-152)